The Doctor and the Athlete

# The Doctor and the Athlete

Second Edition

## Isao Hirata, Jr., M.D.

*Director, Student Health Service*
*University of South Carolina*
*Columbia, South Carolina*

## J. B. Lippincott Company
*Philadelphia    Toronto*

ISBN  0-397-50330-X

Library of Congress Catalog Card Number 73-21970

Printed in the United States of America

1 3 4 2

Library of Congress Cataloging in Publication Data

Hirata, Isao.
    The doctor and the athlete.

    Bibliography: p.
    1. Sport medicine. I. Title. [DNLM: 1. Athletic injuries. 2. Sport medicine. QT260 H669d 1974]
RC1210.H5    1974      617′.1027      73-21970
ISBN  0-397-50330-X

# *Preface*

Since the 1968 appearance of the first edition, the mushrooming interest in sports medicine noted therein has continued apace. At the same time the need for a volume directed toward the team physician and his problems, both general and specific, has increased correspondingly. It has been gratifying to note the nationwide acceptance of the first edition by team physicians. From both oral and written comments from readers throughout the athletic world, including coaches, trainers, physical education students, medical students, and, most important, physicians directly associated with organized athletic programs, it is apparent that the objectives outlined therein were in large part attained. Furthermore, it is of interest to note that, in those peak years of radical emergency knee surgery that coincided with the appearance of the first edition, much critical reaction was heard from those orthopedists who believed that the conservatism espoused therein was entirely wrong; yet rereading of the text in the light of accumulated surgical experience since that time indicates that there has indeed been a swing back toward a more conservative handling of knee injuries, so innocuous is the content today.

Because of the general and critical acceptance of the subject matter contained in the first edition—the one notable exception being at an institution famed for its bitter rivalry with Yale—few changes have been made in the text other than for the purposes of clarification. Supplementary material has been presented to make note of the increasing drug problems in athletics, and certain additions have been made to correlate the text with the needs of grant-in-aid athletic programs, which are by far predominant throughout the country; in this respect advantage is taken of the author's latest position at the University of South Carolina with its "big-time" grant-in-aid athletic program. Finally, a previously published statistical summary of five years of Yale Intercollegiate Football Injuries (compiled during the author's eighteen-year tenure as Yale athletic surgeon and team physician for Varsity football) is included, exactly as presented to the American College Health Association Meeting in Atlanta in 1972; contained therein is a statistical confirmation of much that is offered in the preceding text.

In conclusion, I would like to add my sincere thanks to authorities at the University of South Carolina, particularly Mr. Paul Dietzel, Athletic Director and Head Football Coach, in addition to all those mentioned in the preface to the first edition. And specific tribute must be paid to the hospitality and assistance so cheerfully provided by Dr. Robert Andrivet of the *Institut National des Sports* (Paris, France) and Dr. Herbert Reindell of the *Lehrstuhl für Kreislaufforschung und Leistungsmedizin* (Freiburg, Germany).

ISAO HIRATA, JR., M.D.

# Contents

*To American athletes,*
*and in particular to Junior Varsity athletes,*
*whose spirit, determination, and self-sacrifice*
*so often go unrewarded*

# Part One

## General Principles

# 1

# *Introduction*

To publish yet another book on the injuries and disabilities of the athlete, be he Little League, high school, or professional, requires some justification. In the past ten to fifteen years book after book has appeared, each purporting to treat authoritatively this very subject, some of little or no practical value, others of truly classic stature. It is our purpose, however, to view the entire field from a vantage point that no other work offers, that of the doctor on the field. For it is here that the greatest help is needed in athletic medicine, and at the same time it is here that the available literature falls short.

With the increasing activity of the Little League and similar organizations throughout the country, sponsoring miniature versions of football, baseball, and basketball, and with the growing impact of the mass media on every facet of amateur and professional athletics, there is an ever growing need for physicians to supervise and provide medical care to competitive athletics at one or another level. Governmental interest in physical fitness, the burgeoning age-group AAU program, as well as the ever growing population and the concomitant increase in secondary schools will further intensify the demand for medical services. There can be no doubt that medicine, whatever its feelings on the matter, must be increasingly involved at the level of direct responsibility.

It matters little whether the doctor be an orthopedist, general practitioner, internist, or even obstetrician, his direct responsibility cannot be evaded for long. The general public, its appetite whetted by universal television coverage of college and professional football, basketball, and baseball, expects its local community to provide proper facilities for these and other sports; at the same time the public expects the medical profession to provide services for these programs. Refusal to participate because of insufficient time, insufficient financial return, or strong convictions against competition among the young will not change these programs or these demands for service. Instead, the doctor may find, as often happens, that his own children have become a part of one of these competitive programs (moral disapproval notwithstanding), and he will then find himself, as a parent, demanding the high level of medical care that he himself had refused to provide. This does not mean that every doctor should cut his practice to become team physician for the local high school; but it does mean that when he comes to terms with competitive athletics—as come to terms he must—he may find that he is ignorant of the field and its problems. For despite the many books and voluminous literature by experts in the field he will find, as I did, that the real problems, the difficulties that plague all doctors working directly in athletics, are either not to be found in the printed word or are hidden in the middle of paragraphs dealing with more "major" clinical problems. A thorough residency training program in general surgery, which included thoracic surgery, orthopedics, and neurosurgery—even 3 years of surgery in the military—failed to prepare the writer for the unique disabilities found only in competitive athletics. It is unlikely that the anxious doctor-father, no matter what his specialty, will be any better prepared.

What can he say, what can he do, when an earnest young sprinter walks up to him and asks innocently: "My hamstring is a little tight today. . . . Should I work out or lay off for the meet tomorrow?"

A frenzied scrutiny of the literature at the nearest medical library or a quick look at one of the accepted classics will avail the doctor nothing. He will most probably find no answer to the question, or, if by luck he does, the boy will long ago have wandered off to ask someone who is very likely to have the answer: his team trainer!

Why should this be so? Why is there such a paucity of accurate medical information on this level? Why is so much written about the proper timing of major knee or shoulder surgery on this or that professional star and nothing written that could answer this boy's inquiry?

The answer to these questions is simple. An overwhelming percentage of athletic disabilities is so minor as to warrant little or no attention from the devoted clinician who deals only with "serious" conditions. A sore hamstring, asymptomatic except when a boy really "pours it on," is hardly worthy of notice; there is no real disability, the boy can continue to go to school, he is not in pain, so why worry about it? The soreness will surely disappear if the part is adequately rested, will it not? Given sufficient time and rest, the complaint cannot fail to disappear!

But view the problem from the boy's standpoint. He has worked hard to make the track squad, at training that with a college runner may be measured in years. By "training" we mean hours of practice at middle distances, short distances, interval repeats, time trials, and all the other drudgery that goes with building up one's neuromuscular and cardiovascular systems to the highest possible peak. Yet with his complaint all is in danger of going for naught, because a sprinter who can't sprint is as truly crippled as one who has a fractured femur. To consider this complaint as subclinical and therefore unimportant is to be unwittingly contemptuous of everything the boy has accomplished up to that moment!

Here lies the key to the problem. To the average follower of sports athletic injuries include all injuries suffered in athletics, thus cover the entire gamut of traumatic surgery. Although this is true semantically, a fractured femur is a fractured femur, no matter what the cause. Proper treatment thereof in no way differs from that afforded any person so injured regardless of the circumstances of the injury. Rehabilitation in the athlete must be carried beyond the usual definition of full function, but otherwise a clinical injury is a clinical injury, whether the victim is an athlete, a bank president, or a housewife. However, such truly clinical problems, the diagnosis and proper disposition of which are perfectly straightforward, constitute less than 5 per cent of the total injuries in an average intercollegiate athletic program. They are, from the standpoint of the team physician, the most clear cut and least problematical: he knows what to do and whom to call as consultants. But what of the remaining 95 per cent?

Athletes and coaches fully and justifiably expect serious accidents and disabilities to be treated with efficiency, dispatch, and skill. Beyond this, however, they expect that *any* disability—no matter how minor—will be treated with the same efficiency, dispatch, and skill, simply because the demands that they place on their bodies are such that the slightest handicap has serious consequences. They appreciate this and expect their team physician to appreciate it too. It is therefore the obligation of a doctor with direct responsibility in athletics to eliminate the words "subclinical" and "temporary" from his vocabulary. All disabilities are important and must be dealt with vigorously.

Furthermore, all disabilities must be dealt with individually, not by delegation or by rote, and each disability must be dealt with equally, not according to whether the injured athlete happens to be a star or not. This last bears repeating, for there is an all-too-human tendency among doctors to be impressed by the "star" athlete and the publicity attendant upon his injury. Thus, a minor disability in the "star" will be given the "red-carpet treatment" with press conferences and the like, while the lowly fourth-stringer with an identical injury is neglected. This same human tendency leads to the publication of scientific papers based on three or four cases of no statistical value whatever but somehow blessed with special significance because the three or four cases were champion athletes! Such articles are mentioned only to be condemned, yet the inference drawn by such writers cannot fail to disturb the critical reader, namely that, because the subjects of the report are truly outstanding in their field, there can be no doubt that the writers by association are equally great in the medical field!

To consider the foregoing as purposely exaggerated in order to make a point would be a great mistake. Unfortunately, the author's responsibility has placed him in an advantageous position, the better to view this all-too-common pattern of behavior as it affects athletes from every corner of the country.

Through all of this the athlete remains steadfast: his is a disability he knows exists, whether the doctors make little or much of it, and, "red-carpet treatment" or not, he awaits results. Prompt, efficient attention and a sympathetic ear are all he asks. If undue favoritism is shown or if compromises are made, he will know it and so will his fellow squad members.

Consequently, the doctor should check each complaint thoroughly and fairly, begin treatment promptly, and above all prove correct in his diagnosis and prognosis. For here we touch upon the keystone of any controlled athletic medical program: confidence. The athlete and his coach must know that the doctor understands his problem and is just as interested in returning him to competition as he himself may be. If there is a good reason for prolonged disability, the athlete will accept it. However, if he suspects that the doctor is "burning feathers," is temporizing because he is unable to make an accurate diagnosis, or is "going through the motions" for lack of interest, the doctor will lose his cooperation. And without voluntary communication, the physician will be reduced to the status of an ambulance driver, splinting obvious fractures and dislocations or dispatching the seriously injured athlete to the hospital for specialist attention. For no rule has ever been promulgated that will force an athlete to confide in a doctor, nor can regulations force an athlete to accept treatment from a doctor in whom he has no confidence. Furthermore, no administrative rules or closed panels can force an athlete to accept care from a consultant if he has no confidence in the referring doctor, the team physician!

On the other hand, athletes as well as coaches are more than anxious to find a doctor who looks at their problems from their point of view; once they find him, their friendship and cooperation are assured. It is difficult to recast one's thinking and look at all problems in this different light, yet such must be done. One need only look as far as the team trainer to appreciate this. To many doctors the functions of the trainer are of no great importance, but if questioned most of them could not describe these functions. Nevertheless, it is because of the widespread refusal of the medical profession to take part in a coordinated program at the level of the athlete and coach that trainers have become an integral part of the athletic scene. The need of the athlete for care in conditions that fall short of the textbook definition of disability together with the doctor's lack of involvement on this level created a therapeutic vacuum early in this century as competitive athletics began to establish themselves. The trainer filled this vacuum and continues to do so. A skilled trainer can handle most athletic problems far better than a doctor unfamiliar with the care of athletes. It would be easy to brand the sprinter with a sore hamstring as badly misguided in seeking medical advice from his trainer, but, if we as doctors cannot give him the answer, where else can he turn?

It is toward this end, then, that this book has been written. The orthopedic surgeon, the neurosurgeon, the thoracic surgeon will find nothing here that will change his outlook in his chosen specialty; the internist will find no formula to cure the athlete who presents with a hacking cough. All doctors, however, can profit from experiences in our program, a program of medical care over the entire spectrum of intercollegiate athletics, a program that may seem far removed from clinical practice, yet through counterpart programs in every community and secondary school may be as close to them as their own families.

Accordingly, no attempt will be made to debate the advantages or disadvantages of this or that knee incision or this or that repair of a recurrently dislocating shoulder. Exposition and discussion will center instead on the physician on the field, without the dry and trimmed x-ray in his pocket, without the lab reports before him, but working with the tools that physicians have used since time immemorial—eyes, ears, and hands. The problems with which he must deal will be discussed at length as well as the treatment of choice. The need for prompt referral to consultants will be discussed in relation to specific conditions. Comment will be made when germane on certain clinical procedures in terms of athletic performance before and after such procedures. By and large, however, the focus will be on that same doctor to whom our young sprinter directed his "innocent" question.

# 2

# Basic Requirements of Proper Medical Management

To organize an overall medical program that will fulfill the needs of the athlete, one must first assess the social content and importance of athletics, and then incorporate this assessment into a basic medical philosophy, applicable to all sports and to all athletes.

## The Value of Competitive Athletics

First of all, let us consider the basic morality of competition. Many pediatricians and psychiatrists feel that competition between youngsters and between young men is neither desirable nor healthful, and they are probably correct in the case of pre-school and grade school children. But to carry this philosophy to the level of secondary school and above is to ignore the realities of modern life. Competition between peer groups exists at these levels, whether it is approved or not, and it affects every facet of life thereafter. There is competition for academic marks, social popularity, status symbols—even competition to be the least competitive! To deny the existence of this drive, simply because it would appear to be the root of all evil, will not make it disappear. It is there, and nothing on earth can change it. Thus we see children racing against one another to see who can run the fastest. Given a bat and glove, they will vie against one another to be the better baseball player. Given a heavy stone (or shot put, if you will), they will grunt and groan, striving to heave it as far as possible. Even proper young ladies, given a jump rope, will strive to outdo one another in fancy maneuvers, new chants, or sheer endurance.

If competition is thus an inextricable part of human existence, what then of competitive athletics? Would not the energy poured into sheer physical competition be better applied to more peaceful and intellectual pursuits? Here again we encounter an immutable truth: Those of us who are blessed with better-than-average neuromuscular strength and coordination cannot be prevented from pitting these attributes against others so endowed; similarly, those of us who are primarily introspective, contemplative, and sedentary will find others of like mind and vie with one another also, (perhaps to the extent of sneering at any and all accomplishments of the more athletic group). One needs only to overhear a group of intellectuals, striving to insert some obscure reference and quotation from Hegel or Schopenhauer into a heated discussion, to realize that they, too, are pitting their strength against their peers. Authorities, therefore, who favor intellectual pursuits to physical ones as being more peaceful and constructive, had best take a closer look at themselves.

## The Value of Contact Sports

Let us accept the inevitability of competitive athletics in our way of life and turn to consideration of the various sports themselves.

The first differentiation to be made is between contact and non-contact sports. According to the criteria applied at most schools contact sports include football (the one primarily so considered but actually, as Michigan State's Duffy Daugherty has said, a "collision sport") as well as soccer, basketball, hockey, wrestling, rugby, lacrosse, and to a lesser extent baseball; all others are considered non-contact activities. A number in this list, such as hockey, rugby, and lacrosse, are obviously violent, and body contact is not only uncontrolled but quite legal, but other sports are included that do not normally come to mind as contact sports. Thus, surprisingly, basketball, in which there are numerous rules against contact, is definitely on the list: Knee and ankle injuries, usually suffered when returning to the floor after a high jump and landing on someone's foot, severe contusions from inadvertent collisions, and back and kidney injuries from flying knees and elbows "under the boards," all are commonly seen during an average basketball season despite the rules. Similarly, baseball contains certain contact risks aside from the inherent dangers of the swung bat and a rapidly moving, almost rock hard ball: Catchers are exposed to violent collisions both with determined base-runners and the unyielding stands behind them on foul pops; ardent outfielders also risk collisions with walls or fellow fielders, as do shortstops and second basemen on the double-play ball.

From this list it is easy to see that contact sports include virtually all those athletic activities most enthusiastically supported by athletes and spectators alike, and it becomes immediately apparent that included therein are those sports that enjoy the greatest financial success in the professional field, with multi-million dollar contracts, television packages, and nationwide press coverage.

It is not surprising, therefore, that critics, who favor gymnastics, swimming, track, tennis, and other non-contact sports, find themselves mere voices crying in the wilderness in any discussion of athletic injuries, particularly fatal ones. Many of these critics contend validly that contact sports are not necessary to the growing youth and do not create finer physical specimens than, for instance, Yale's own Don Schollander of swimming fame. They advance the equally cogent argument that elimination of contact sports would eliminate serious injuries and fatalities. Nevertheless, a majority of the American people consider their view unacceptable. Contact sports have become too deeply entrenched in our way of life to permit blanket abolition, nor do we recommend that such a radical and unenforceable step be contemplated. For, if the truth be known, the type of youth that engages in vigorous contact sports, whatever his deep psychological motivation, considers these activities a necessary part of his life, and, given no opportunities to satisfy his need by officially sanctioned activities, he will find equally dangerous pastimes over which medical supervision is impossible.

## A GUIDING MEDICAL PRINCIPLE

With the role of competitive athletics so firmly established, how can the medical profession best exert meaningful control? How can the team physician best fulfill his role?

The physician must demand a degree of overall control commensurate with his responsibilities, and his decisions must be ruled and accepted as final. Nothing short of this will suffice, for he must be in a position to apply his philosophy at all levels without exception and without compromise. Above all there must be no deviation from one all-important basic principle that must underlie each and every decision, large or small: *No athlete can be permitted to risk permanent aggravation of existing disability whatever the circumstances.*

Application of this principle can be a team physician's most difficult task, and to employ it honestly and universally without modification requires a coordinated program and control far beyond the usual game-day team-doctor arrangement. Certainly many doctors fully appreciate this need, but are unable to establish such a program. Nonetheless, such a program is the ideal in medical care for the athlete and thus should be a constant objective for all doctors.

## THE CONTROLLED MEDICAL PROGRAM

The need for finality in medical decisions, commensurate with the responsibility that any physician assumes when he steps on the field, would seem to be too obvious to require mention. It is the keystone to doctor-patient relations, and without it there can be no relationship at all. Every practicing physician appreciates this fact and is constantly aware of it each time he deals with patients. The only contradictions and criticisms he accepts are those from other members of the profession. Consequently, he cannot be held at fault if he assumes that his medical decisions will always be treated with respect by the non-professional. Unfortunately in athletic medicine he will find that such is not the case. Much to his chagrin and disillusionment he will find that his decisions are subject to wholesale criticism, not only from his colleagues (all of whom would have succeeded in returning that injured athlete to the fray in one half the time) but also from every layman who cares to read the sports news. And, far worse, he will find that some coaches and athletes may simply go their own way without the slightest regard for his opinion if it disagrees with theirs.

The establishment of an atmosphere of mutual respect and confidence is paramount in ending this dangerous situation; beyond that the doctor must be assured of administrative support and a degree of authority certifying that the final word is his. It is naive to assume that he can charm the entire coaching staff of a large athletic department as well as each and every athlete and thus obtain their cooperation. A small percentage may not choose to cooperate, and the doctor must be forearmed with a modicum of administrative power to enforce his decisions. If this is impossible, each disagreeable decision he makes will be met with ever increasing subversion to the extent that his efforts to provide reasonable medical care are largely nullified.

Over and above the basic need for physician control of final medical decision, however, an ideal medical program for the athlete must carry such control several steps further. The medical care program required by the injured or ill athlete is significantly different from that required by the rest of the student population. The reasons for this difference can be attributed to a number of factors, the most important of which are: first, the publicity surrounding diagnosis and case disposition;

second, demands of both coaches and fellow athletes for an accurate prediction of potential disability, demands which are justifiable because of the team adjustments required. These factors admittedly cannot and should not alter a calm, deliberate, painstaking diagnostic work-up and treatment program, but they are factors that must be recognized and accepted.

## CENTRALIZATION OF MEDICAL CONTROL

To best provide for these factors, there must be established a centralized overall medical control, toward which trainers, coaches, and the athletes themselves will turn voluntarily for information and guidance as treatment and rehabilitation progress. Such centralization eliminates the inevitable bugbear of conflicting opinions and conflicting statements from this specialist or that consultant, usually delivered orally to an already confused athlete. Centralization thereby eliminates the misunderstandings that so often negate the efforts of all concerned.

Furthermore, it fosters the immediate reporting of all injuries by the athlete and by the coaching staff as well as prompt referral of every disabled athlete by the coaching staff, be the disability medical or surgical. The deplorable delays in diagnosis and treatment that result from ignorance and self-care are thus eliminated.

Centralized control should be a day-to-day control, not just week-to-week, providing thereby a continuously available authority to which the athlete can turn, and at the same time providing an authority through which individual programs of rehabilitation can be checked to assure the early return to participation of a fully conditioned athlete.

Lastly, such centralization can go far in eliminating the willful use of contradiction and confusion by the athlete himself. By way of explanation, it must be pointed out that any modern program of medical care must provide specialists and consultants of every description. Disagreements and differences must be expected, therefore, and these become even wider when dealing with an athlete. Although professional disagreement can and does result, it can be controlled by centralization of final authority.

Over and beyond this honest professional confusion, however, is the confusion that a single, crafty young man can produce with surprisingly little effort, shrewdly directed. It is no secret that doctors disagree. Knowing this, a young man can go from doctor to doctor at will, giving whatever historical data he feels will garner the most sympathy, in the sure knowledge that his complaint, stemming as it usually does from some particular athletic activity that is very likely outside his listener's personal experience, will provide him with the recommendation he is looking for. If he is sufficiently alert—and all such young men are—he will be certain to vary his approach, visiting first this doctor then that one, compounding confusion atop contradiction until no one, not even his coach, dares tell him what he can or cannot do: no one, that is, except himself, which is precisely his objective.

Obviously, such behavior cannot be tolerated, but there is only one way it can be neutralized. That way is to assure that such a boy can neither begin nor continue such "medical shopping" without the full knowledge of the doctor in overall control. He is then presented with an organized medical structure instead of a series of uncoordinated fragments, a structure whose solidity will usually prove too imposing to warrant his effort.

## A RATIONAL ATHLETIC POLICY

The application of sound medical principles, the establishment of a controlled overall medical program, and a centralization of medical authority are pivotal parts of any conscientious effort to provide the best care for the athlete, and these are the precise areas where the interested physician can accomplish much by his own efforts. However, beyond his control and overshadowing all his endeavors is one key requirement: a rational, overall athletic policy. If understanding prevails among the high-level policy makers, all will be well. Certainly, if a doctor has been successful in establishing control and responsibility for the medical care of athletes, he can justifiably hope for the best, but a specific statement of aims in athletics, such as the President's Agreement among the Ivy League schools, is the only ideal assurance that his efforts will not be in vain.

For, in those unfortunate instances where winning is the one and only justification for the existence and expense of competitive athletics, the athletes become professionals, hired to win. If it be a school, the alumni and/or administration become the arbiters of what constitutes proper medical treatment; if it be a professional franchise, the owners, the ticket buyers, and the injured athletes themselves become the arbiters of medical competence. In such surroundings the physician finds himself compromised before he starts, his decisions tempered by considerations that a sensible athletic policy would never require.

Yet it is intriguing to note the ready acceptance by otherwise critical physicians of recommendations by doctors caring for professional athletes. In particular there is a dangerous trend toward the adoption of standards of treatment and of disability evaluation used by professional franchises, simply because these franchises are champions in their conference, division, or league. One cannot honestly fault the doctors who find themselves trapped by such a distorted policy. It is only when their personal opinions and judgments are presented as oracular pronouncements and disagreement discouraged, that a plea for caution must be made. For in this situation the medical profession is split by unnecessary confusion and controversy, and, more serious, many athletes and their families accept these distortions as truth and demand identical treatment.

## A SYMPATHETIC MEDICAL APPROACH

The need for sympathetic understanding of the athlete and his peculiar problems has already been mentioned, but beyond this the physician must be interested in all sports, no matter how doubtful their value may seem to him. Some doctors prefer football, others gymnastics, yet, when functioning as a physician to athletes, personal preferences cannot be allowed to color professional decisions. To many the concept of hordes of brawny enthusiasts, chasing pell-mell after a small rubber ball while committing mayhem on one and all with a hardwood stick, borders on the ridiculous—to these earnest young men, however, this is the noble sport of lacrosse. All too often, purely medical decisions are modified, compromised, even vitiated, because the doctor is an enthusiast of a particular sport or, conversely, regards it as suicidal, hence an activity from which any participant should be barred on general principles regardless of the actual disability. Thus, a lacrosse player may find himself "on the shelf," because his doctor neither understands nor appreciates the game and, hence, sees no reason to hasten rehabilitation. Much worse, a player may find himself urged to "get back in there, I played with worse" by one who used to be a player himself.

### Differentiation Among Athletes

As sports differ, so do athletes, and it is equally important for the doctor to acquire an accurate insight into each one, not just as another case in a squad of 50 but as a real person. If a physician is unable to generate enthusiasm about people and their motivations—in short, if he lacks interest in personality and, if you will, psychiatry—

he will find himself floundering. Athletes, even more than the average human, are subject to unfathomable quirks and psychosomatic symptoms. In the crucible of varsity competition many find themselves unable to excel or even survive; some cannot face defeat; others welcome it. In general, this is most prominent in the so-called individual sports, such as track, in which inadequate performance is painfully obvious to even the rawest novice. The hypothetical young man in the preceding chapter might represent such a typical problem, since the "sore hamstring" is a favorite gambit among runners. Thus, he may have seen the last 220 time posted by his rival on the morrow and wants no part of the race; on the other hand, he may be the typical boy who simply needs reassurance. Even worse, he may be the not uncommon type who hates to run and, having spotted a new doctor, proceeds to "con" him into an excuse from practice. To navigate in this sea of motivational cross currents, to separate gross exaggerations from the real thing, to eliminate "con-artists" and yet encourage the frightened boy is far from easy. It requires above all a personal acquaintance with every boy, which, although apparently impossible, can be accomplished by sincere effort and honest concern.

## Differentiation Among Sports

Having achieved an accurate picture of injury or disability, the doctor must also differentiate among the sports involved. External otitis in a football player, though uncomfortable, is hardly disabling; whereas for a swimmer it is a sheer disaster. Similarly, coryza and a slight cough without fever does not hamper a football player, even on a muddy field and in a cold rain; whereas it would prevent a two-miler, running indoors in a dusty arena, from reaching the finish line. Needless to say, differentiation to this degree requires a detailed knowledge of the mechanics and demands of each individual sport, to a total of 18 sports in an average collegiate program. However, with diligence and above all personal interest in the contestants, it is not as difficult as it might seem.

Similarly, disability must be measured against variable factors within each sport as well as from sport to sport. A mild sprained ankle will hamper an offensive center very little, but a sprained thumb, secondary to its effect on the snap-back for punts and extra points, can result in 10 to 14 days of disability. On the other hand, an offensive guard with identical injuries must be judged from an entirely different viewpoint; a mild sprained ankle to him is a major disability as he pulls out and cuts for an offensive hole, but a sprained thumb strapped into his fist does not hamper him at all.

Finally, disability varies from person to person, and the team physician must appreciate this. Motivational variations have been touched upon, as they affect complaints of disability, but beyond that identical injuries and disabilities vary in their effect on different types of athletes. Some are inherently cautious, even hypochondriacal, and they nurse an injured part with loving care, never under any circumstances risking its aggravation. Such a boy can be allowed to name his own day for return to full activity without the slightest concern that he will prematurely aggravate his injury. On the other end of the spectrum, some boys have no concern whatever for their physical well-being and will, in coaches' parlance, "run through a brick wall." These athletes cannot be trusted and require a watchful eye at all times. In one such instance, when contact work was contraindicated but general conditioning desirable, we removed every piece of padded equipment from the young man's locker. Despite this the moment we turned our back on him on the practice field, he tried to enter a skeleton scrimmage without pads or helmet. When ordered out, he proceeded, muttering imprecations, to the bucker, still without pads or helmet, and then lacerated his right ear against the rough canvas padding on the bucker upright!

## COOPERATION WITH ATHLETIC STAFF AND PRESS

### Doctor—Trainer Cooperation

The place of the team trainer on the athletic scene is as firmly established as that of the team physician. In many schools, in fact, his place in athletic tradition reaches back into the dim past, whereas a dozen team physicians may have come and gone. He is part of the athletic staff on an equal footing with the coaches, and his entire professional life is devoted to athletics. The author has been singularly fortunate in having been associated with a head trainer who is universally considered as one of the best. Consequently, ours was a gentle initiation into a most difficult and poorly documented area of medical responsibility. Potential pitfalls were gently pointed out, divergent requirements were tactfully outlined, and basic philosophical principles were molded in long hours of patient discussion. Many physicians, particularly those at the secondary school level, are not so blessed and must struggle alone. This is unfortunate, because to fulfill the medical needs of the athlete without the aid of a good trainer is virtually impossible.

The reason for this are numerous, and only a few of them will be touched upon. By and large, however, there is one common denominator: the true caliber of the trainer in fulfilling his duties. Thus, he must be an expert equipment man, able to cope with the countless details of ordering, evaluating, fitting, and maintaining proper equipment for all sports. He must be able to design and construct legally sanctioned pieces of special equipment to order, such as hockey masks and injury pads. He must be expert in the field of physical rehabilitation and physical therapy. He must be expert in all the intertwined by-ways in that veritable jungle of controversy, physical conditioning. He must know nutrition, particularly as it applies to what an athlete will or will not eat regardless of the mineral or protein content. He must be expert in the application of splints, slings, bandages, dressings, and other first aid measures, as well as the host of specialized taping maneuvers used only in athletics. He must be expert in the mechanics and maintenance of heavy ancillary equipment used in the various sports. He must be expert on field maintenance and what constitutes a good turf for football, a good infield for baseball, and so on. He must be expert in his handling of the varying temperaments within any large coaching and training staff, advising and counseling, compromising and criticizing, all at the same time. Most important of all, he must be the father-confessor of each troubled athlete, the one man to whom they will turn for help and advice on study methods, organization of work schedules, financial difficulties, as well as the entire gamut of medical and sociological problems every young man encounters.

It is this last function that renders a good trainer truly invaluable. All other functions can be rendered by others, though only with the greatest effort by the physician, and even then not nearly so well: thus, when the Olympic Games deprived us of our head trainer for 6 weeks, we were able by expending much time and effort to limp along until his return—however, the one function that proved impossible to fulfill involved his insight into the physical and mental well-being of the football squad as a whole, insight which only an alert and capable trainer can provide. The hours that a good trainer spends in the training room are filled with the banter, personal exchanges, shop talk, and mutual confidences of virtually everyone on several squads, talk that is freely given and received within a purely athletic framework, talk that no doctor in any official capacity would be allowed to enter. Personality quirks, candid opinions of fellow athletes, and personal anxieties can provide the experienced listener with an amazingly accurate insight into the doubts, motivations, hopes, and, in fact, capabilities of a team. As an integral and accepted part of this athletic scene, the trainer in turn can provide the doctor and coach with an accurate insight into many problems as they develop, insight without which many of these problems would remain a complete enigma. Without an alert trainer no one, not even the coaches, will gain a glimmer of this all-important aspect of athletics, for no coach, any more than a doctor, can enter a training room without himself sensing an immediate change in atmosphere.

These, then, are some of the qualities a good trainer can bring to any athletic medical program. Naturally, trainers vary in ability, and many of these qualities may be lacking. The physician must, therefore, work very closely with his trainer until he can judge how far short of the ideal he may be. A careful evaluation of how he fulfills his varied functions is a necessity, and the degree of delegation of duties and responsibilities only then decided upon. Such delegation must be discussed and clearly established by mutual agreement and not by pronouncement; no trainer should be laden with responsibilities that he does not welcome, regardless of his capabilities. At the same time delegation, once clearly established, should be respected in all instances. The doctor who runs out on the field at the slightest provocation on heavily attended game days, but leaves the trainer to sink or swim during week-day practice, may impress the crowd and himself but certainly not the trainer or the team. Far worse, he exhibits little respect for the trainer's integrity and in turn will receive very little.

Similarly, areas of special trainer skills should be as carefully respected as purely medical areas should be by the trainer. The doctor who can tape an ankle or knee properly is a rarity indeed, and to apply tape as expertly as an experienced trainer is little short of impossible for most doctors. This being so, there is little justification for a doctor to enter a training room, extract the number-one quarterback or All-American lineman, and tape him as a personal gesture.

Without mutual respect there can be no mutual confidence, and a tragic breakdown in communication may result. And without communication the physician will find himself working under a self-imposed handicap. For despite his efforts and despite the confidence athletes may have in him every team physician will find that there are many small injuries that never reach his official attention. This is perfectly understandable from the athlete's viewpoint; to his way of thinking the risk of a possible 1 day absence from practice on medical advice may be too horrible to contemplate. Consequently, he will slip in quietly to the trainer, confide in him, and thus avoid the risk. A good trainer will evaluate this worried boy and his injury and, if it is sufficiently minimal, reassure the boy without calling the doctor, thus respecting the boy's confidence without neglecting the injury. Such a minimal injury can then be reported orally to the physician, who in turn can respect the confidence in which it was given and simply make a mental note of it or, if by mutual agreement further evaluation is necessary, accomplish this as tactfully as possible. At the same time more significant injuries can be examined together with the trainer, and a treatment plan formulated jointly that will fit the planned squad workouts, the practicalities of special added equipment, the legalities involved, and all the other specialized knowledge a good trainer has at his fingertips. Progress reports can then be exchanged daily on each disability on the squad with information flowing in both directions.

By such means an integrated effort can be exerted to the best interests of the athlete, the squad, the coach, and all others concerned. This integrated effort obliterates the not unusual schism in athletic medical care, the schism between a trainer loyal to the athletic department and a doctor aware only of medical responsibilities. And it is this schism that athletes and coaches will gladly widen if it is to their own advantage, thus nullifying the best intentioned medical program.

## Doctor—Coach Cooperation

The concept of mutual respect as it applies to the trainer applies equally to the coach. The coach's lot is not a happy one, and the team physician is often just one more cross he must bear, because only rarely does the doctor bring him anything but bad news. Granted, there are degrees of bad news, but those instances in which anything medical must be discussed that will better the coach's situation are difficult to imagine. Be that as it may, a coach should be informed of diagnoses, prognoses in particular, and rehabilitation progress. It is his job to make adjustments based on these reports, and he cannot do his job without accurate information. Preparations for a long or short disability, maintenance of team morale in the face of a key injury, shifts of personnel based on accurate medical prognosis, all are the task of the coach. It is clearly an arduous one.

All information given to the coach must be accurate, and despite the difficulties of accurate day-to-day or week-to-week prognosis on any given disability such predictions are precisely what the coach needs above all. Anatomical and physiological details and medical polysyllabism do not accomplish this end, nor do detailed explanations as to why accurate prognosis cannot be given. The coach wants to know how bad the disability is, if it is permanent, and, if not, how long before it will be well—no more but certainly no less. He will not be happy (and who would be?), he may argue for a while, and he may mention some professional athlete who "never missed a practice." In the end, however, he will accept accurate information calmly given. (Of the many coaches on the large staff at Yale, all were ready to accept accurate information, disastrous though it might have been to their plans, just so long as it was accurate.) A constant effort must be made to avoid inconsistency or uncertainty. Obfuscation in the face of confusion is readily penetrated by these former athletes and once the coach's confidence is shaken the entire medical program hangs in the balance.

Coaches, for example, are blessed with exceptionally long memories, particularly with regard to injuries within their sport. A 20 year veteran can probably recall in detail just what was done for a certain injury 20 years ago, how long the boy was out, and whether he was as good a performer when he returned. If modern medical methods cannot improve on such recollection, modern medicine is in trouble; if modern medicine cannot do as well, the physician is in trouble! Similarly, a coach can be depended on to recall just how long an identical injury and disability lasted in an athlete in some other sport in such and such a year; if his boy is going to be disabled for longer there had better be a good reason! None of these problems is insurmountable and cannot be easily overcome with forthright honesty and logical reasoning, but a doctor in athletics must be prepared to deal with each and every one of them. If he is fair and honest, does not favor one sport over another, does not become personally enmeshed with one coach among the others (only to find himself "obligated" to bend his principles for his friend), and remains strictly neutral in his medical position, not only from sport to sport and coach to coach but also from "star" to lowly fourth-stringer, he can be assured of every cooperation from all coaches.

This cooperation is the keynote of any successful medical program in athletics. With it the coach will modify plans for future contests on the basis of medical indications, and, equally important, will make minute-to-minute changes in an athletic contest on the same basis. Without it he will go his own way. A truly coordinated effort results in immediate on-the-field adjustments in personnel, removing an athlete whom the doctor observes to be nearing the borderline of physical disability. It allows the doctor to check such boys and recommend either an immediate return to the game or possibly a rest of 5 minutes or a quarter, all with the sure knowledge that his recommendations will be respected. The game then remains under medical control, without seriously interfering with the myriad other problems that weigh upon the coach.

Further, cooperation serves to maintain the mutual respect that must characterize doctor-coach relations. The coach may occasionally try to penetrate into a purely medical area out of sheer enthusiasm, but, if he is given cogent reasons for medical decisions, he will return to his own field. By the same token the doctor should never invade the coaching field. Each is an area of complexity that must be respected. Cooperation between the doctor and the coach assures the best medical care for the athlete, but confusion accomplishes just the opposite.

After years in a particular sport the doctor cannot help but gain considerable knowledge of the techniques, tactics, and other "inside" matters that will enable him to understand the complexities of that sport often to a greater extent than the layman or sports writer. He may even feel quite capable of assessing talent in an athlete and how it should be handled. If the reader doubts this, he need only observe and listen to doctors who have recently become officially associated with a football staff. Their mastery of the jargon, their judgment of squad members in coaching terms, and their views of tactics and strategy are so professional as to be intelligible only to those in the sport!

However, insight into the personality makeup of an athlete is not the same thing as having a coach's viewpoint. The particular insight that is valuable to the doctor should be used for his own medical needs, not to criticize the coach's methods with a player. Often the athlete, who medically is "tough as nails," who complains only when something is wrong, and always gives the doctor an accurate clinical picture, lacks some basic ability that the coach is able to detect; whereas another "problem" boy, the type that causes trainers and doctors to look heavenward for help each time he approaches with a wounded look on his face, may possess just those qualities the coach wants. We should not allow our medical "insight" to color either our treatment of the boy or our respect for the coach.

The complexities of coaching, despite the ease with which the more superficial aspects can be acquired, are such that these men devote their entire lives to it. No doctor can acquire similar knowledge unless he wants to coach (which some have done), but he cannot be a doctor and a coach at the same time. Certain dangerous techniques and customary practices can be criticized from a medical standpoint, but only to assure a healthier team, not a more expert one. The latter is the job of the coach and should be left to him. By the same measure the doctor must never leave a medical decision for the coach to worry about. A boy sent back to practice at "full go after the coach thinks it's OK" burdens the coach with a responsibility he does not want and should not be asked to assume. He has his job to do and so does the doctor; to each his own.

### The Doctor and the Press

One of the most striking differences between the care of athletes and of patients in the average clinical practice is the disproportionate publicity associated with everything in sports. The doctor in athletics therefore finds himself in close contact with the sporting press. Since it can be assumed that he is honest and forthright, there would seem to be little need for guidance in this area. Most doctors have on occasion cared for patients who have attracted the attention of the local press, although such instances are probably few in number for each physician. In athletics, however, the doctor discovers that he is dealing with patients who attract daily local press coverage and frequently that of the nationwide wire services.

In coping with this publicity, the doctor must recognize that his is a unique position. He will be personally known to every local reporter, each guided by his own personal standards. He will find himself being quoted out of context, paraphrased by laymen, and, far worse, judged by his own medical colleagues on the basis of completely inaccurate news reports. That the latter is deplorable and grossly unfair does not alter the fact that by and large doctors are sports fans first and critical readers second. Considering their limited experience with the press, this is certainly understandable. Nonetheless, any doctor directly concerned with athletics must remain aware of this unjust but ever present factor and temper his actions and words accordingly.

The doctor's first concern must be that all gross inaccuracies be kept from the athlete's family, by direct and immediate communication if necessary. Similarly, he must provide each disabled athlete with as much information as he can absorb, so that regardless of what appears in print the athlete knows the truth. Lastly, he must assure that the news that reaches print is as accurate as possible. At the same time he must keep temporary disabilities out of the press (opposing coaches also read the papers).

To accomplish these ends, circumspection is the byword. Certainly there should be no difficulty in keeping the athlete and his family informed, as in any clinical practice. To do so is a medical obligation regardless of the press. If anyone should have access to accurate medical information, the immediate family should. However, the problem often is to convince both athlete and family that what they have been told by the doctor is really the truth and that what later appeared in the press is inaccurate. As for the rest much will depend on the type of reporter involved, something over which the doctor has little control. Thus, some reporters strive to check and recheck every item for accuracy and will approach the doctor merely to confirm information they already have; others find it easier to fill their column with a "complete medical report" on the entire team, a medical report gleaned from talking to the athlete, his teammates, maybe a roommate or two, and the coach. Since there are usually a few athletes who are hobbled by minor injuries early in a football week, this gambit is sometimes used weekly as a column filler, without once speaking directly to the doctor or head trainer. To hope for even the slightest accuracy under these circumstances would be optimistic, and at times we have been flabbergasted by such reports. Inaccurate though they are, these reports gain wide publicity and are usually accepted as fact by the majority of readers.

The doctor in athletics soon recognizes these types of journalists, and he may advantageously impart accurate information to the first type in order to counteract an inaccuracy by the latter. By and large, however, information should be given sparingly and with the condition that no names will be used. (A general term such as "medical department spokesman" is sufficient.) This last is of some importance. Not giving a name emphasizes the team approach, including the trainer, the team doctor, the radiologist, the orthopedist or internist, all of whom may play a role. Of equal significance, such "ex cathedra" pronouncements will keep other inquiring reporters from harassing the team doctor, reporters who may not yet be aware of the overall medical program.

On rare occasions such impersonal releases may be inadequate, owing to rumors and speculation concerning what has not been said or done. At such times it may be necessary to resort to a direct quotation attributed to the physician. If the doctor has no access to a professional press-relations man, he is advised to seek out the reporter whose sense of responsibility and propriety has proved most dependable and request that the release be quoted in its entirety for both local and wire service distribution. The release in turn should be so succinctly worded that quotation out of context and/or paraphrasing will render it unintelligible, thereby assuring that quotation out of context will not be attempted. The exact wording, therefore, is best decided upon in close cooperation with a professional newsman or public information officer.

Beyond these efforts there is little more the physician can do. The power of the printed word is truly awesome, and never will the physician be more aware of this than in athletics, where poor, inaccurate reporting can do more to destroy a team, a coach, and even a medical program than any other single factor. Good reporters realize this and try their best to rectify the situation, but whether their efforts are successful is debatable. The mass media have also entered the fray with more "inside" reporting, much of it romanticized and packed with technical coaching terminology to impress the readers. These media take positions and make judgments in keeping with their "expert" rank in every phase of athletics, whether it be coaching, playing, doctoring, or all three at once, while at the same time they are exercising their real forte, mass circulation.

## INTERCOLLEGIATE ATHLETICS AND THE CONTROLLED MEDICAL PROGRAM

In order to review briefly how the foregoing requirements can be applied in an overall program of medical care, we shall summarize the program developed at Yale University. We do not mean to imply that this program is superior to any other, but it serves as a practical demonstration of what can be accomplished by coordinated effort.

Competitive athletics at Yale has constituted a vast program, designed to offer some type of physical activity to every student no matter what his talents or inclinations. There are several levels of competition in every sport: the intercollege (or intramural), the freshman-intercollegiate, and the usually-thought-of varsity and junior varsity intercollegiate athletic squads. Although every student is eligible to compete at any level, movement from one level to another in the same sport is controlled by rulings designed to prevent an intramural team from suddenly acquiring athletes of varsity caliber for a crucial contest. The available selection of sports is roughly equal on all levels of competition, including tackle football, and equipment and playing areas of equal quality are provided by the University.

In a program as sprawling as this with some 300 boys in one or another level and type of sport vying against some 300 like minded Harvard students on a typical traditional football weekend, some attempt at differentiation had to be made in medical service. This, plus the lack of a central diagnostic and treatment area near the playing fields, necessitated a separation of medical services into two distinct channels: one for intramural and one for intercollegiate and freshman-intercollegiate. In addition, this differentiation was maintained throughout the central downtown medical facilities, to preserve some semblance of order and to assure that doctors assigned to the intramural field-work saw the same injuries on subsequent visits to the central facilities. At the same time, all serious freshman competitors, as well as varsity and junior-varsity level athletes, were seen by only one athletic surgeon, both on the field and in the field house and central Health Department.

### The Grant-in-Aid Scholarship Program

In contrast, the Grant-In-Aid Scholarship Program is predominant nationwide among the "big time" powers in intercollegiate athletics. As at the University of South Carolina, most beneficiaries of these programs are housed, fed, and supervised apart from the rest of the student body and are in fact distinctly separable therefrom. Moral objections aside—and these are many—such programs certainly simplify centralization of medical authority as well as centralization of medical services and the delivery thereof. All that is required is specific agreement with the Athletic Director and all else falls into place, no matter what resource is footing the medical bills. Medical care can be prompt, efficient, and totally arbitrary and should accomplish its end with far less controversy and far less effort than in equivalent Ivy League programs. However, it should be noted that with these advantages there is one distinct disadvantage, namely that self-motivation of the athlete, so much a part of Ivy League athletics, cannot be as blithely taken for granted in these more rigid programs; because the athlete is trading on his athletic prowess in a "strictly business" arrangement, problems of the sort more often seen in industrial medicine can be anticipated and are indeed more often seen. In short, athletes in Grant-In-Aid Programs are in general less likely to "play with pain" since it is hardly in their interest to do so—as long as they are willing to keep their end of the bargain and play when they are well, why should more be expected of them?

## A Central Athletic Clinic

Over and above attendance on the field it is necessary to maintain a central focal point on a daily basis. Accordingly, an athletic clinic should be held daily in the central Health Department, with x-ray and physical therapy facilities immediately available (7 mornings a week during the football season, 6 days a week for the remainder of the year). The hours chosen for the clinic should allow any student to get in between classes in the morning. The time and place of the clinic should be formally announced to all squad members by every varsity, junior-varsity, and freshman coach. Thus, every athlete knows where to go and when, and with the coaches' cooperation it is rare that problems are missed that were noticeable in the morning but unnoticeable the previous practice or game day.

Attendance at the clinic must be constant. The athletic surgeon and the head trainer of the athletic department must work together daily from pre-season football through the last baseball, track, and crew sessions in the spring, thereby assuring a continuity of control and a constant personal contact with all intercollegiate athletes. Equally important, at precisely the same hours an internist should be available to see all medical problems, and an orthopedist should be on hand for direct and immediate consultation. Both should be, by their availability and by design, best prepared to deal with athletes. Thus, the personal insight of the athletic surgeon and the head trainer into basic personality, motivations and ability, all of which is necessary in dealing properly with the competitive athlete, as well as their special knowledge of the sport concerned, position concerned, and coach concerned can be shared directly. Decisions concerning disability and limitations can then be reached by mutual agreement as a single, unified medical team.

## Disability Evaluation

To further assure that recommendations from the Medical Department are properly carried out, the head trainer should inform the coach directly, thereby placing no dependence on what the athlete may or may not choose to tell his coach. At Yale, the athlete's name was entered on the disability list (revised daily), a copy of which was forwarded weekly to the Athletic Department. The list provided each coach with an up-to-date written record of the medical status of each of his boys. If disability was such that the athlete could not report to practice, he was listed as on "full disability"; whereas, as was more often the case, if disability was not sufficient to bar an active rehabilitation program on the field, limited participation in some activities was permitted by placing his name in the "competitive disability" category. The latter barred by official directive any participation in intrasquad or outside scrimmages or contests. Moreover, by the on and off dates in each category an attempt could be made to predict return to full activity for those vitally concerned.

| Name | Class | Sport | Full Dis | | Comp Dis | | Diagnosis |
| | | | On | Off | On | Off | |
|------|-------|-------|------|------|------|------|-----------|
| Jones, J. | 68 | Fball | 9/15 | 9/17 | 9/17 | 9/20 | blanked on athl Dep copy |

In those sports in which the athletic surgeon is also the team physician, further accurate control is exerted by on-the-field follow-up. Equal control in the many other sports underway simultaneously can be accomplished through the cooperation of the coaches and the assistant trainers, through whom the head trainer can act by delegation.

In addition, every incoming freshman should be thoroughly reviewed for pre-existing disabilities that could compromise his college athletic career (about which more will be said in a later chapter). Such a review must extend to a proper and permanent categorization of disability, to be applied throughout his college career. Thus, some sports are barred, while others are permitted, as medically indicated. Such categorization requires knowledge of all sports, and should therefore be the added duty of the athletic surgeon, again aided by the same medical team. This assures that baseline evaluations and subsequent follow-ups are carried through by the same doctors, who, working as a team, can then modify their recommendations or maintain them. Again, lists of such permanent disabilities and sports prohibitions should be made available to all coaches of all sports without an accompanying diagnosis, and by departmental regulation the coaches should be responsible for checking through all squad rosters to assure that no such candidate appears upon them. If the coach has any questions about a particular disability or would like a review of an initial decision, the head trainer and athletic surgeon are then in a position to deal with the situation without confusion or misunderstanding, to the maximum benefit of all concerned.

It is obvious that our overall program at Yale was short of ideal, but, considering the basic requirements listed in the foregoing pages, it did accomplish something of what all physicians in athletics are striving to achieve. Better geographical centralization and improved physical facilities would have eased the task, and certain doctors remained convinced that changes in the medical team in their favor would have solved all problems.

At the University of South Carolina, in contrast, the structured scholarship program and its strict control by the Athletic Department vastly simplify the entire problem, requiring only that all Grant-In-Aid recipients be thoroughly examined annually and followed closely thereafter, with direct communication and control through their respective coaches requiring little administrative effort because of the centralization inherent in the program. The rare "walk-on" candidate is known to all at the outset and is easily dealt with medically and administratively from the start.

# 3

# The Physical Basis for Exclusion from Athletics

Discussion of such a broad subject, covering as it does the entire range of human pathology, must necessarily be incomplete. However, certain basic principles can go far in creating order out of chaos.

## CARDINAL PRINCIPLES

Above all, the paramount consideration is that *no athlete can be permitted to risk permanent disability whatever the cirmumstances.*

Secondly, all decisions must be based on an impartial view of all sports, without the preconception that one sport is safer or saner than another. Every effort should be made to assure an athlete's participation in the sport of his choosing, just so long as he can participate in all aspects of practice and competition without danger to himself or to the team. Accordingly, no special conditions on the type of practice and type of intra-squad activity should be made for medical reasons; either he is to be a candidate for the squad on an equal footing with everyone or he is barred from the sport. By keeping this last precept in mind, the physician avoids the not uncommon problem presented by parents or family physicians who are willing to have a candidate risk permanent injury so long as he is "on the varsity" and not in "some useless junior-varsity workout." Similarly, no medical differentiation can be made between competitive levels within the same sport in the mistaken belief that potential dangers increase as the level of competition rises. This is simply not so, for intramural competition with its wide disparity in native ability, conditioning, and muscular development is by far the most dangerous level in any sport. Such qualifications to medical clearance burden the trainer and coach with a problem that shackles them in their handling of the athlete and in turn affects the moral of the team faced with this "special case."

Thirdly, differentiation must be made between disability in one sport as against another. The specificity of disability in each sport and the specific mechanical demands in each must always be considered before an accurate decision can be made on sport disability. Thus, crew and polo are similar in that lower limb disability is of equally lesser importance than in the running sports. However, ligamentous instability in the knee, barely noticeable in the straight-line flexion and extension necessary in working the slide of a racing shell, is a dangerous disability in polo, in which nearly all stresses to the knee are absorbed with the knee in a partially flexed position; the hooking of stirrups in frequent collisions exerts a tremendous torsion force, transmitted through the boot to the already weakened knee.

## MEANS OF EVALUATION

With these basic principles firmly in mind the actual means of discovering and evaluating physical disability must be assessed.

**Clinical History.** For accurate evaluation a precise clinical history is an absolute necessity. However, the physician must remember that he is dealing with persons quite different from those seen in his office practice. The average athlete is not ill or in pain when he is under survey for sports eligibility. The doctor, to whom he is giving the history, represents a very significant threat to participation in his chosen sport rather than a friend who can and wants to help him. Consequently, athletes distort, conceal, even deny significant items in their past history. More distressing, parents of athletes often aid and encourage such evasions. Furthermore, family doctors and even specialists may support these distortions. Finally, it is not uncommon for athletes to invent or magnify insignificant historical items in an attempt to gain sympathy from the medical department and from teammates and coaches. They use this as an emotional "crutch," upon which they can lean should their abilities be found wanting. In short, the physician must be perpetually aware of many pitfalls in evaluating any athlete's clinical history, straightforward though it might seem at first glance.

**Physical Examination.** The second integral part of any medical evaluation, the physical examination, cannot be depended upon to eliminate every candidate who should be disqualified (despite the confidence placed on pre-season physical examinations by the sporting press and public). The questionable value of mass physical examinations is apparent to anyone who has been in the military service, yet an impatient squad of some 90 to 100 football candidates cannot be handled in a single day in any other manner. It has been of interest to observe the results of routine, thorough physicals performed annually upon our varsity football squad by competent and interested physicians, examinations that are compartmentalized to assure skilled evaluation within each specialty. Despite the care taken it is rare that problems of long standing (known to us by virtue of our close association with each athlete) are ever uncovered either by history or careful physical examination. Furthermore, the complete evaluation of a back or a knee as carried out by an orthopedic surgeon or the complete neurological evaluation of lesions involving that specialty cannot be carried out on everyone. They must be reserved for those in whom such an examination is indicated. Nevertheless, this thorough an examination is the only standard by which any potentially disabling condition can be evaluated fairly. A responsible decision in each case is far from easy, since it requires the detection of a truly significant historical item as well as its evaluation through thorough and accurate functional anatomical tests.

## DISQUALIFYING PHYSICAL CONDITIONS

When the difficulties enumerated above have been overcome and a true clinical evaluation has finally been attained, there is a large number of conditions that are disqualifying for the contact sports if not for all sports. Although it is not possible to list every clinicopathological problem in its relation to sports, a number of general rules apply.

### Congenital Disabilities

There are numerous congenital defects that may be encountered in an average school population, and candidates with congenital defects producing a gross disability in normal activity should be barred from contact athletics regardless of how well they may have compensated for the disability. For example, deformity, malfunction, or absence of a limb should be obviously disqualifying, yet we know of an instance in which such a disability in an upper limb was not considered so by the candidate, his parents, or his doctor despite the dangers inherent in tackle football. (They thought that it would have a damaging effect on the boy's morale to recognize the defect.) At the same time there could be no objection if the same boy were to compete for track or any of the individual non-contact sports.

Similarly, the survivor of severe infantile hydrocephalus with marked deformity of the calvarium but without brain damage may be encouraged to compete in any of the non-contact individual sports, but certainly must be barred from such sports as football, basketball, or baseball.

Congenital cardiovascular defects must be recognized. If surgical repair has accomplished full compensation and restored normal cardiac reserve, there is no reason to bar any type of sport. Written clearance, however, should be obtained from the cardiovascular surgeon concerned before sports participation.

As to congenital defects that are not disabling at any particular time serious consideration must be given to the risk involved in any contact sport and the potential injury that may result. Unilateral kidney malformation or related pathology should be automatically disqualifying for contact sports, as should a single descended testis, a single eye, or the like no matter what the efficiency of the functioning part. Our concern is over the dire result of future injury to the remaining functioning organ. Such a decision seems clear cut enough but can become quite difficult when one is faced with an aggressive young man who has been allowed to play 4 years of tough high school football with one eye correctible to no better than 20/400 and normal 20/20 vision in the other. He may have from his ophthalmologist a letter describing the pathology and its permanence and the impossibility of any further damage to the virtually sightless eye; therewith granting full clearance for all sports (and with full agreement from the parents). Yet what of the consequences of violent and extensive ocular injury to the 20/20 eye? No sport is worth the risk of nearly total blindness.

Omitting detailed consideration of other congenital defects, it is sufficient to say that adherence to basic principles can be the only guide-line. Thus, spondylolisthesis without spondylolischisis and without symptoms is no bar to contact sports competition, but even without demonstrable spondylolischisis spondylolisthesis with low back symptoms of a chronic variety is disqualifying. Boys with congenital or acquired blindness may be encouraged to try such sports as wrestling, but they should never be allowed into a swimming pool unless under continuing close supervision. Through thorough consideration of the dangers in each sport and constant concern for the well-being of the athlete each case can be evaluated and the best decision made.

## Acquired Disabilities

Acquired disabilities far outnumber congenital defects. They can be divided into surgical and medical categories.

**Surgical.** Traumatic or surgical loss of any one of an organ pair or loss of a limb must be considered totally disabling for contact sports. Far more difficult to evaluate are those old injuries which despite the difficulties in both history and physical examination have finally come to light. Recurrent glenohumeral dislocations, for example, are not uncommon and present a significant problem in contact sports though less so in the non-contact sports. Such candidates may be allowed to continue in competition only after thorough evaluation both anatomically and functionally; a final decision must be rendered as to the necessity of external support by cuff and chain or internal support by surgery. Even postoperatively such shoulders continue to present difficulties—the position played may not allow the practical use of cuff and chain, and the surgeon may not care to risk his operative result with or without external support.

Acromioclavicular separation with demonstrable laxity and separation should be considered disqualifying unless the candidate and his parents are fully aware of the likelihood of a complete separation. Complete orthopedic evaluation should include serious consideration of surgical fixation; however, recommendation of internal fixation merely to "settle the mind," without persistent symptoms, would seem questionable. Wires break and screws bend or break under the stress of full-scale contact.

Of even greater difficulty is the post-traumatic knee, of which we see so many. In general, our policy is: firstly, to allow continued participation in all sports as long as there is true stability; secondly, to support mild anatomical instability in the collateral ligaments by external means, should such instability be insufficient in degree to be functionally noticeable on the playing field; thirdly, to bar participation in contact sports to any boy with an instability that is symptomatically noticeable either on the field or elsewhere. By these criteria any significant extent of cruciate damage with anteroposterior instability is disqualifying, as is any postoperative knee with persistent instability. Such functional disability must be viewed as permanent, and any risk of further injury must be avoided.

Many successful athletes in the professional field would be barred from contact sports if these rigid standards were universally adhered to. But our interest is in the present and future physical well-being of all our athletes. We do not feel that a permanently disabled knee, persistently unstable and prone to early traumatic arthritis, is a fair price to pay for the sake of athletics.

The same can be said for all chronic joint problems, where limitation of motion, early arthritic changes, recurrent swelling, and persistent pain accompany every effort to compete in a chosen sport. Whether the picture is the result of an earlier fracture, fracture-dislocation, dislocation, or simply of repeated and incessant small traumata, such disability must be viewed as permanently associated with the particular sport and further participation barred categorically. We are seeing more and more college students who have graduated from the baseball Little League program as promising young pitchers, 17- or 18-year-olds who already have arthritic changes in the elbow and old, poorly healed avulsion fractures or periostitis of the medial humeral epicondyle. Should we inject these elbows with cortical steroid and novocaine, bathe them in ice, and encourage these young men to go on pitching despite the pain? It is better to suggest that they find another sport that is not as progressively damaging.

In like manner, problems in the general surgical field must be evaluated carefully and individually. Inguinal hernia is frequently encountered, preponderantly of the indirect type. The repetitive, straining nature of football leads to progressive enlargement, possible incarceration, beyond the obvious risk of direct injury to hernia sac contents despite the "cup" jockey. Therefore, that sport should be categorically barred until repair has been performed and an adequate rehabilitation program of at least 3 to 4 months completed. Equally contraindicated is weight lifting and all sports that include weight lifting in their program. Since this includes virtually all the sports—even crew, swimming, and other seemingly innocuous ones—unrepaired inguinal hernia or any other type of abdominal hernia is by and large disqualifying for all sports.

Major surgery of any kind must defer active participation in athletics; firstly, until the causative factor for the surgery is uncovered and evaluated; secondly, until an adequate period of recovery has passed to insure solid wound healing in the face of stresses that far outstrip those encountered by the average postoperative patient. Careful consideration must therefore be given to the type of incision and its inherent strength, the type of sport and its demands both in body-building weight training and actual competitive stresses. A routine appendectomy for acute appendicitis without perforation or peritonitis, performed through a muscle-splitting incision, presents a different problem than does a complicated appendectomy, involving drainage, through a right rectus vertical incision. Following the former, a boy could return to active general conditioning in 3 weeks and full weight training and non-contact competition in 4; whereas, following the latter, he would require months of careful reconditioning. Postoperative cases with chronic fistulae, sinus tracts, or surgically created ostomies of one or another sort are also disqualified. In general, the reasons for the drainage, surgically intended or not, suffice to discourage competitive athletics. However, a chronic draining pilonidal sinus, either pre- or postoperative, is judged separately from an ileostomy for ulcerative colitis. The former can be weighed against the particular sport in question; the latter is disqualifying for all but the most undemanding sports (rifle shooting or the like). This is the case because of the nature of the primary disease itself and because of the complications inherent in any ileostomy that is exposed to possible direct trauma or prolapse from maximal muscular effort of any kind.

There are countless problems that may be encountered. They must be solved individually by: (1) a combination of expert evaluation in the indicated surgical specialty or subspecialty and study of the demands of the sport involved; (2) a unanimous decision; and (3) administrative control that insures that this decision cannot be altered by unqualified medical or lay opinions.

Insistence on unanimity and finality may seem rigid, but it has been our experience that nothing less will suffice. For instance, a boy with severe ulcerative colitis, presumably cured by total colectomy and ileostomy, was given written outside medical clearance to participate in contact sports, because he had never been allowed to believe that he was not completely normal; it was thought that a different attitude might cause him to become depressed and unhappy. To cite another example: A lacrosse player who underwent intracranial surgery elsewhere for a large subdural hematoma was given verbal permission by his neurosurgeon (without any written record) to return to school and to lacrosse 5 weeks following the operation!

**Medical.** Any acute medical problem, such as infectious mononucleosis, pneumonia, acute nephritis, and the like, will probably prevent a candidate from reporting. If it does not, the physician is faced with the fact that such illnesses may be difficult to detect once they have run their course. Nonetheless, accurate appraisal of recent acute medical disease is an absolute necessity, because such a weakened candidate cannot hope to equal his healthier compatriots and must suffer injuries sooner or later. Moreover, there may persist despite an apparent overall recovery such specific problems as hepato- and splenomegaly after infectious mononucleosis, clearly a potential danger.

As to more chronic problems general overall condition in terms of muscular strength, coordination, and above all endurance must be the deciding factor. Thus, young men with chronic cardiovascular disease of any kind should be discouraged from competition, because of the excess demand placed thereon by any vigorous sport. Any other chronic medical disease with which a boy is essentially in equilibrium should not be disturbed by excessive demands on strength, cardiovascular efficiency, or endurance.

Periodic recurrent problems, requiring considerable individual attention and evaluation, are also encountered. Idiopathic epilepsy, providing it is completely controlled (without a single escape episode over a period of years), should not be disqualifying. On the other hand, if control is so borderline that episodes of grand mal or petit mal seizures occur even as infrequently as once a year, the unpredictable nature of these episodes and the complete helplessness of the individual at such a time could lead to serious consequences during a scrimmage or game. Such a boy should be categorically disqualified not only from contact sports but even from entering the swimming pool alone. Paroxysmal auricular tachycardia should be categorically disqualifying for all competitive sports for precisely the same reason: Such attacks are no more alarming than the periodic fainting of the Stokes-Adams syndrome (once the diagnosis has been established and the possibility of more serious basic pathology ruled out); however, such attacks are totally unpredictable. When they occur, they demand special attention from the victim, possibly at the precise time that his attention must be turned elsewhere for self-preservation. This is to say nothing of the effect such attacks have on the coach, trainer, and other athletes on the squad if the doctor is not present at each episode.

What about concussion or a history thereof? A very sensible rule-of-thumb is that recommended by Thorndike of Harvard: "Three strikes, and you're out." If we know that three clinically recognized concussions have occurred in a boy's competitive career, he is disqualified from all contact sports. However, clinical judgment must be focussed upon each case: Two concussions, each severe and lasting for more than a minute and followed by any sequellae whatever, are sufficient for disqualification; whereas three momentary "stuns," barely qualifying as concussions, are not equally significant. Furthermore, this general rule is well known among athletes at all levels. For that reason we are hard put to extract any history of past head injury from most football players. Even worse, it is not uncommon to receive our first definite information about previous concussions from parents only after one occurs under our direct jurisdiction—a factor which is understandable though no less regrettable. Equally regrettable is the fact that, although an athlete may feel perfectly well with every bit of muscular strength, coordination, and endurance that he has had in the past, he may find himself facing total and permanent disqualification from contact sports. His mother will most likely agree wholeheartedly with such a decision, but the reactions of the father are often as vehement and vociferous as his son's. To bolster his own position, the physician can point to very little concrete evidence with which to turn aside the wrath of son and father; nonetheless, he must maintain his position according to his conscience.

## RISK OF PERMANENT DISABILITY

Similar difficulty should be anticipated with each disqualifying factor alluded to above. By and large, however, straightforward honesty and logic usually prevail. After that unassailable administrative finality must prevail. For regardless of the means *if there is risk of permanent disability of any kind either now or in the future under any and all practice and game conditions, that athlete should and must be kept from the playing field regardless of objections from him or anyone else.* To uncover clinical evidence that can lead one to such a decision may be difficult, and to maintain such a decision may be infinitely more difficult. Nevertheless, it is a responsibility that must be accepted by every physician in organized athletics.

# 4

# *General Conditioning*

We certainly cannot cover the subject of physical conditioning and training in a single chapter. Many books have been written upon this subject as a whole and upon its specialized aspects. It is sufficient to say that coaches, trainers, and athletes have been the most directly interested, and despite the many medically inaccurate beliefs that have developed their conclusions generally must be considered as valid. This is true despite specific criticisms that will be mentioned in the following pages, because medical science is still far from being able accurately to measure potential, ability, endurance, and neuromuscular coordination; therefore, existing knowledge must remain empirical and in the hands of those most directly involved.

## Medical Research Findings

Current physiological research involves the most sophisticated microanalyzers, analogue computers, cardioscopes, and the like. Nonetheless, when dealing with the microseconds of neuromuscular coordination, balance, and strength that spell the difference between, for example, a Mickey Mantle and a Class D .250 hitter such research falls short. In the Soviet Union and Eastern Europe doctors are currently using every known physiological and chemical parameter to chart the conditioning progress of athletes, and with the accumulated data they are trying to predict future performance which they claim to be able to modify through their position of co-responsibility with the coach. Notable is the work of Professor H. Reindell of the Sports Medicine Research Center in Freiburg, Germany. As a leading cardiologist directly associated with German international athletic teams since 1936, he has accumulated an overwhelming wealth of data on the cardiovascular system under stress conditions, including serial chronological records on many surviving former competitors from prewar years. Some doctors in this country are in pursuit of similar objectives. But we must remember that failure to recognize the limitations of our means can lead our research into often erroneous conclusions. In short, if the physiological index used is insufficiently accurate to differentiate between, say, an experimental medical student, a routine plodding competitor, and a champion, conclusions drawn are likely to be of little practical value to coach, athlete, or trainer.

## Relative Nature of "Good" Condition

To be in good condition is to be equal to the neuromuscular demands, the necessary strength, and the requisite stamina of the sport in question. To be in good condition for football is not the same as being in good condition for competitive swimming: Entirely different muscles are brought into play and the demands are dissimilar. Therefore, what constitutes a good training and conditioning program for one does not for the other. To take a specific example, football is a running, collision type of game, and football players must be able to run. However, some players can run like scalded cats; others can barely keep themselves warm. Nevertheless, in regard to physical condition, both are tip-top: the former, probably a back, is expected to run fast and "run all day"; his practice is spent running back-squares, pass patterns, and punt returns. The lumbering lineman must be equally prepared to accelerate his bulk into violent motion on every play, but will rarely be called upon to "sprint" at his best speed for more than 10 to 15 yards. To take another example: A competitive swimmer, who has geared his conditioning program to the 500 yard and 1000 yard events, is rarely capable of competitive times in the 50 or 100; even more rarely can a sprinter go the longer distances without "dying."

Despite the foregoing, if these young men are matched against average, non-athletic students, their endurance and stamina, their strength in single effort or in repetitions, and their total performance will be more alike, one to another, than in comparison to the non-athlete. Exceptions usually involve borderline athletes.

It is therefore virtually impossible for the physician in athletics to contribute much in regard to conditioning programs. The intricacies of interval training, "fartleck," overdistance work, and the intermingling of all these and many others are what a professional coach has to offer, and it should be neither surprising nor humiliating to the physician that he is beyond his sphere of competence. What he *can* attain is an understanding of the physiological principles behind these training programs. If they make physiological sense and the results are valid, then they are good; if not, why not?

**Planned Program**

A planned program of conditioning, embarked upon long before any particular sport season, should be insisted upon. This is more easily accomplished in football, conditioning for which begins at the end of the summer vacation after a period of relative freedom and before classes begin. One such typical program, beginning with a June letter, followed by prescribed exercises for each month to assure a return in September in good "football" condition, can be found in *Athletic Training and Conditioning* written by the head trainer at Yale, Mr. O. William Dayton (Ronald Press, New York, 1960). The series of exercises outlined, although they represent the bare minimum of what is expected, would seriously tax the strength or ability of the casual non-athlete. Significantly, each exercise is calculated to strengthen just those muscle groups that are the most important in minimizing subsequent injury. By demanding this minimum of physical preparation, the coach, the trainer, and the doctor can feel more confident that the candidate will possess at least enough strength and stamina to protect himself. He will also have subjected himself to more than a little self-discipline and thus will be better prepared for the grueling weeks ahead.

Once the official season has started, other considerations come into play, built upon the basic conditioning accomplished in the preseason period. Accordingly, it is up to the coach to decide where any candidate will best "fit in" and to design, with the trainer, his practice sessions in such a way as to assure that the physical and mental demands of each position are fulfilled. Thus, the football lineman spends much time everyday "hitting the bucker" to strengthen himself for incessant, repetitive, explosive acceleration; his sprinting is usually limited to a maximum of 20 to 25 yards. On the other hand, the defensive back will sprint the length of the field time and again in addition to the constant running necessary to learn his assignments.

Certain exercises should be discouraged regardless of the sport. The worst of these are the so-called deep-knee bend, still used by many in the belief that it strengthens the quadriceps, and the "duck-waddle" which has for generations been used in the football conditioning program. Both are mentioned only to be condemned, because the stresses these exercises exert on the knee and in particular the cruciate ligaments far outweigh any value to the quadriceps muscles.

In each instance the physician has little if any role; these are technical considerations that each coach must assess in terms of his own knowledge and his own approach to coaching. If they are overly demanding to a few on the squad because of medical deficiencies, the doctor should never have allowed them to compete in the first place. We emphasize that medical clearance to compete in any sport must include consideration of all the demands of that sport—the conditioning work and the practice drudgery as well as the games themselves. The doctor must know these demands ahead of time, not afterwards. If he does not, the candidate finds himself inadequate in the face of demands that his teammates readily fulfill. It is far less kind to force a medically handicapped young man to drag himself off the practice field a physical failure, than to bar him at the outset as medically unable to withstand the rigors that the physician should know are required.

## INTERVAL TRAINING

Few activities in athletics more graphically emphasize the rigorous demands of competition than does interval training. Sports such as track and swimming may seem healthful and innocuous, yet nothing could be further from the truth. The demands on strength, endurance, and the ability to withstand self-imposed pain are maximal in these sports, and it is in these sports that the most minor physical ailment can have serious consequences. The contests to which spectators are admitted are only the smallest portion of what each athlete goes through day after day and week after week. With the advent of interval training, the days, weeks, and months have become even more grueling.

A brief review of the history of this training concept is necessary. Its development began back in the early 1940's, when all conditioning programs called for overdistance work, interminably repeated. The basic concept then was that with greater distance and therefore greater endurance the shorter distances could be traversed that much faster—certainly a sound physiological program. Swimmers and runners would labor daily to "get in the miles," secure in the knowledge that their specific competitive distance would then be child's play, as indeed it was. However, the endless drudgery of those "miles" could be disheartening, particularly when the competitive times at the shorter distances failed to improve at a rate commensurate with the drudgery. At this point the Swedish distance runners (as typified by Gunnar Haegg) began an assault on records that was noted throughout the world. Their "fartleck" system emerged as a revolutionary training idea and the source of their amazing success.

In essence, "fartleck" means spurts of speed work "for fun," sprinting at full speed for brief periods, resting, then jogging greater distances, resting, then sprinting again. This concept was adopted and adapted by the English distance runners, notably Roger Bannister, who recognized the key importance of the speed work done at intervals and began to run full-speed quarters and halves, repeated again and again, while retaining the traditional overdistance work on alternating workouts. The result is history, and interval training has since been adopted by the entire track world.

Swimmers, faced with the same drudgery of overdistance work, also turned to interval training, with results that have been incredible. So deeply has the concept penetrated that it is used with little modification in the nationwide age-group AAU swimming program from 8-year-olds on up. World records now are continually being set, broken, and set again by 14- and 15-year-old competitors.

What of the physiological effect of this training program? It consists of repeated, staggering demands on cardiovascular efficiency and reserve, not muscular endurance. Consequently, overdistance work remains an integral part of the overall conditioning program.

To take an example: 25 to 27 seconds is no longer a competitive time in the 50 yard freestyle at the college level, yet to cover the distance in this time still requires considerable effort. This is true even for the college swimmer who can cover the distance in a "one-shot" sprint in 22 seconds or less. As a consequence, he and his fellow sprinters may be required to do ten 50's at 35-second intervals without getting out of the pool. Since he is deprived of a flying start, he will have difficulty doing 23 seconds "all-out," and with ten 50's to do he will be wise not to go "all-out"; on the other hand, if he tries to save himself too much, his time will fall to 30 or 32 seconds, giving him only 3 to 5 seconds to catch his breath before he must go again— not once but 10 times.

When one realizes that this is only one small part of a swimming workout, taking exactly 350 seconds, one can appreciate the staggering load even one 2-hour workout can place on the cardiovascular system. Multiplying this by the days, weeks, months, and years that go into the making of a champion swimmer, it is no wonder that the resting pulse rate and the pulse rate after clinical exercise tests (that send average rates to 160 or more) remain a steady 40 to 45 in virtually all swimmers and runners.

Many authorities have become concerned about this and have predicted a dire fate for the "athlete's heart." Over the years, however, no dependable study has indicated any lasting ill effect from such exercise. If one could see the host of AAU age-group 8-, 10-, and 12-year-old swimmers who thrive on this program and cover distances in times that would have been nationally competitive 30 years ago, there would be little concern about physical damage. This is not to say that *psychological* damage does not occur in this intense competition, but the methods of training, especially interval training, must be accepted as physically valid and effective.

It is obvious that such demands posed on anyone who does not have a normal cardiovascular system may lead to sheer disaster. The general advice of cardiologists that exercise is good should not be interpreted to include such rigorous competitive swimming or running. The written advice of a cardiovascular surgeon that no exercises should be barred cannot be interpreted to include such a regimen unless the surgeon knows precisely what his patient may have to undergo just to make the team. In short, final medical clearance must be the responsibility of the athletic physician; he is best situated to appreciate these rigors, and he must be prepared to accept the responsibility.

## CALISTHENICS AND THE WARM-UP

Questions are often raised concerning the value of calisthenics in a conditioning program. Certainly, veterans of World War II do not look back upon those hours of mass calisthenics with longing, but the basic principles and logic behind the program are unassailable.

Calisthenics properly designed and properly performed call into action muscle groups that are little used, isolate them effectively, and strengthen them by reasonable demand and controllable repetition. Analysis of the kinesiology of the "side-straddle hop" or the "squat jump" is not within the scope of this discussion and can be found in any physical training manual, but it is sufficient to say that these exercises are within the reach of everyone. By judicious control over the number of repetitions they can increase muscular tone and gradually build up cardiovascular efficiency. These exercises can be used as the ground work for any physical training program and, combined with an intelligent running program, can be integrated into a broad, increasingly demanding and successful system.

Before endorsement of any such program some further assessment is necessary, particularly of the home programs that have become so popular. The Royal Canadian Air Force Program, not particularly different from any of the many available, has recently become popular; men and women of all ages have tried it. One principal feature, the fact that no special equipment is necessary and therefore that it can be carried out in one's home, has contributed to its popularity.

Judicious control is an integral part of conditioning, however, and this and other programs fall short in this respect. Without supervision the eager subject is likely to overdo some of the exercises; the soreness, the strains, the discouragement that result cannot be measured, and it is certain that far more people have started and then abandoned this and other programs than have persevered. Secondly, as with all similar programs, it is hard work when properly done and is "not very much fun." The reward of a better conditioned body always impels the question: "What for?" If the program is used by the subject for a season of skiing or swimming or squash, all well and good; but to immerse oneself in the drudgery of an increasingly demanding program of exercises without some objective closer than the remote prospect of greater longevity would seem inherently discouraging.

Athletes have much more specific objectives, and the rewards of such drudgery are much closer at hand. An intelligent program of calisthenics, specifically designed to increase strength and endurance in those muscle groups necessary for a sport, forms a basis on which other skills and strengths may be built. The difference is in degree: The calithenics in general programs would be too easy for the average trained athlete; so for him the degree of demand is set high at the beginning and increased more rapidly. The principles remain the same, however.

The same basic calisthenics, still on a level that would tax the average person but insufficient to accomplish more with the athlete than "work up a sweat," are used for the pre-practice and pre-game "warm-up." Some authorities have questioned the value of the "warm-up," and in physiological terms there is little to justify it. Theoretically, by gently exercising a part blood flow is increased thereto, and muscular efficiency and tone is thereby increased, resulting in greater efficiency of the entire part. However, figures on actual blood flow, oxygenation, and the like are not available in the trained athlete, except for data gained under the most artificial circumstances. They are not likely to be available in statistically accurate form for several reasons: Firstly, the means of obtaining samples are artificial and far from pleasant to undergo; secondly, the actual blood flow and oxygenation to the precise muscle group in question cannot be accurately measured in an athlete performing at top speed (the sole measure of the efficacy of warm-up); thirdly, it is possible that the athlete himself despite his willingness to cooperate will "tie up" because of the artificiality of the experimental situation.

Conclusions concerning the efficacy of "warm-up" must therefore be empirical and must be based on sufficient years of observation to render the total sampling statistically significant. In these terms, it is the general consensus of coaches, trainers, and associated physicians that the overall incidence of muscle strains and "pulls" is distinctly increased when there has been an inadequate "warm-up" period, a period that may vary with the athlete, the sport, or the external temperature.

## WEIGHT TRAINING, ISOTONICS, AND ISOMETRICS

### Weight Training

In view of the increasing use of weight lifting and other adjuncts in athletic training programs some estimate of their value is in order. The value of progressive resistance in physical rehabilitation is unquestioned; however, as it applies to athletics and athletes, much controversy exists. The use of weights in physical training has its adherents as well as its opponents, each side with graphic examples that purport to prove their point on an empirical basis. Yet, as with so much in athletics, the true value lies somewhere between the opposing claims.

The concept of weight training has been distorted by the widespread belief that weight lifters are "muscle-bound" and that the entire concept is therefore worthless. Yet any attempt to determine the exact meaning of "muscle-bound" leads into a maze of varying assessments, none of which can be evaluated accurately. This being the case, it is common for opponents of this training method to point out some heavily muscled weight lifter, his arms and chest bulging, who is visibly awkward and ungainly. However, no one is able to say whether that same individual was *ever* well coordinated and graceful —weight lifting aside.

Such erroneous logic is common in athletics, where "post hoc, propter hoc" reasoning rules supreme. Nonetheless, critical evaluation of the weight lifter reveals a number of striking characteristics. First of all, the typical weight lifter is extremely muscular, to a degree that is difficult to believe at first sight; so no one can deny that weight lifting builds muscle. The next logical question is *why* the young man wants to build muscle, and here we encounter the real basis for the controversy. For the motive that drives him to the truly eye-bulging efforts demanded by weight lifting must be a powerful one indeed, while the ultimate objective is not at all apparent. He labors endlessly over repetitions, grimly increasing the weight with each set of repetitions, carefully using this and that particular lift again and again to build one or another group of muscles, devoting 2 to 4 grueling hours a day—and toward what end?

In my opinion the conclusion is clearly indicated. The typical weight lifter, the individual whom coaches and athletes consider "muscle-bound," may very likely be pursuing an attainable objective in lieu of one that he cannot attain. He may be devotedly building his body into a mountain of rippling muscle because he was not particularly muscular before and, more important, did not have the innate neuromuscular coordination of the true athlete. It is no wonder that, when such a young man tries to throw a ball or attempts any of the commonplace but complex movements of his better coordinated athletic colleagues, he is clumsy and ungainly. Then purely muscular strength avails him little, then the body beautiful helps him not a bit, but that does not prove that weight lifting is solely responsible.

What, then, of weight lifting? Can it be applied judiciously? The answer is again obvious. Weight lifting programs, carefully designed to strengthen those muscle groups most needed in any particular sport, are now an integral part of every training program. The use of lead-weighted anklets and lead-weighted jackets to strengthen basketball players and track men merely indicates the extreme to which some coaches will go, once they become convinced that a concept is valid. Nonetheless, such examples of questionable application should not be used to negate the value of the program. Swimmers can use overhead pulleys or 50-pound weights in each hand, while duplicating the motions that propel them through the water; wrestlers can use 50-pound sandbags in grueling drills to the same end; track men, particularly long distance runners, can use light weights, incessantly repeated, to strengthen their arms; crewmen can use the weighted bar to strengthen wrists, upper arms, and shoulders; football players can use the weighted bar to strengthen upper body muscles, to better handle blockers and ball carriers: these athletes profit from judiciously selected weight work and are better competitors for it. But theirs must be a continuously reinforced objective—to excel in their sport, not at weight lifting.

A further analysis of weight lifting is necessary to properly assess the nature and value of related isometric and isotonic exercises. Weight lifting, using the usual bar and weights, requires a maximum effort at the outset of any exercise in order to overcome the inertia of the bar and weights. This is true whether one is doing the usual military press, the so-called clean and jerk, or straightforward curling to develop the biceps. In the former movements, the barbell is moved from the floor to an overhead position according to certain prescribed rules; in the last, the barbell is raised repeatedly from a dependent position in the hands to a position under the chin by simple flexion of the biceps. Regardless of the rules that apply, once the mass is set into motion and accelerated, the demand on any particular muscle group falls off to a significant extent, while neuromuscular adjustments are made to catch and hold the moving mass at the next desired position. It is true that every weight lifter should try to perform each motion as slowly as possible to gain the greatest benefit in muscle building and strength, but the explosive initiation of action is still a necessity.

## Isotonic Exercises

In contrast, isotonic exercise, by using friction or spring devices, maintains a constant measured resistance against motion. Because such an apparatus cannot be heaved into accelerating motion, it is considered far more beneficial. One such device, which uses an adjustable friction resistance, has become a routine training adjunct in professional football and has, therefore, become quite popular on the college level; its value as a muscle builder when properly used is unquestionable. We might ask, however, whether this simple device is the real reason the pros are as good as they are.

## Isometric Exercises

The same can be said for isometric exercises. Maximum muscular effort is directed against an essentially immovable object, be it a bar sunk in cement or the side of a building, and this maximum effort is exerted for from 6 to 12 seconds. The effect on the systolic blood pressure of this exercise must be seen to be appreciated, but its many proponents emphasize the more rapid increase in muscle strength and bulk by this means as compared to any equivalent form of repetitive drudgery. To many, therefore, it is an attractive short cut to strong muscles. Business executives have been urged to strain against the office wall or door, to pit their biceps against the bulk of their mahogany desks, and so on—all for a 3- to 5-minute period "between appointments"—with the confident assurance that they will be stronger men. But stronger for what? For heaving bulky desks, for pushing down a wall or door?

The only sensible conclusion is that conditioning exercises of any kind are beneficial when directed toward some logical end. If it be to produce stronger, better athletes, all well and good. For, in truth, most capable athletes view ancillary exercises as sheer drudgery, to be avoided whenever possible. The weight room has its earnest devotees during the winter and spring, but aside from the formal weight programs designed and supervised by coaches for their particular sport, attendance is poor at best. Competitive athletes want to excel in their sport, not engage in feats of brute strength, and their musculature, ofttimes the equal of a "Mr. America," is only a means to an end.

## HEAT AND HEAT STROKE

As part of general conditioning, some mention must be made of the effects of heat on the competitive athlete, particularly in view of the occasional fatalities and serious illness attributed to heat. Much research is being directed toward this problem in the hope of minimizing these tragic occurrences. In addition, many authorities have formulated rules and regulations for football teams, that include indices of wet and dry bulb thermometer readings, proper clothing, and the like, rules and regulations that if rigidly applied could end pre-season practice and much of the football season for many teams in the deep South.

Football, as a rigorous, demanding fall sport, requires pre-season practice that cannot be carried out in gym shorts. Profitable working practice in football demands contact with sleds, with buckers, with each other, and contact requires pads—all of them. As doctors, we can deplore the necessity of vigorous muscular exertion twice a day in the heat and humidity of an early September day. It would clearly be more healthful for all (including the doctor) to rush off to some nearby beach and lie in the sand. But the necessary work must be done thoroughly, or the first game in September will be a travesty, and, more important, injuries will fill the infirmary beds. In terms of condition and the sport those hot September days must be filled with vigorous, demanding work.

The physician, trainer, and coach must work together to produce a practice schedule that accomplishes the necessary work, assures the necessary buildup of physical conditioning, yet does not endanger a single squad member. Thus, salt in enteric capsules must be available and each squad member instructed to take at least two per practice or four a day during the double sessions, as well as salt his food liberally. Each squad member must weigh in and weigh out upon each practice session, recording the data on a posted sheet by the scales so that the head trainer and doctor can check the weight loss each session and, more important, check on whether the weight loss is made up by the next session. If a weight loss of over 10 pounds is recorded for any session, particular attention is paid to that athlete's returning weigh-in figure; if there is a persistent loss, he is checked for unusual fatigue, headache, listlessness, and other signs of early salt depletion and dehydration. Even if these are not present, he is watched constantly during the next few practice sessions for the slightest sign of neuromuscular slowing; the coach is forewarned of these same signs, and, when any candidate appears the least wobbly or clumsy, he is immediately referred to the doctor and trainer. Such athletes are taken out of the hot sun, cold towels applied, sweaty clothes loosened, and the recumbent position assumed. Return to practice is based entirely upon full recovery of brightness, eagerness, and rapid, normal conversation. If these do not return, the athlete does not resume practice until they do. On the other hand, if there is no specific instance of alarming persistent weight loss but instead a series of hot and humid days leads to steady overall weight loss in the squad with an accompanying detectible sluggishness, the pattern of workouts can be altered to allow for a non-contact session or two in shorts.

By using these empirical methods and by keeping in mind the early danger signs, our program has been successful since its inception. There have been no instances of heat cramps, much less heat exhaustion, and despite the fact that heat in New England is not nearly as severe as the heat of September in the deep South similar programs in the latter region have yielded comparable results. This is not to minimize the efforts of researchers who have concluded that heavy muscular work requires at least a liter or 2 of slightly saline water by mouth to assure good hydration. To this we heartily agree, and we always offer water on the field at regular "water breaks" during every practice session as well as iced soft-drinks afterward. The truth is, however, that under the demands of any average pre-season practice each candidate is continually working at the very border of nausea. Consequently, any bulk in his stomach will more often than not re-emerge within 10 minutes regardless of experimental figures on gastric absorption of fluid. Is it any wonder, then, that our squads prefer to rinse out their mouths and pour the rest of the water on their heads? The advent of the pre-packaged and pre-calculated electrolyte mixtures for oral ingestion has not altered these basic points; these solutions have indeed proved most useful in maintaining electrolyte equilibrium among those athletes who find their flavor not unpleasant, but there remain many athletes who simply cannot stomach them and must subsist on the measures outlined above. Reasonable care in the overall handling of any squad is worth more than any rigid ruling concerning the THI (temperature-humidity index) and/or mandatory electrolyte intake; these latter measures are admittedly helpful but must supplement rather than replace the careful medical management of an entire team, particularly those members who, for example, cannot or will not take the particular electrolyte and/or those whose electrolyte loss may exceed by far that predictable by certain arbitrary indices.

# 5

# *Diet and Habits*

Nowhere else in athletics can be found the incredible variations that abound in the area of diet and training rules. A physician entering the athletic field is utterly bewildered by the amount of misinformation and the number of conflicting "authoritative opinions" that surround every facet of this subject. And it must be remembered that it is this area that most directly affects the athlete in his life away from the practice field; it is here that he find himself most often at odds with his non-athletic colleagues. Because he must control this area himself, he must both understand and be convinced of the validity of all its tenets. If what he does and believes is foolish, who is at fault? The physician should try to understand the reasons for the often mysterious rules and thus better advise players and coaches of the true rationale behind them.

To evaluate this subject, one must first review its origins. As illustrated in Sir Adolphe Abrahams' book of common-sense physiology, *The Human Machine* (Penguin Books, Hammondsworth, Middlesex, 1956), the origin of many current beliefs dates back to the early days of bare-knuckle prize fighting in England. By and large the fighters were professionals, sponsored by titled patrons, and, as hired men of violence, were customarily drawn from the lower classes. Preparing such men for prize-ring contests that at times lasted over one hundred rounds was no small task no matter what their natural strength or bulk. With the large wagers that were made much rested upon success, be it rational or empirical. Certainly, gin and similar intoxicants had to be eliminated, although moderation in drinking was not the temper of the times. An adequate diet, possibly the first such men had ever seen, might be expected to do wonders and very likely did. Unquestionably, consorting with women of the type such men might find in those times must be barred at the outset.

Here, then, we have the rudiments of a training program: no drinking, a regular diet, plenty of exercise, and no women. That each of these tenets remains an integral part of any modern training program is not to ridicule them because of their primitive origin. But it does help one to understand why there still are coaches who equate marriage with the end of a promising athletic career.

## TRAINING RULES

Age-old customs aside, a more objective scrutiny of training rules confirms their basic validity. In all competitive athletics we are concerned with activities that place a premium on mental and physical ability. Consequently, any measure that enhances these qualities is advantageous. Conversely, any factor that demeans these qualities must be avoided. Rationalizations and criticisms of the rigid standards fail to face this central issue. Thus, every athlete hears again and again that the "pros smoke," "the pros drink," that this or that championship team trained on beer, that so-and-so, Champion of the world, was a "lush and a chaser," all in an attempt to discourage him from his self-imposed regimen of "no smoking, no drinking, and sexual abstinence." This is not to deny that such instances occur. There is no question that a well coordinated 250-pound football player, who can run the 100 yard dash in 9.8 seconds, stands six-foot-five in his stocking-feet, and "eats nails for breakfast," will be able to drink, smoke, and carouse and still beat an average 6 footer of 200 pounds who has never run the 100 yards in less than 12 seconds. Such instances, however, despite wide circulation among those who seek some rationalization to break training are very rare and are very short lived. Sooner or later such a man will meet one of equal size, strength, and speed who has been sufficiently determined to keep himself in training: The result of such a meeting need hardly be questioned.

Medical science is unanimous on the harmful effects of smoking with regard to damaging vascular effects and potential lung cancer, and there is nationwide interest in the subject. Of more immediate importance to the athlete is the effect of smoking on the "wind," for it is well known that the small percentage of carbon monoxide in the smoke inhaled effectively "ties" an equally small but fixed percentage of oxygen-carrying capacity in the erythrocytes. This miniscule proportion is barely measurable under normal laboratory conditions, but in the area of oxygen debt (wherein virtually all competitive athletes operate) such a difference can mean everything. Similarly, a little alcohol cannot be considered harmful, but how does one determine moderation as it applies to one or another athlete? Similarly, if sex means staying out night after night to all hours in pursuit thereof, it cannot help but affect athletic performance.

No training regime can make a small man bigger or a fourth-stringer a star, but it can make each athlete better, while at the same time inculcating habits of self-discipline and dedication that may last throughout his life. To see a determined young man, his athletic ability so clearly limited that he and everyone else knows that he will never be a "starter," punishing himself day after day to help the team is to see dedication and self-discipline of a high order. There are many more "bench-warmers" than there are stars on every athletic squad, and to each of these boys "staying in training" is a self-imposed burden for which there is little reward. In athletics this is part and parcel of what is called, for the want of a better term, "guts."

## DIET

Let us accept, then, that smoking, drinking, and "chasing" are not beneficial to the competitive athlete and turn to the one remaining cornerstone of training—diet. This is the most difficult to discuss with clarity despite the fact that the subject is basically simple: The competitive athlete needs a good, balanced diet, as does every other human being, the difference being that in his area of activity he needs a lot more of it.

### Special Requirements

A balanced diet of protein, fat, and carbohydrate, sufficiently assorted to provide all essential minerals and vitamins, seems reasonable enough. The need to increase the total amount and caloric content, to compensate for the extreme physical demands of athletics and the natural needs of growing young men, seems perfectly straightforward. But what about vitamins? Shouldn't athletes have extra vitamin C, so they won't catch colds and won't get bruises? Shouldn't they have extra vitamin $B_{12}$ for extra energy, since $B_{12}$ shots help people with pernicious anemia and give them energy? Shouldn't they have red meat to build muscle and blood? Shouldn't the meat be nearly raw, so nothing essential is destroyed? Shouldn't they drink six times as much milk as anyone else, since they will then be six times stronger? (Look how babies grow on milk.) And doesn't the athlete need lots of quick energy available as immediately as the demands; in other words, shouldn't a sprinter need a quicker source of energy than a plodding football tackle? Honey is a natural food and has natural sugars, so wouldn't it be the ideal source of quick energy for all boys? And fat—shouldn't you stay away from fat because it weighs you down, and shouldn't you stay away from buttered toast, maybe even burn the dry toast a little?

The list of questions grows longer and longer as the years pass, with no end in sight. Humorous though such questions may seem, they have demanded logical, reasoned answers time and again. The physician finds, however, that with or without his professional approval athletes continue to eat what they think is best for them.

**Pre-Game Meals.** A case in point is the "pre-game meal," as it has developed since the earliest days of football. From the beginning without guidance from nutritionists, physiologists, or doctors the football world—professional, college, and secondary school—gradually fostered the "steak and eggs" concept by following certain "logical" progressions. Energy and muscle power were needed in prodigious amounts in the afternoon, but a heavy lunch usually ended up on the playing field; hence, the only answer was a heavy breakfast. That a large beefsteak was included should be no surprise, since beefsteak has always been the epitome of good eating in this country (and eggs were included merely to identify the meal with breakfast). Any young man provided a meal such as this—at bargain rates thanks to the football department—could hardly be expected to push it aside. However, in the face of the emotional tension that builds steadily before game time, the gastric emptying time of any meal is certain to be prolonged; consequently, the nutritive value of such a meal is limited. In fact, researches have shown that the meal still may be in the stomach 2 hours after the game is over.

**Liquid Meals.** Liquid meals can be the ideal solution to the pre-game feeding problem. Modern preparations in palatable form contain easily digested dietary, mineral, and vitamin ingredients equal to the best breakfasts, and absorption is efficient and rapid. Much consideration was given to the introduction of such a regimen, when these preparations first became available. But such a regimen had to be on a purely voluntary basis. A very few football players did take the liquid meal, among them some who habitually vomited before every game. Of these some continued to vomit, some spent game day on the bench, while others ate the steak and eggs and the liquid meal as well!

In contrast, the liquid meal has proven popular on the track squad, for runners are typically more knowledgeable about the workings of their anatomy and are eager for any nourishment likely to stay within that anatomy for a profitable period of time. Other organized squads have also adopted the meal particularly for road trips. One can therefore safely predict that its value eventually will be recognized. Its adoption must be voluntary, however, and according to circumstance: As far as his food is concerned, the athlete feels the way he thinks he should feel; if a steak makes him feel stronger, then by all means give him steak.

**Vitamin Supplements.** There is no real need for supplementary vitamins in any balanced diet, but, if the athlete believes that he cannot perform without some oral supplements, they should be supplied within reason; without them he is very likely to perform badly. Control should be exerted, because to most athletes a little good from a little amount automatically means tremendous good from a tremendous amount; the total intake can be quite staggering if uncontrolled. So long as the amount taken is not harmful, however, greater harm can come from banning it.

This last is the keynote to the confusion that surrounds this subject. A basic, adequate diet has already created and nurtured every athlete up to and through his previous athletic career, and he should continue to be provided with nothing less, prepared the way he prefers it and not the way some dietitian thinks is best. Fancy dishes that stray from the "meat and potatoes" line, elaborate salads to increase his intake of greens, "foreign" dishes that might add some desirable ingredient go untouched, while he sprints down to the nearest hamburger palace to eat gargantuan amounts of what he prefers. But he will thrive on simply prepared food in adequate amounts and, most important, will feel that he is well fed.

Common sense, then, is the most important factor a physician can contribute to this field, debunking where necessary but compromising within reason when physical well-being is not at stake. At times it is difficult to maintain professional equanimity when faced with some of the more ludicrous extremes encountered. It profits little, however, to exert medical pressure to reform details that are largely of little importance in the long run. Thus, the athlete who gulps honey by the spoonful for its quick energy and digestibility only to vomit it up just as regularly is an object for sympathetic understanding, not ridicule. If he prefers it this way rather than regurgitating a heavy meal, who is to say he is wrong? And, if an athlete believes that wheat germ and other vegetarian products are the source of his strength and skill, we should not force him to eat meat.

## WEIGHT CONTROL

Much has been written about the problem of weight control, particularly in those sports where competitive weight is the arbitrary measure by which contestants are matched one to the other. As might be anticipated, abuses of the most flagrant variety have been and are common in these areas of athletic endeavor, and much of the criticism is well deserved. Many measures have been suggested; the most valuable hinges upon a voluntary cooperation on the part of both coach and squad member by using such self-measured objective indices as skin-fold thickness to determine optimum weight for competition, thereby hopefully eliminating the deplorable starvation and "sweatbox" routine occasionally encountered. However, it must be pointed out that all such measures depend on wholehearted and honorable cooperation by all concerned, a rare commodity when driving a squad toward a winning or championship season where just a little manipulation could be pivotal. In truth much of the problem lies within the very rules of the particular sport, since the actual determination of competitive weight must be done at some arbitrary period before competition begins, an interval not infrequently measured in hours, even in days! Under such circumstances it is relatively easy to "make weight" with the secure knowledge that immediately thereafter the contestant can gorge himself in a frantic effort to recoup his lost strength and endurance. That such last minute efforts frequently end in failure does not deny the fact that on many occasions such measures accomplish exactly what they are meant to do, that is, matching a larger and stronger contestant against a smaller one by "bouncing" into a lower weight for that one moment of arbitrary measurement. Yet, generally speaking, only in the case of flagrant abuse should the physician interfere on purely medical grounds. Surely he should guard against medically harmful practices, but he cannot enforce morality! Certainly, the prevalent custom among wrestling coaches of taking down a boy's weight to the next lower weight class in order to strengthen the lineup must be condemned. Any boy who has to starve himself throughout the week to make his weight on match day clearly belongs in another weight class. By the same token, however, any boy who can thrive on grueling wrestling workouts day after day and still win his share of matches is not the drained starveling that some might suspect. The fact is that a well conditioned, muscular wrestler in his proper weight class is equal to demands as great as any in competitive athletics, but, if he is carrying the least bit of excess fat, he will tip the scales into the next higher class and find himself against another who is all muscle and no fat—hardly a fair beginning. Consequently, the physician must keep an eye on the squad, particularly through the training staff at the weigh-ins. Obvious cases of gross weight abuse are then easily detected.

In an analogous manner there has been in recent years an alarming trend among weight lifters, hammer throwers, shot putters, and the like to indulge heavily in anabolic steroids in the hopes of gaining muscularity, muscular strength, and weight. There is no question but that large dosages of anabolic steroids will indeed lead to electrolyte and water retention, hence a measurable gain in total weight. However, whether this leads to any actual increase in muscular strength has never been proven and carries with it at the same time the distinct risk of an artificial hormonal imbalance that could conceivably lead to secondary gonadal atrophy, something which no athlete in his right mind would intentionally risk. It remains only to be condemned, yet the widespread practice does and will persist. Again, the physician can only make strong recommendations as well as point out the objective risks, since these athletes have apparent access to limitless supplies of such steroids regardless of medical disapproval. The threat of significant gonadal changes would appear to offer a telling argument to bolster medical disapproval; this has certainly been our experience.

**Oxygen Supplements.** The use of tank oxygen as a vital supplement must be condemned. That oxygen is beneficial is beyond debate in those instances in which oxygen depletion is apparent at the intrapulmonary gas-blood exchange membrane. However, if true oxygen debt is secondary to excess muscular demand, pure oxygen will not significantly improve oxygen saturation, which is already at a maximum. These are physiological facts, yet oxygen tanks may be seen as routine equipment next to many team benches. Perhaps they do have some salutary effect, particularly psychologically, but the concomitant spread of acute respiratory illnesses through the common mask far outweighs any such advantage. Such equipment *is* of inestimable value at high altitudes and low oxygen pressure, but, barring such special conditions, there is no excuse and little justification for its use when the disadvantages are so numerous (e.g., spread of disease, respiratory acapnea).

## DRUGS AND ERGOGENIC AIDS

The entire subject of drug use in athletics has become one of increasing import in the past few years. This should not prove surprising in view of the increasing drug problem as it applies nationwide. It should not be unexpected that the same specious philosophy, which has spawned the "acid-freak" and the drug-oriented hippy culture, should have touched even lightly athletes of that same generation. The pernicious use of anabolic steroids by weight men has been mentioned above, while the use of various stimulants, mood modifiers, tranquilizers, and the like has reached such proportions that international athletic events have been forced to take specific measures against such abuses. The confusion that results from the misuse of this broad spectrum of drugs has been highlighted by several highly publicized incidents in the recent past, revolving around urine tests for drug metabolites, exactly as such tests are used in horse racing. For the same reason the American College Health Association and the AMA Committee on the Medical Aspects of Sports have both passed recent resolutions condemning the "non-therapeutic use of drugs."

Worse yet, the problem of such purposeful drug abuse by athletes, aided and abetted by coaches, trainers, as well as by overly enthusiastic physicians, has at the same time been aggravated by a significant incidence of "hard drug" usage among athletes. This again should not be surprising in view of the far greater problem as it applies to the entire younger generation of today. Nonetheless, it must be recognized. The increasingly efficient athletic recruiting now penetrating into "ghetto" areas has brought many teen-agers from such deprived backgrounds to college campuses all over the country, bringing with them habits of drug abuse that were rarely if ever encountered before on the college level. Team physicians throughout the country have recognized this unfortunate trend and, faced with individual instances thereof, have been forced into many agonizing decisions. Suffice it to say, such decisions must be based on the individual incident and the effect of such an incident on the athlete as well as on the coach and remainder of the squad and cannot be dismissed lightly as a regrettable sociological phenomenon. Direct medical steps must be taken to help each such individual overcome his addiction, while at the same time maintaining the strictest confidence between doctor and patient that can only under the most unusual circumstances be broadened to include the affected coach.

It is deplorable that these problems should have arisen in the past few years, and to hear "responsible adults" encourage and extoll on purely philosophical grounds the use of hallucinatory drugs to "better one's inner-self" is more than a little distressing, when one is faced with a pathetic, once promising athlete who has failed to understand that athletic competition is by definition a contest of neuromuscular skill, strength, and/or coordination under specific rules, which contest rewards the best which can be *naturally* attained. His misguided attempts to rationalize the self-administration of this or that drug for this or that ad hoc effect to attain that "Nirvana" of personal success have cast him into the vortex of that same ideological maelstrom that has already irreversibly swallowed so many of our younger generation!

In summary, sound handling of this fascinating field involves one principle: that the rationale of any regimen be physiological and that the psychological aspects of harmless variations not be ignored. Nothing more is necessary; nothing less will suffice. One illustration will serve to highlight this truth. It concerns a product that was first brought to our attention by a runner (who later went into medicine), an intelligent and serious middle-distance man who was always up on the latest adjuncts that might ease the track man's thorny way. The product was a candy bar whose ingredient list could have come from a textbook of nutrition—ingredients in a variety that fulfilled every known dietary need and in amounts that were a safe multiple of minimum daily requirements. One had only to smell the bar to know that the vitamin B complex was unquestionably a prime constituent. Its odor was not at all appetizing, and it was therefore forgotten until we received a report from Tokyo and the 1964 Olympics that the candy bar was distributed free to all athletes. The athletes promptly gave the aromatic bar to clamoring Japanese children, and according to reports these crafty gamin just as promptly threw the uneaten bars into the street!

# 6

# *Proper Playing Conditions*

Of all the important factors in a coordinated medical program in athletics the most easily controlled is the physical environment in which a sport is played. The beneficial results of such control may be impossible to demonstrate in any concrete way, simply because their efficacy can be measured only in preventive, rather than therapeutic, terms. The physicians in athletics must, therefore, make absolutely certain that his recommendations, his demands, his minimum standards are known in every instance. Should he be ignored for reasons of economy or because of long-range projects of greater importance and the like, his position should remain unchanged—a steadfast insistence on nothing but the best in equipment and playing conditions for each and every athlete!

In short, if any school, college, or professional franchise cannot fulfill the equipment requirements for a given sport, it cannot afford that sport. The responsibility for making these requirements known is the doctor's and his alone, but the ultimate responsibility must lie with that school, college, or professional franchise that chooses to ignore these requirements.

## THE PLAYING FIELD

Although rules and regulations cover the dimensions, type of surface, and markings of the field of play in every sport, fulfillment of technical requirements does not render a field playable. A football field that is studded with rocks and "gopher holes," broken glass and litter does not deserve the name, nor does a basketball court with rigid structures within inches of the baselines, or a swimming pool without underwater lights or adequate underwater lane markings. All are playing fields, and as such should be arenas where the athlete can prove himself at his sport and not his ability to survive dangerous physical facilities.

## Turf Sports

Every sport played on turf should be played on *turf,* not on sand, coal dust, or the like. The turf should be level over the entire field and kept evenly mowed and rolled. It should be clearly marked with non-caustic material, and all sideline markers should be collapsible. Equally important, there should be adequate level turf on all sides of the field to allow speeding athletes sufficient room to hurtle out of bounds without encountering any rigid structure. Lastly, the turf should be kept free of contamination with horse manure, which despite its excellent fertilizing effect contains high concentrations of tetanus and gas-bacillus organisms and spores.

**Artificial Turf.** In recent years there has been an increasing trend toward the installation of permanent playing surfaces of artificial material, totally synthetic and of a consistency and color to suggest, if not resemble, grass. These artificial surfaces have been installed over a base, which has varied from installation to installation and from various points in time since the original development of said surface. Consequently, there are many different artificial playing surfaces manufactured by one of several predominant manufacturers, which surfaces are placed over a base, which may vary from a rock solid asphalt construction in accordance with the local highway surface regulations to, in one instance, an actual dirt base. The advantages of such surfaces from an administrative viewpoint, namely ease of maintenance, uniformity of surface, uniformity of bounce characteristics, and savings on laundry bills, must be balanced against what is undoubtedly a much harder surface to impact upon as well as certain individual characteristics of the artificial turf involved, such as inherent abrasiveness, local heat retention—which in some instances can be of alarming significance—and an extraordinary loss of traction under wet conditions. Since all such surfaces require special footgear to avoid damage thereof, a further complicating variable has been introduced into the shoe playing surface interface, which last must be considered pivotal in the production of knee and ankle injuries. The principal objections of many medical authorities to the rock hard consistency of some artificial playing surfaces, hence to the increase in painful contusions and strains secondary thereto, must therefore be considered variable in view of the marked differences between "early generation" surfaces installed with minimal padding as against "late generation" surfaces installed with an inch to an inch and a quarter padding, a significant contrast. On the other hand, uniform to all surfaces is the acute problem of skin abrasions, which may be so extensive as to require skin grafting in some rare instances. There is, therefore, considerable controversy as to the relative safety of these surfaces as contrasted to normal turf, and no blanket statement can be made to cover all the varying factors involved. Suffice it to say, abrasion of exposed surfaces can be anticipated, as can be severe contusion of elbows and knees—e.g. by long sleeves, mandatory elbow pads, etc.—as well as aggravated joint injury from "cleat hang-up" in the woven surfaces which do not "give" like natural grass. Athletes can learn to avoid or control these factors, hence the increasing popularity of these surfaces. Nonetheless, those athletes who compete on these surfaces on rare occasions must anticipate such difficulties as are mentioned, difficulties which those accustomed to competition thereon may no longer appreciate.

**Track and Field Sports**

In the track and field sports there should be enough space to allow safe separation of one from another: The sight of javelin throwers, and hammer, shot, and discus heavers launching their lethal missiles while runners circle the track in the immediate vicinity is a familiar sight to many track fans. It is only the rarity of injury that has enabled this dangerous practice to continue. The high-jump pits, the pole-vault landing area, the long and triple-jump pits, all should be of adequate size and well cushioned. On the track itself lanes should be clearly marked, rigid curbing eliminated where possible, and ancillary equipment such as hurdles should be of the latest resilient style, constantly maintained to guard against splintering.

**Court Sports**

In court sports such as squash and handball the athlete is surrounded by rigid walls, with which he must learn to contend as part of the game, but basketball would do nicely with no walls at all; a player racing in for a layup usually crosses the baseline at full speed, his attention still directed upward, and, if there are rigid bleachers extending to the baseline or an unpadded or even padded wall mere feet from that baseline, the result can be bone shattering. Similarly, the common practice of bringing audience seating within 2 or 3 feet of the sidelines may increase gate revenues, but it will not benefit a basketball player in pursuit of an errant ball.

## Swimming

Swimming, in contrast to the above sports, would seem to offer few problems, since the standard pool should suffice. However, even the so-called standard pool may prove dangerous. The deep-diving end should be deep enough (12 feet for three-meter, 16 to 18 feet for tower diving), because there have been instances of significant injury from striking the bottom off the high board. A competitive pool should have surface lane markers, underwater lighting, and underwater lane markings, in order to prevent head-on collisions between swimmers in adjoining lanes. Each pool entrant must have taken a thorough soap shower immediately before, to minimize contamination of the water. The water itself should be adequately filtered, circulated, and chlorinated. Failure in any of these measures leads to increased contamination and cross-infection, which could affect an entire swimming squad.

## Wrestling and Other Sports

*Wrestling* offers a particular problem. The mat is the playing field, and it should be the best available regardless of cost. The mat and all clothing must be kept scrupulously clean, not only for matches but also during practice. The dangers of impetigo and herpes simplex are such that whole squads have become infected and matches have been cancelled, all because of a direct spread of these maladies through direct contact from person to person, to mat, to clothing, and back again.

*Other sports* offer other problems to be solved individually. A *baseball* field should have adequate room behind the catcher and outside the first and third base lines to provide a safe area for the pursuit of foul pops. Some type of palpable surface change, bordering all rigid walls and similar structures, should be installed to act as a warning to fielders as they approach these dangerous areas. Bases should be firmly but not rigidly anchored to protect the sliding base-runner, and home plate should be carefully countersunk to keep the rigid margins from catching cleats.

*Hockey* in a standard-sized rink offers only those hazards that are part of the sport, and, aside from assuring that the ice is even and uniform most protective measures are for the benefit of the spectators, who should be shielded from flying pucks and sticks.

All these requirements are costly and demand constant maintenance. Although they are outside the physician's technical sphere, it is his responsibility to require that they be fulfilled and, once fulfilled, that they be maintained to satisfactory standards. Such responsibility can be delegated to a good trainer, but, lacking one, the physician must assume it himself. Otherwise, serious and even fatal injuries can result.

## PROTECTIVE EQUIPMENT

A glance at any equipment catalogue from a major sporting goods manufacturer reveals the plethora of protective gear for every sport that has been developed over the years. The conflicting claims, the variety of styles, the different price ranges are confusing, and the superiority of one product over another may become a matter of subjective preference and brand loyalty. A good trainer can thread his way through the forest of claims and counterclaims with the instinct of a cat, but what of the physician lacking a trainer's expert advice and counsel?

Our advice is to trust in the pressures of an intensely competitive market. There is a powerful "grapevine" in athletics, and equipment failure rapidly becomes so widely known that no reputable manufacturer dares risk any new product or style of product without a thorough preliminary testing for fear of failure in this very specialized market. The top manufacturers offer competitive lines of equipment on every level and, in fact, may relabel the top line of another in order to offer a complete selection; hence, there is little difference between top-quality equipment of comparable price regardless of the label. Cheaper lines are inferior regardless of their manufacturer, and the lowest price line is the most inferior. Despite the risks bargain priced, poor quality equipment is frequently used by teams with limited budgets; such equipment cannot hope to provide adequate protection, when even the best occasionally fails.

### Football

**The Helmet.** Turning to football equipment, the most elaborate and cumbersome of all protective athletic equipment, let us consider the helmet. Despite the criticisms of many writers the modern football helmet is a masterpiece of engineering. It is constructed on the multiple-impact principle; that is, it is built to withstand multiple stresses and impacts (as contrasted to the "single-impact" motorcycle crash helmet, which combines a suspension principle with a crown, which by crumpling reluctantly on impact further absorbs and dissipates that impacting force). The football helmet fulfills its role with an effectiveness that has surprised its many medical critics. It has withstood G-forces that no one except those working in the field believed possible. The plastic shell has also been severely criticized and has even been called an offensive weapon. One popular model uses a layer of softer plastic material over the crown to neutralize this defect, but it does so to only a limited extent.

Although proponents of this latter model include two leading colleges, the trend has been toward the suspension shell-helmet, which has become almost universal since its first appearance in the era of Doc Blanchard, Glenn Davis, and the West Point teams of World War II. This suspension model has undergone numerous minor modifications, but the principle behind it—a canvas web suspension, supported at lateral points by rubber shims, inside a square-browed plastic shell—has remained unchanged. In the past 10 years the added face bar, at first a plastic single bar for backfield men only, has become a standard helmet attachment, varying from the "birdcage" type used mostly by linemen to the double-bar type used by ball handlers (because the clear space provides a maximum of visual field).

When this combination of suspension-helmet shell and face bar was indicted by one author as the cause of serious and fatal hyperextension neck injuries (by no means confirmed), the manufacturer added a protective pad under the posterior rim of the helmet shell. Our helmet-of-choice at the time was another model, which incorporated a combination of suspension together with heavy foam rubber padding, thus dissipating impact through the suspension and absorbing the remainder by padding, a combination not found in the pure suspension model. This helmet offered another advantage in that unlike the universal square-browed models it was off the brow. As such, one of the main criticisms of the pure suspension model was avoided; namely, the tendency of the helmet shell to swing over on its suspension, forcefully impacting the square browed rim onto the nasal bridge and inflicting soft tissue and occasional bony damage on our more Grecian profiles.

However, the square brow is now the only model available in any line. As a result, all helmets damage the nasal bridge, provided it is high enough. Because of this we have gone back to the universal shell-suspension model. Withall there has been no discernible difference in the incidence of concussions, no serious head injuries, and no hyperextension injuries of any kind. The added posterior cervical pad has been found completely unnecessary, since we have not been able despite vigorous effort to demonstrate any guillotine effect by hyperextension, even exerted through our most protruding type of face bar. Fingers inserted under the posterior-cervical helmet rim are barely pinched even with effort, and the secondary mechanism postulated, namely, the effect of the chin strap breaking, has simply removed the helmet from the head, damaging the external ears but not the cervical spine. At the same time the protective advantages of the present face bar and helmet have been most striking. Soft tissue and bony facial injuries have dropped off precipitately, and the formerly routine dental injuries have dropped to a negligible minimum.

The present face bar and helmet may in fact be too efficient! The increase of so-called "pinched nerve" incidents (about which more will be said later) may be due to the fact that the protection afforded by these two pieces of equipment is so complete that present-day players are recklessly using head and face in ways inconceivable ten years ago, thus exposing themselves to greater torsion forces than ever before. The deplorable development of the present day "stick" tackle, the technique of putting one's head "through the numbers," could never have taken place were it not for the remarkable protection afforded the face and head. The manner in which players are now throwing themselves head-first into trouble typifies the paradoxical effect of too effective protective equipment.

(The use of cervical collars will be discussed in direct relation to cervical injuries, as will all special appliances for specific injuries.)

**Shoulder Pads.** The shoulder pad is another complicated product of engineering research, with top line models comparing in quality across the board. The "inside" cantilever and "outside" cantilever models, the "low-profile" models, the externally padded models, and the internally padded models, all have had their share of praise or criticism. Advantages and disadvantages must be balanced against individual needs. Thus, all shoulder pads are designed to provide impact protection to the clavicles, acromioclavicular areas, and with their epaulettes the deltoid areas. Similarly, all shoulder pads extend down onto the anterior chest and posteriorly, rest over the scapulae. In athletes the latter is almost uniformly a deep bone, covered by thickly developed supra- and infra-spinatus muscles, rhomboids, and trapezii. Since it is the anterior chest and scapular areas that receive the transmitted blows from the shoulder—by planned dissipation through the pad structure—the scapula could conceivably suffer injury therefrom, were it the usual protruding subcutaneous bone seen in females and non-athletic males; in fact, scapular injury involving the body of the bone is practically never seen in football. A high cantilever pad could, therefore, be of advantage in protecting a bruised distal clavicle.

Of even greater value, however, is the "big boy" or "linebacker" model, which carries the rigid molded pad structure further down on to the rib cage on all sides and thereby transmits and dissipates even greater forces over the entire chest and upper back. Its bulk, on the other hand, is a distinct disadvantage, so much so that its originally intended use, to protect the lower ribs, is better accomplished by a separate set of rib pads; on canvas webbing, these hang from the shoulders to surround the lower ribs as a separate entity from the regular shoulder pad. In all instances, individual needs and requirements must determine the proper selection of models.

An increase in cervical problems has been attributed to the low-profile "pro-style" pads now in vogue. Though the theory of this mechanism seems logical enough, it has been our experience that the so-called "pinched nerve" must be examined in other ways. For these "injuries" have increased at Yale to a similar extent as elsewhere, yet we neither like nor have adopted "pro-style" pads. Our objection both to this and to the special "quarterback" model (now used by most professional quarterbacks) is the minimal protection offered in exchange for a saving in weight and bulk, a bad medical compromise.

**Hip Pads.** Similarly, the ultra-light, scaled down "pro-model" hip pads sacrifice too much protection for the sake of lightness, particularly since the ideal hip pad must cover the trochanters and trochanteric bursae laterally, the sacrococcygeal area and the posterior iliac spines posteriorly, the entire iliac crest laterally, and the anterior iliac spine anteriorly. Painful injuries are common in each of the areas named, and adequate protective padding for all these areas is necessarily bulky. The fact that many "pros" have completely dispensed with hip pads and instead tape pieces of sponge rubber here and there, does not alter the fact that all these areas must be protected and that the conventional hip pad, despite its bulk, does the job admirably. It must, however, be fitted and worn correctly with the iliac crests completely covered, which creates bulk around the waist (where all athletes wish to be sleek and speedy). Possibly for this reason most football players must be continually reminded to pull up their hip pads. Doing so hikes up the shell pant (because of the built-in belt groove), tautens the latter material, and better fixes the thigh pad in its proper place. Despite these interrelated advantages a painful "hip pointer" is ofttimes required to fix this necessity in a player's mind. One can always spot such an athlete by how high up his hip pads are and how sleekly his pants seem to fit.

**Thigh and Knee Pads.** As to the thigh pad and knee pad, each do their job well if the pants fit properly; otherwise, they slide around and do no good at all. External adhesive tape helps but should not be necessary if the pants fit properly and the hip pads are high enough to keep the pants from sagging down. Some people have inquired as to why padding is not provided for the lateral and posterior aspects of the thighs. To do so would add an encumbrance and would only afford a protection that is not as necessary as it might seem. This knowledge is a result of years of experience and development, empiricism that has demonstrated that direct impact to these areas is neither frequent enough nor disabling enough to warrant the added bulk.

**Shoes and Cleats.** Renewed interest has been focused on the shoe and the cleat used in football. The high top model shoe has now been replaced almost universally by the "low-cut" model, although the high lace, high top affords added protection against ankle injury. This last was graphically demonstrated in our experience when an obvious bi-malleolar fracture-dislocation of the ankle occurred in a practice scrimmage: The injury was prevented from compounding only by the external support provided by the high-top shoe, which we had insisted be worn in practice. Nevertheless, all football players insist that the "low cut" is lighter (½ ounce by weight) and therefore faster. Most important, "the pros wear them." Fifteen years ago, our runners, backs, and ends were the only players who clamored for "low cuts" to give them speed, and we were forced to compromise by permitting their use on game day. Little did we realize that we had opened the "flood gates." Linemen soon began clamoring for the same privilege, admitting that theirs was not a question of more speed but simply a matter of allowing a better demonstration of what little speed they had! We remain unconvinced, but our players feel speedier with "low-cuts," and maybe they are.

Much has been said concerning the role of the normal cleat in knee injuries (through straight torsion on a fixed foot without impact). We remain unconvinced despite the logic behind the theory, simply because every instance of significant knee injury in our program over the past 15 years has come as a result of impact—with other added factors—but always with impact. Although the round cleat that appeared about 20 years ago as an analogous answer to torsion ankle injuries was a practical failure, we tested the oval, specially sited cleat to evaluate its true efficacy in minimizing similar knee injuries.

To confuse the issue even more, the advent of artificial turf, as produced and advertised by several major manufacturers, has brought with it the mandatory cleated shoe of an entirely different configuration. With teams not infrequently practicing on grass with normal cleats then switching to special cleats for artificial turf during games, the statistical significance of all studies has been further vitiated. Of additional significance, the careful study of Philadelphia High Schools by Torg has led to a shortening of all cleats no matter the surface, with an added effect on knee and ankle injury which has yet to be determined. Now Cameron and Davis are advocating an entirely revolutionary concept, revolving cleat plates, and have mustered impressive statistics in support of their new design vis-à-vis knee and ankle injuries. What with this last as just one more factor, suffice it to say there is specific agreement that the key to the problem is the interface between the athlete and the playing surface and that modification of this interface must of necessity affect both knee and ankle injuries. Beyond this little more can be said until many more controlled studies have emerged that can overcome the confusion of the moment (e.g., first-, second-, third generation Astroturf as an additional variable); until such statistical proof is available, a continuing vigilance on the part of the team physician for that which is sensible and logical must suffice. (Fuller discussion of the mechanisms of knee and ankle injuries must be deferred to a later section, detailing specific regional disabilities.)

**Other Sports.** Protective equipment in the other sports is as uniquely adapted to particular needs as is football equipment. It receives little public attention, because injuries in football are the more numerous and dramatic. In the other sports equipment quietly accomplishes what is asked of it. The catcher's pads and mask, the hockey goalie's bulky padding are easily recognized. Because they do the job for which they are intended, there is no medical controversy over the modification of some detail in their construction. In the same category are the shin pads used in soccer, the fencing mask, the seemingly flimsy helmet and face guard used in lacrosse (flimsy only in comparison to the counterpart football equipment), and the equally flimsy yet effective shoulder and arm guards in the same sport, designed to protect these specific areas from intentional and unintentional battering by opponents' and teammates' sticks. The relatively new batting helmet in baseball merits special mention for its effectiveness both in professional and school play. And the fiberglass goalie mask used in hockey, a rarity 10 years ago, is now a routine sight on college rinks, though its fabrication requires a painstaking custom-fitting that only an expert trainer can manage.

In summary, all protective equipment of first quality is well constructed and particularly designed to accomplish particular ends. That injuries occur despite such equipment does not mean that it is inadequate, that it is poorly designed, or that any doctor can blithely design a better device. If, after acquiring a thorough grounding in engineering, plastics, fabrication, and why and how a particular piece of equipment has been developed, that doctor still believes he can design a better device, all well and good. Unfortunately, events as described with regard to the plastic-shell suspension helmet and face bar are more typical. Medical criticisms of the helmet, its construction, its design, and its appearance became widespread throughout the nation. In the face of this condemnation objective research not only vindicated but by careful electronic telemetry proved that the helmet was vastly superior to anything that researchers or critical doctors believed possible. The company engineers knew this, and team physicians, who had seen player after player scramble up without the slightest sign of discomfiture after head-on collisions audible one hundred yards away, knew it too. The concerned neurosurgeon who evacuates a subdural hematoma on one football player in 10 years may be convinced that the helmet is inadequate, but, when collisions such as described occur at least once a day throughout an average football season, the helmet does not deserve such condemnation.

This is not to say that present equipment is so perfect that nothing more need be done. Improvement is always possible. But improvement should be based upon a calm, logical assessment of all that has gone before as well as future needs. Qualities that merit preservation should be recognized and retained, not obliterated by radical changes no matter how laudable the objective. Continued reappraisal is going on constantly within the specialized competitive market of the sporting-goods manufacturers, since any true advance in the field, reasonably based on previous functional quality, reaps the financial reward of market domination. It is not surprising, therefore, that each manufactuter continually offers improvements, all carefully tested for market worth, nor is it surprising that these improvements are the result of hours of painstaking research and design. It is the athlete who profits most from this competition, and it is his safety and well-being that lies at the heart of the matter.

# 7

# Injury: Pathology and Treatment Principles

Before discussing specific injuries by region (Part II), we shall review basic pathology and general treatment principles. This is necessary, in order to assess factors common to all acute injury and to develop a basic rationale of treatment, that can with logical variation according to anatomical and functional differences be utilized throughout this vast field.

## THE ACUTE INJURY

### Definitions

How might we define *injury?* For our purposes injury may be considered an abnormal disruption of normal tissue continuity, microscopic or macroscopic. So defined, all injury can be roughly equated no matter what the extent and no matter what the force, be it external or internal. Similarly, viewed in this manner, injury becomes an independent entity, with variations being secondary to the actual tissue disrupted, rather than a series of separate definitions for this or that injury in this or that anatomical area.

Accordingly, a specific condition such as hematoma becomes a disruption of vascular continuity sufficient to cause extravasation, which then becomes of itself a gross finding. Contusion becomes a local crushing of tissue, at least sufficient to disrupt continuity of blood vessels with resultant extravasation of blood, if not further continuity of tissues in the impacted area. A fracture becomes a disruption of bony continuity with an almost inevitable disruption of contiguous structures—such as periosteum, neighboring muscle, vascular bundles, and the like—either microscopically or macroscopically. Dislocation becomes a disruption of capsular elements and supporting tissue fibers (depending upon the location and direction of force but a disruption nonetheless).

A further advantage of this definition is the enforced recognition thereby of the infinite variations possible in the degree of microscopic or macroscopic disruption of tissue continuity. Thus, a sprain of the ankle does not automatically become a complete or partial tear of one specific ligament with specific clinical rules of treatment to be applied "by the book"; it becomes an infinitely variable disruption of continuity, that is reflected in degrees of immediate or delayed pain, degrees of swelling, degrees of response to local treatment, and degrees of healing per unit of time. At the same time such a basic definition requires that the doctor know the microscopic and gross anatomy of the area traumatized, in order to be able to visualize the actual tissues involved, their relative vascularity, their relative functional strength. Prognosis and treatment response can then be accurately extrapolated from these factors, without resorting to blanket statements of disability that are rigidly applied in all instances of this or that specific clinical diagnosis.

**General Treatment Plan**

Let us now relate our definition of injury to a general treatment plan, the rationale of which is equally applicable. First of all, disruption of tissue continuity can be likened to that accomplished by surgery and the surgeon's scalpel with the obvious difference between clean incision and forceful tearing. In both instances, the most immediate and most striking result is bleeding. This bleeding can be quite brisk without any specific blood vessels in sight; in fact, anatomically named vascular channels are rarely dealt with in surgery without specific reasons and specific technical steps for their control. In like manner traumatic bleeding results from the disruption of myriad unnamed vessels—venous, arteriolar, and capillary—and must accompany every instance of injury. In equal measure, then, swelling accompanies all injury; it reflects the injury and is no more than an expression of the underlying damage. To become overly concerned about the degree of swelling and to modify one's efforts on the sole basis thereof is to lose sight of the real problem. Rapid and gross swelling may indicate simply that a local venule may be involved in a very minor overall injury; on the other hand, it may signify extensive tissue damage, whichever the case may be as indicated by entirely separate criteria of pain, spasm, functional loss, and instability.

**Control of Bleeding.** Treatment of injury should be directed first toward measures that control the bleeding or minimize the swelling. To accomplish this, some external means must be employed in just the same manner that a surgeon places hemostats in an operative wound. Certainly heat, which dilates vessels and increases bleeding, is not the proper means. On the other hand, *the use of cold,* which only now is becoming a matter of routine throughout the sporting world, offers a number of obvious advantages. It causes a local vasoconstriction, which, despite experimental work indicating local vasodilatation as an inevitable "rebound" phenomenon, can be maintained as long as desired. Secondly, it is easily transportable and applicable via ice bags or special cold packs. Thirdly, it has a numbing effect that greatly reduces the athlete's discomfiture.

Such logic may seem elementary, but the use of cold in acute injury is an innovation in athletics. Similarly, such elementary logic places the use of ethyl chloride in its proper light, branding it for what it is: the totally unphysiological application of an agent simply because it feels cold. Ethyl chloride does cause local vasoconstriction for the brief seconds it takes to volatilize on the skin, but in seconds there is visible capillary flare that graphically demonstrates the "rebound" phenomenon. To stop bleeding effectively, more than a few seconds of very superficial vasoconstriction is needed, and the subsequent vasodilatation is surely an undesired effect!

How long should cold be applied? Because of the likelihood of recurrent hemorrhage, regardless of how minimal, cold should be continued for 24 to 48 hours, even 72 hours in those specfic injuries that are prone to recurrent hemorrhage. Prolonged over this period of time, it assures vasoconstriction for a period of time sufficient to assure a firm organization of intravascular clots in the area.

Contrariwise, exposing the injured area immediately thereafter to heat through the use of infra-red lamps, hot packs, or hot whirlpool baths stimulates widespread vasodilatation of those vessels, dislodgement of clots, and recurrent bleeding. It has been argued that such local stimulation is necessary to encourage the earliest possible healing, by dilating the vessels and accelerating the pick-up and elimination of waste products and detritus in the area and thus facilitating an orderly commencement of normal healing processes. We have no argument with this concept, but external stimulation should be delayed at least until such time as the danger of further extravasation of blood is past, for nothing will delay normal healing progress more than accumulated blood and blood products, of an amount visible or palpable.

It has been also argued that prolonged application of cold leads to local "frostbite" and other manifestations of cold injury. This is a cogent contention and has some theoretical basis, but the simple expedient of requiring some intervening material, be it an elastic bandage or a pants leg, between the cold vehicle and the skin has eliminated this as factor in our experience. Our one episode of true "frostbite" occurred only after prolonged application in violation of these rules and with a moist icebag. That there is a consequent loss of some local effect particularly to the superficial layers of dermis cannot be denied, but these layers are almost never the objective of treatment and the cold still manages to penetrate to the areas desired.

Simultaneous with the application of cold, other measures are instituted, still directed toward the one controllable factor common to all injury, extravasation of blood. Some type of *local pressure* should be applied, and maintained for a period of time sufficient to assure lasting hemostasis. If the area is large, and the injury is diffuse, general compression with an elastic bandage will suffice; if it is a superficial hematoma, a sponge rubber pressure pad is even better.

**Elevation and Immobilization.** Consideration must also be given to those factors that caused the tissue disruption both in terms of the anatomy involved and the measures necessary to neutralize such forces and prevent further tissue injury or further bleeding. Hence, *elevation and immobilization* of the part make up the third integral part of a proper treatment regime, eliminating dependent rubor and dependent edema and, most important, placing that part at rest. Immobilization can be obtained by skillfully applied tape, elastic tape, Unna's paste, or even plaster casts and should be in the most comfortable and functional position, thereby apposing the margins of tissue disruption as ideally as possible without direct surgery. Whether this last has anything more than a salutory effect on eventual healing is questionable, but certainly judicious positioning prevents further injury.

This, then, is the initial treatment regime that has proved itself time and again. *I*ce, *c*ompression and *e*levation—I-C-E—not a new concept, not a revolutionary concept, but a logical and rational concept nonetheless. It is simple to apply, so simple that many of our athletes have picked it up and now apply it themselves automatically out of season, when we are not directly supervising their care. The rationale behind it coincides with the microscopic and macroscopic circumstances within the injured area itself. It makes anatomical and physiological sense, and it works!

## THE HEALING INJURY

To form a sound basis for treatment and rehabilitation of injury once the acute stage is past, one must return to a consideration of the progressive steps in microscopic healing. After bleeding has stopped resolution begins, organizing the minute thrombi so important in hemostasis and creating a granulation tissue rich in capillaries from which pass acute inflammatory cells and macrophages to digest the detritus of devitalized tissue and extravasated blood elements. On the background network of fibrin within the traumatized area move other tissue cells, the fibroblasts, to begin the process of active repair. In addition, depending on the particular tissue involved, further regeneration of injured tissue elements occurs, culminating in a fibrous scar of a size and extent proportional to the injury, with some persistent chronic histiocytes and lymphocytes, few if any acute polymorphonuclear leukocytes, rapidly disappearing granulation tissue, and overall a steadily diminishing vascularity.

All these stages take place consecutively in all injuries, merging into one another with a rapidity that varies from tissue to tissue and with the extent of injury but overlapping in time in different areas of the same injury. In a clean surgical wound research has shown healing with good fibrous union is nearly complete within 10 to 12 days with very little increase in strength beyond that time. Closed soft tissue injuries are far from analogous but are usually more sterile than the cleanest surgical wound. As such, tissue repair progresses without infection and at a pace that may be quite rapid.

**Treatment During the Healing Process.** What would be a rational approach to treatment of injury in this healing stage? Certainly nothing should be done that might aggravate the healing tissues, disrupt this complicated process, and restimulate bleeding. Since normal body processes are striving to heal the injury at maximum speed in response to inherent local stimulation, how much more stimulation is necessary? It is our contention that no profit can be gained from stimulating an already complicated process that needs no stimulation and that hydrocollators, whirlpools, massage, infrared, ultrasonic, and other modalities available in physical medicine are, in a sense, whipping an already laboring horse. To carry the analogy one step further, shooting the area full of enzymes, which were first developed to dissolve clots in inaccessible areas (such as the pleural space), or hormones, which are anti-inflammatory in action (when healing is an inflammatory process), is akin to shooting benzedrine into that same hapless horse; if the poor horse collapses, who is at fault, the horse?

**Appraisal of Healing Progress.** A conscious attempt should be made to provide every opportunity for natural local processes to assert themselves, by purposeful anticipation of each step in resolution and healing. In most instances of injury in athletics the involved area is accessible to inspection and palpation; hence, *continual inspection and palpation,* daily and sometimes twice daily, is the keynote to an accurate appraisal of day-to-day progress. Every doctor who treats athletes directly should take advantage of this unique opportunity. Under such close scrutiny it is possible actually to feel and observe the various stages of healing, from the initial control of bleeding, through the inflammatory absorption of blood and blood products, to the stage of fibrous deposition and chronic inflammatory reaction. The initial stage is one of swelling with little increase in local tenderness provided steps have been taken to assure local hemostasis. The second stage is characterized by a slight increase in local heat and redness, simultaneous with a moderate increase in diffuse tenderness over this area of reaction; the third, by a palpable thickening and brawny induration that becomes progressively painless.

Variations in local findings in each of these three stages can be evaluated as to their specific meaning and treatment varied accordingly. If a more than usual amount of bleeding has occurred, for instance, one may anticipate that the inflammatory reaction that follows will be more acute and more diffuse. Similarly, the extent of brawny induration and fibrous thickening that follows in such an instance can be expected to be more extensive, and it always is.

### Active Rehabilitation

Regardless of local individual variation healing progress takes place in logical sequence in every injury. Consequently, a logical series of treatment steps can be developed, taking advantage of this knowledge. The resolution stage must be supported by external measures that provide continuous support to the disrupted tissues yet neither aggravate nor impair its necessary sequential completion. *External support* by means of splinting tape and elastic bandages should be continued, but, as with even the most extensive surgical wounds, *active motion* can be started in a series of gently progressive steps. *Repeated inspections* of the injury site throughout this program must assure that activity is never locally injurious. Increased local swelling and tenderness always indicate such an untoward effect; conversely, their absence will signify an almost incredible acceleration of the entire healing process. In short, if proper local support is provided for the injured area, a graduated rehabilitation program can be initiated as soon as bleeding has definitely ceased, following which the inflammatory reaction of the resolution phase of healing will be seen to subside even more rapidly than usual and to merge into the phase of fibrous thickening. (See Figs. 22–1 to 22–4.)

As soon as the stage of fibrous thickening supervenes, as indicated by inspection and palpation, progressive rehabilitation can be accelerated. It is surprising how such a program is reflected by an equally accelerated subsidence of both swelling and tenderness, to a point that nothing but a history of recent injury remains and full athletic effectiveness is restored. Brawny fibrous induration, an inevitable accompaniment of acute ankle injury when it is treated by complete immobilization for 10 days, appears and disappears by the 6th to 8th day when such a case is subjected to a regime of early rehabilitation under close supervision with the added advantage that atrophy and weakness of surrounding muscles does not occur.

The greatest argument against such a regime is its effect on tissues that cannot possibly heal in the short time allowed and the accompanying certainty of permanent damage therefrom. In answer, we must return to the initial evaluation at the time of the injury and the consecutive findings thereafter. The evaluation must have been accurate and confirmed by subsequent developments before activity is initiated. Obviously, injuries that have involved joints or bones cannot be so accelerated to a healed state. Bone takes weeks to heal and must be immobilized, and unstable joints need support far longer to assure subsequent stability. These are clinical injuries about which there can be no argument. The "hamstring pull," the muscle contusion, the minor sprained ankle need *not* be treated the same way. Each may be treated as intensively and as individually by certain logical rules here outlined. Constant reinspection and reevaluation of such cases has failed to reveal permanent damage from too early activity. On the contrary, full and complete recovery has been attained more rapidly and more satisfactorily than by any other method. (See Chapter 23)

The second argument pertains to local pain and its necessary relief. It is the contention of many that extensive and prolonged immobilization is the only assurance of a painless recovery regardless of the concomitant atrophy and fibrosis (which always occurs and must always be overcome by an additional period of rehabilitation). Local pain from an injury can always be best controlled by total immobilization in plaster, as anyone who has experienced a broken bone can avow. In the injuries with which we are dealing, however, pain has been less than anticipated—even during the first 24 hours and progressively less so thereafter. In fact, aside from major clinical injuries (i.e., fractures) we have never needed more than a mild analgesic for our athletes. Pain is after all a relative thing and the most difficult to evaluate objectively. All athletes contend with pain of a degree that is difficult for the non-athlete to understand, and this is no more true of the contact sports than it is of the non-contact sports. The average athlete is far more stoic about his injuries than others, and accordingly he is prepared "to pay the piper" in terms of local discomfort. His concern is not with the pain of the moment; it is: "How long will I be out?" This is not to say that haste should supersede medical judgment for the sake of returning an athlete to the playing field, but, if relief of tolerable discomfort is the chief justification for a treatment regime that delays a return to full function by a week or 10 days, there are few athletes who will not choose the more uncomfortable road to an earlier return to the field.

**Anesthetic Injections and Pain.** Injections of local anesthetic are not only unnecessary but must be openly condemned. Pain or tenderness is a prime means for gauging recovery progress in our program. Together with local swelling it provides us with an infallible index of functional recovery. If, for example, the injured area is more painful and swollen after a single controlled workout, too much has been done too early. Without this guide the entire program is lost. Local anesthesia, in turn, creates local swelling and destroys pain sensitivity, hence destroys all guide-lines for the logical control of rehabilitation. This alone should suffice to rule out its use, without even considering the calamitous prospects of uncontrolled stress on an injury-weakened, completely benumbed part!

But, it might be contended, if pain is to be such an important guide-post to healing and rehabilitation, then it must be objectively assessed repeatedly, and, as we have admitted, this can be most difficult. To answer this criticism, we must return to the basic requirements of medical management (discussed in an earlier chapter). An injured athlete is not a stranger with unknown stress tolerance and pain-threshold, as is most often the case in clinical practice. He is known to the coach, to the trainer, to his teammates, and to the doctor, and it is at this juncture that the direct and continuing familiarity with the athlete is most decisive. If the doctor knows and understands the injured boy, if he knows how he has reacted to pain in the past, if he knows all the cross-currents of motivation and desire that apply at this moment, he is able to accurately evaluate not only initial pain but local discomfort during recovery. Pain may be excruciating before a large audience and virtually absent in the dressing room. Pain may be totally absent during examination on the sidelines, yet necessitate a monstrous "gimp" immediately upon return to the big game before admiring thousands. Pain may cause one boy to shriek and pound the earth from an injury that another will not even bother to report. Pain from a dislocated finger, promptly reduced, may disable one boy totally for 2 weeks, another for 2 minutes. In each instance, however, there is a certain individual consistency which affords the doctor the necessary information he needs. Careful assessment must include all these variables from the beginning; no mean task, but one that is part of the doctor's job.

## ADVANTAGES OF ACTIVE REHABILITATION

Some of the advantages gained by a program of early active rehabilitation have already been touched upon, such as its salubrious effect on both the resolution and healing phases of injury recovery. When judiciously controlled, there are many other advantages.

**Maintenance of Conditioning.** Most important is the maintenance of overall conditioning, something of small note to the non-athlete, but representing an investment of months of grueling effort by the athlete; not something to be thrown away lightly. For example, a 2 week layoff to recover from an injury, the last 10 days of which might have been spent on an active program, exercising all other uninjured parts and maintaining cardiovascular efficiency, is time lost that can never be recovered. On the other hand, a combination of vigorous exercise of all but the injured part and a progressively demanding and simultaneous rehabilitation of that part assures that both will "peak" at the same time, thereby returning a fully conditioned athlete to full activity without a single day's delay.

**Optimal Resolution and Healing.** Another advantage is more direct, consistent with the accelerating effect of controlled activity on both resolution and healing of an injury: the prevention of fibrous tissue adhesions in the area. It is a situation analogous to the postoperative wound, upon which enforced inactivity usually produces a thick, indurated cicatrix, its anatomical layers densely apposed in a mass of fibrous tissue that is equally adherent, layer to layer. Such a wound will be tight and uncomfortable for months or years. In contrast, an un-complicated appendectomy scar, following active ambulation from the first postoperative day, will be soft and mobile, with layers sliding freely upon one another and with no "tightness." In much the same way, a minor ankle sprain, tender at the outset at a 5.0 to 10.0 mm. spot in the anterolateral ligament (such remarkable localization is routine in athletics, where on-the-spot examination is possible seconds after injury), treated "by the book" with a paste boot for 4 days, ra-diant heat and whirlpool baths thereafter, crutches for the first 6 to 7 days, and continued physical therapy for up to 14 days, will present a brawny, indurated, "leathery" appearance, with motion limited in all directions, a visible limp on walking, and a total inability to run with-out an obvious "gimp," all of which may take an additional 2 weeks to a month to overcome. In contrast, such an injury, strapped and iced initially for 1 or 2 days, started on supported walking the 2nd day, jogging and running to tolerance the 4th day, will by the end of the 5th to 6th day present an entirely normal appearance, with all landmarks visible, no visible or palpable edema, subsiding tenderness only in that one original spot, and, with support, the capability of fulfilling all athletic demands. Overabundant scar tissue is characteristic following necessary immobilization in major joint and skeletal injury and must be accepted as inevitable. But minor injuries similarly treated (long-term sling or crutches as the case may be) will also develop the most remarkable masses of scar tissue, masses that can permanently hamper performance. This need not be accepted as inevitable. Active rehabili-tation, judiciously controlled, can result in a return to full function with little if any palpable scar, a worthy objective in any case but mandatory in the athlete. Can this be criticized because it is too de-manding of the athlete? We think not.

**Team Participation.** Finally, active rehabilitation allows the injured athlete to remain a part of the team rather than a discarded alien brooding in his room. He can carry out his assigned program under direct supervision, and the coaches can continue his nonphysical train-ing. He keeps up intellectually, while he catches up physically. When he is finally ready, he is ready in every respect. In the meantime, his teammates and coaches have never lost sight of him, nor he of them, and continuity is thereby maintained, each to the other. There are those who prefer to play the "wounded hero" among their less athletic classmates, eschewing the monotony of practice workouts and the par-ticular drudgery of a graduated rehabilitation program directly under the demanding eye of doctor and trainer. There are those who by nature refuse to move a muscle until convinced that they are absolutely well. And there are those who welcome the opportunity to absent themselves from a sport that deep within themselves they actually dislike. In each instance, however, the program plays an invaluable role, offering the willing athlete an indispensable adjunct to recovery and the unwilling one an opportunity to uncover and face his problems. Response to injury is a universally recognized factor of key importance in athletics, one that the shrewd professional franchises now specifically inquire about, one that is expressed in curt euphemisms such as "tough," "plenty of guts," "plenty of desire," and the like. And it is the active rehabilitation program, directly related thereto, that offers opportunity for a truly meaningful contribution by the medical staff to the benefit of the team, the coaching staff, and to both the physical and mental well-being of the injured athlete.

# Part Two

## *Specific Injuries and Disabilities*

# 8

# Intracranial and Visceral Injuries

Specific athletic injuries will be discussed in relation to the anatomical regions in which they occur, and each region will be discussed systematically and consecutively in logical sequence from above downward. However, this opening chapter to the regional approach includes three separate anatomical regions and may be considered to supersede all others in overall importance. We are concerned here with those regions that contain vital organs, pivotal to life itself, and therefore with problems that are the most dangerous of those encountered in athletics. We are concerned here with injuries that every physician must keep uppermost in his mind whenever he runs onto the field, whenever he examines even the slightest injury, and whenever he questions a complaining athlete. These injuries have the most insidious beginnings, the most protean manifestations, the most disastrous potentialities. These are the injuries that before all else must be ruled out, yet at the same time are the most difficult to rule out. Fatal injury in athletics occurs almost exclusively herein, and crippling injuries, usually permanent, occur with distressing frequency herein. The injuries and problems discussed in this chapter comprise the most difficult and challenging that the athletic physician will encounter, and, no matter what his particular training, he must be thoroughly prepared to cope with them. Management of major fractures, dislocations, and even gross muscle and ligament tears are as child's play compared to the diagnostic skill and judgment demanded by these injuries.

## INTRACRANIAL INJURIES

Intracranial injuries have contributed preponderantly to the overall death rate in competitive sports. This fact has been used to condemn contact sports, and the prohibition of some, football in particular, has been recommended. A cursory glance at the statistics might seem to confirm a rising death rate from head injuries. It must be pointed out, however, that the rising numerical death rate from head injuries is more alarming than real; a proper correlation with the greatly increased number of total participants in the sport reveals a steady drop in incidence to a present low. Though certainly not acceptable, this low can be viewed as reasonable. Study of the statistics reveals that the percentage incidence of fatal head injury, most often quoted as exhibiting a frighteningly constant rise over the past 20 years, is actually a statistical distortion. The percentage incidence of fatal abdominal injuries, the other principal killer in football, has at the same time dropped off remarkably (as a result of early diagnosis and surgical treatment). Obviously, if one percentage figure falls in relation to the overall 100 per cent, the other major figure must rise to maintain the mathematical equation. Furthermore, study of the individual cases in recent years reveals a real possibility of further improvement through the employment of more intensive clinical supervision by a medical profession made increasingly aware of the disastrous potential of all head injury, particularly on the secondary school and "sand-lot" level. Nevertheless, head injury remains the primary killer, and the reason for this is easy to find when one attempts to define a logical formula for prompt diagnosis and therapy, applicable in every instance of possible intracranial trauma.

**Major Head Injury**

There are rare instances of *massive head injury* that are obvious from the moment of impact, such as a hard-hit baseball smashing into an unprepared fielder's skull, or a helpless hockey player cannoning off a rigid goal upright with the side of his head. Loss of consciousness, even deep coma, may be apparent from the start. There is extensive soft tissue damage overlying the calvarium, and a depressed or compound fracture of the skull may be grossly evident. Treatment is perfectly straightforward: immediate transportation by stretcher and ambulance to the nearest hospital, treatment of traumatic shock, immediate skull x-rays, débridement and/or intracranial surgery as indicated—all are logical and sequential steps, to be carried out without delay. Required are a rapid, skilled neurological examination, diagnostic lumbar tap, funduscopic evaluation of physiological cupping of the optic nerve disc, and close inspection of the skull films to ascertain depressed or linear fracture, and, in the case of the latter, to determine whether the fracture line crosses the course of the middle meningeal artery, with its added threat of epidural hemorrhage. All these are diagnostic and clinical appraisals that must be made quickly by a physician best qualified by training and experience. It is equally clear that such examinations and evaluations differ in no way from those applied to every case of major head injury admitted to a hospital emergency room. The magnitude and severity of the trauma is grossly apparent, and every effort should be made to assure that the best specialist attention is obtained.

It is not within the limits of this book to summarize traumatic neurosurgery. This is a field of infinite complexity and belongs within the province of the trained neurosurgeon. The reader may consult any standard neurosurgical reference for such information. More important, the training of the physician in athletics is unlikely to extend into this specialty to any significant depth, and, by being the first to admit it, he can make certain that a trained neurosurgeon is always reasonably available. Even a limited formal experience in this specialty, as part of a general surgical training program to assure satisfactory performance of the more limited intracranial procedures under the most pressing circumstances, did not provide the author with more than a wholesome respect for the entire field and a desire for the closest possible cooperation with these specialists. Only the trained neurosurgeon can provide the necessary care in these major problems both in the long run and from the very beginning. The team physician must not attempt to carry the responsibility.

## Minor Head Injury

In fairness to the physician in athletics, instances of major head injury are quite rare. He is faced instead with a procession of minor incidents, individually differentiated by infinite variations but possessing the common denominator of impact, variable degrees of "blackout," and/or headache. These cannot be referred to the neurosurgeon, who could not begin to cope with more than a small portion of the total. It is, therefore, the responsibility of the doctor in athletics to formulate a means of handling these problems that will assure that potential dangers are anticipated, while truly innocuous incidents are recognized as such.

In order to accomplish this, one must return to the basic characteristics of head injury. The major traumas within the calvarium are lacerations or contusions of brain substance, hemorrhage epidural and/or subdural, and skull fracture with displacement of fragments. Aside from the direct effect of injury on function (e.g., the motor area, the major tracts, the medulla), the principal dangers are hemorrhage and/or edema within a closed space, hemorrhage and/or edema that may be rapid or insidious. Direct injury to functioning tissue is recognizable from the outset, but the early detection of bleeding and/or edema is often difficult. One must review the clinical means of detecting the latter developments and how these means can be best employed. In the first place, it is apparent that initial loss of consciousness is of no significant diagnostic value. Secondly, an initial negative examination is valueless without a carefully formulated and thoroughly applied follow-up program with the physician alert to the earliest warning sign.

**Clinical Approach.** It is essential, then, that there be some clinical "starting point," following which such a thorough observation regime can be instituted automatically. Clincial developments in head trauma are such that certain easily performed procedures can establish clear guidelines as to progress, but the "starting point" presents a problem, simply because this regime cannot be employed indiscriminately on all headaches that occur in a multiple-impact game such as football. Headaches, in fact, are general on every football squad, once active body contact begins. They may be secondary to slight dehydration in the heat, sinus troubles on changing from home to school environments, or tension from the competition. On the other hand, *headache that persists* without change beyond the usual 3 to 5 days certainly qualifies as a "starting point." Also, *loss of consciousness on impact* must be considered a "starting point" regardless of its lack of value per se. Loss of consciousness is a direct reflection of influences within the calvarium and is therefore a mirror of what injurious physical forces may have penetrated the total brain substance; the deeper the loss, the more intensive the possible damage. It is well known that loss of consciousness does not necessarily precede the subsequent development of a *subdural hematoma,* and it is not uncommon that the initial head injury in such cases may be so insignificant as to be forgotten by the patient. Similarly, *epidural hemorrhage* is classically characterized by the "lucid interval" prior to catastrophic developments thereafter. One must accept the fact that impacts sufficient to cause subdural hematomas occur repeatedly throughout an average contact practice day, particularly in football. Every candidate on the squad could be considered suspect for subdural hemorrhage and might even justifiably undergo daily skull films to check on the equally dangerous second possibility—early epidural hemorrhage. Loss of consciousness, on the other hand, is not a common occurrence, and, because it reflects a total jarring of the intracranial contents, it can serve as an empirically satisfactory clinical "starting point."

But how does one differentiate between the momentary "stuns" that occur 3 or 4 times a day, instances in which a boy typically shakes his head, blinks his eyes, and gets up a little slowly, but is within moments completely normal? Or those occasional bone jarring impacts, in which both parties lie motionless for up to 30 seconds, slowly but steadily gathering their wits? What constitutes a "loss of consciousness" in these instances?

There can be no accurate answer to these questions, only an empirical approach. In our experience an arbitrary definition has become necessary. If by the time we arrive at his side, in an average of 20 to 30 seconds, the injured athlete is awake and thinking, recognizes us, and can talk to us, he has not had a true concussion. If he is still out of contact with his surroundings, he *has* had a concussion. In the former instance, careful cranial nerve tests, close questioning, tests on his positional responsibilities in play after play by fellow squad members—all provide the guidelines to determine whether he can return to action or should be followed closely. In the latter instance he will play no more that day or for 10 days thereafter; he is admitted to the infirmary for constant pulse and blood pressure recordings, and tests of verbal response, orientation, and sensorium; his fundi are checked daily or even more often as indicated; subjective headache is followed closely until it disappears (usually in 1 or 2 days); finally, all reading is barred until the headache does disappear.

This arbitrary *10-day period of observation* is admittedly a compromise, since a subdural hematoma can take longer than 10 days to develop. By and large, however, it is a safe period of observation, particularly since it is terminated only if the athlete is and has been completely clear of headache or any other significant complaint for at least half of that period. If at the same time daily neurological examination, funduscopic inspection, and verbal response tests are performed, these, combined with the blood pressure and pulse record, should afford the earliest detection of any untoward change. By the thorough application of this clinical routine any change is noted immediately and prompt neurosurgical consultation thus assured. Routine cerebrospinal fluid tap is not performed, nor are routine skull films obtained. They are not necessary in the majority of instances and can be safely delayed until such time as neurosurgical consultation is indicated by clinical progress.

Such a routine is not possible without the immediate availability of a general hospital and an experienced neurosurgeon, particularly with respect to the omission of routine skull films and spinal tap. If general hospital facilities and neurosurgical consultant care are more than minutes away, these latter measures should probably be carried out.

*Retrograde amnesia* for the causative impact, another clinical "starting-point," can be serially evaluated during this same observation. It is interesting to note the frequency with which such amnesia slowly expands to include subsequent events that were at the time apparently fully recognized and alertly handled by the injured player. Uniformly accompanying this amnesia is an apprehension, which must be dealt with by constant reassurance until the memory loss begins to clear (though rarely completely). By this close a follow-up the boy is constantly supported through a frightening experience, while any rise in blood pressure, blurring of sensorium or cerebration, or any other neurological hint of deterioration is apparent immediately.

*If symptoms, particularly headache, persist* beyond this arbitrary number of days, the period of observation must be prolonged to include further detailed serial studies—such as EEG's, multiple skull films, and any other tests advised by the neurosurgeon. If there is *still* question, then further contact sports should be permanently barred. *Post-traumatic headache* as a sequel to head injury is disbarring for all contact sports according to our criteria, and this disqualification lasts for the remainder of the athlete's school career. The crippling effect of such post-traumatic headache must be seen to be appreciated, and contact sports do not justify the risk of permanent disability. By the same measure a series of *clinically defined concussions* (arbitrarily, 3) is also permanently disqualifying for precisely the same reason.

Individual variations make enforcement of these arbitrary measures quite difficult, but the physician must be guided by basic principles and maintain his ground. There will be clear-cut instances of "play-acting," in which the injured athlete exhibits behavior that is uniquely bizarre, acting out the role of the disoriented movie prize fighter yet characteristically inconsistent in his response to questions. Some football players complain of severe headache during practice yet have no complaints on game days. Others complain of headache until they are finally told that they must give up the sport, a decision which for reasons of their own they seize upon gratefully. In each instance an inner need is being fulfilled, and the physician is well advised to go along despite his personal suspicions—with the sole qualification that under no circumstances can such a complaint be used to avoid practice yet permit games. Complete neurological workup and prolonged observation may seem excessive in these not uncommon cases, but how can one be certain?

Finally, consideration must be given to the significance of *past intracranial surgery* no matter what the cause. Despite the phenomenal progress of neurosurgery, intracranial procedures are never undertaken lightly, hence the reasons they have been performed are usually sufficient to bar contact sports. Moreover, even in the case of exploratory burr-holes adequate to drain very small subdural collections, thorough evaluation and judgment should be exercised before contact sport clearance is given. A skull with burr-holes or, worse, a bone flap is not a normal skull no matter how complete the recovery.

## INTRATHORACIC INJURIES

Although infrequently encountered, intrathoracic injuries can lead to disastrous complication. Such injuries threaten two vital functions —respiration and cardiac integrity—so must be viewed as potentially catastrophic, and every effort must be made to recognize them immediately.

### Airway Obstruction

Gross airway problems, although easily recognized when sought for, may lead to early fatality pending recognition and treatment.

**Larynx Injuries.** The most common airway problem seen in the contact sports (and occasionally in non-contact sports) is *the bruised larynx,* following a direct blow from elbow, fist, racquet, stick, or baseball. Regardless of cause it presents as hoarseness, soreness to palpation of the larynx and the upper tracheal rings, but without airway constriction, hence a simple ice collar overnight suffices.

Nevertheless, thorough palpation and airway inspection are mandatory to rule out the more serious *laryngeal fracture* with accompanying edema sufficient to steadily obliterate the vital airway. That this last is so rare is probably due to the inherent cartilaginous nature of the larynx and upper trachea, which is relatively mobile, is surrounded in the athlete by heavy musculature, and is protected by the drawn-down chin in a split second reflex action. However, laryngeal fractures have been reported (though not in athletics), hence, concomitant *laryngeal edema,* necessitating eventual tracheotomy, is always a remote possibility. Yet, as with so much in athletics, prompt recognition or suspicion will avert panic-stricken emergency procedures; unhurried otolaryngological consultation can then assure the maximum benefit of care. If the latter is not available, indirect laryngoscopy by mirror should suffice to evaluate airway patency, and tracheotomy can then be performed deliberately under optimal controlled conditions.

**Swallowed Tongue.** Of much more immediate import to the airway, though strictly speaking above the thoracic inlet, is the "swallowed tongue." This is a true emergency. It is rarely encountered outside of athletics and fortunately is uncommon even in the most violent sports, but it occurs often enough to demand constant vigilance and a plan of immediate action on the part of any physician in athletics. It is essentially a purely mechanical displacement of the entire lingual mass back upon itself into the pharynx, totally blocking the airway, with immediate asphyxia and cyanosis and, most important, an involuntary yet powerful trismus. It can occur on any type of unexpected impact but usually follows a "clothes-lining" of the victim, suspending and decelerating him by the head and neck in one explosive jolt. As a purely mechanical phenomenon, it can be just as immediately rectified, but one must first be alert to its presence. One must be prepared to overcome without delay the powerful trismus exerted by the cyanotic and rapidly unconscious athlete. Mouth gags, tongue blades, and rigid metallic devices are of little value, and one has no time to break teeth to insert any sort of lever. A hard-plastic "oral screw," based on the powerful expanding-screw principle and with an easily inserted conical tip, affords the ideal means of prying open the teeth to allow a finger, clamp, anything to be thrust into the pharynx to hook the tongue out of its lethal malposition. Relief, needless to say, is immediate and dramatic. Some authorities are convinced that this clinical picture simply does not occur, while others, granting the rare occurrence thereof, recommend that nothing whatever be done, inasmuch as anoxia, cyanosis, and unconsciousness will rapidly supervene, thereby eliminating the need for potentially tooth-damaging measures; however, it will be a rare physician who can stand patiently aside, merely to avert a cracked tooth, while a struggling athlete lapses into cyanosis and coma during an agonizing 1 to 3 minutes.

**Visceral Injuries**

Further discussion of intrathoracic problems or injuries requires a review of the role played by the chest wall in normal respiration, and the proper examination of the entire area and its contents. The "operculum" mechanism of respiration is well known, and the role of the flexible chest wall in this inspiratory and expiratory cycle can be visualized easily. Equally understood must be the degree of internal injury that can take place without significantly distorting or injuring this flexible wall. Thus, the proper examination of any potential intrathoracic injury must include a thorough palpation of the entire wall, which is quite rapidly accomplished. However, the absence of any evidence of rib or costal cartilage damage does not rule out injury. Secondary to this same physiological flexibility, massive displacement and contusion of thoracic contents may have taken place, hence must be evaluated by thorough percussion and auscultation of the entire chest. At the same time cardiac outline should be checked, the character of heart sounds noted, and the trachea checked for midline position.

**Cardiac Contusion.** In this manner *cardiac contusion* can be grossly evaluated, though the extent to which this can be done satisfactorily remains a worrisome problem. When one considers the proven efficacy of external cardiac massage by extrasternal pressure, one can appreciate the extent of potential cardiac damage that can occur by a simple, routine impact on the anterior chest, an impact that must be multiplied a thousandfold to approximate its average frequency throughout a football season. The absence of evident chest wall injury remains of little significance, since, as in the case of therapeutic external cardiac massage, such damage is neither common nor necessarily demonstrable. Consequently, it is not surprising that a report has appeared indicating cardiac contusion as a result of football. But where can one "draw the line," so to speak? Serial EKG's on every instance of anterior chest impact (and they must be serial to be of significant value) are not feasible. Without doubt an athlete who has received a blow sufficient to arouse a desire to be checked should be thoroughly examined before he is cleared to resume his activities. If his cardiac sounds are muffled or distorted, if there is any question of arrhythmia or friction rub, complete electrocardiographic studies should be ordered immediately. If these studies confirm the presence of cardiac abnormality, immediate cardiological consultation should be sought and a clear-cut disability from any athletics established until expert consultation clears the athlete completely.

**Hemoptysis.** Hemoptysis may be the first sign of injury to the pulmonary contents of the chest cavity. Hemoptysis may be so brief as to be limited to a single episode, yet it cannot be ignored. Immediate chest examination may be completely negative or at best may reveal a few sticky rales in one small area. However, barring bleeding from the mouth or nasopharynx (which of course must be ruled out), the diagnosis of *pulmonary contusion* must be made, the athlete admitted to hospital care, serial chest films evaluated, and, if an area of opacity develops, wide-spectrum antibiotics and aerosol inhalations initiated to clear the area before the development of pneumonitis or pulmonary abscess.

**Hemothorax.** If injury has been even more severe, damaging chest wall as well, thorough examination may reveal evidence of fluid, presumably blood, in the pleural space, hence *hemothorax;* or, worse, with hyperresonance and distant breath sounds above the fluid level and shift of the trachea to the contralateral side, *hemopneumothorax.* In either instance, the injured athlete should be hospitalized immediately for definitive care. Intrapleural aspiration should not be attempted in the dressing room unless the tension pneumothorax and shift threaten life itself. Similarly, *spontaneous pneumothorax,* characterized by the same signs of chest pain, hyperresonance, distant breath sounds, and tracheal shift to the contralateral side, is rarely an emergency and should be cared for with deliberate speed under optimal hospital conditions. It is beyond the scope of this book to discuss definitive treatment involving aspiration, catheter decompression, possible thoracotomy to seal a large pulmonary laceration, or decortication to overcome inadequate expansion. These should be performed by a thoracic surgeon, not a team physician. The physician on the spot, however, must be constantly alert to these conditions.

Case 1, J. E.: This 18-year-old defensive halfback was involved in a forceful four-man collision during a defensive play, at the end of which massive pileup he noted severe pain in the left chest area, which, however, subsided to the extent that he was able to continue for the remainder of that defensive series and did not report his problem until on the sidelines he noted persistent pain in breathing, diffusely involving the entire left chest. Examination revealed acute tenderness and crepitus over the left sixth rib in the mid-axillary line, and by that time pain on breathing had become so intense as to be totally disabling. Within 10 minutes of injury respiratory splinting was further compounded by acute pain in the left shoulder and the left upper abdominal quadrant, the latter to such an extent that significant abdominal rigidity was evident on examination. There was no hyperresonance on initial examination and no evidence of hemothorax, but abdominal signs were such that the possibility of a ruptured spleen could not be eliminated. Referral to Yale-New Haven Hospital for further studies confirmed the presence of a displaced fracture of the sixth rib, mid-axillary line, with a 20% pneumothorax but fortunately no further abdominal signs or symptoms. Close observation confirmed a steady resorption of intrapleural air and complete reexpansion of the left lung within 4 days, without requiring thoracentesis. Stabilization of the fractured rib was accomplished with a rib belt and analgesics, and x-rays at 4 weeks and 6 weeks revealed solid callus formation and clinical stability. Active rehabilitation, commencing thereafter and proceeding through increasing physical demand to vigorous contact by the 8th week, was capped by a return to full activity in the last two games of the season.

**Injuries to the Great Vessels.** Even rarer are conditions involving the great vessels within the chest. Massive direct injury simply does not occur under controlled athletic conditions. However, we have seen one instance of *spontaneous axillary vein thrombosis* in a baseball player, the diagnosis of which was perfectly straightforward as soon as we noted the marked venous engorgement and swelling of the affected limb, but the pathophysiology of the lesion remains a mystery. (A detailed clinical summary of treatment and course in this particular instance may be found in a report by Hume.) Disposition in this case was to a cardiovascular surgeon. In the absence of such specialists the team physician may be forced upon his own resources. As with all major clinical problems, however, prompt recognition of the traumatic picture comes first. Thereafter, such major problems should be handled by the doctor best equipped to deal with them.

## INTRA-ABDOMINAL INJURIES

The threat of abdominal injury is everpresent in athletics, though the overall incidence of serious visceral injury remains small. This is particularly evidenced by the fact that, aside from the "chest protector" worn by baseball catchers and the bulky pads of the hockey goalie, there is no formal sport that demands padding over the abdomen. This is not to say that abdominal impact does not occur, nor does it mean that intra-abdominal injury is exceedingly rare, but the performance-hampering effect of bulky padding in this area far outweighs its sporadic need. A hockey player "speared" by an opponent's stick or a football player "speared" by an opponent's helmet could benefit from padding at that moment, but in the meantime how would he move about? The preponderance of blunt trauma to the abdomen, as represented in the literature, stems from automotive accidents—hence a variety of impacting forces that far outstrip any in athletics. Such diagnostic problems as the ruptured duodenum, the torn pancreas and pancreatic duct, the ruptured intestine, the leaking greater vessels need be merely kept in mind as very remote possibilities, while primary consideration is given to the lesser group of common injuries.

The basic factors that provide the evidence of intra-abdominal injury are an initial neurogenic shock from the impact itself (which may be apparent without underlying injury), signs of blood loss (increasing pallor, tachycardia, and hypotension), and the direct findings of local mass and/or direct and rebound tenderness from intraperitoneal irritation. The transient neurogenic stage of abdominal injury is the most frequently seen in athletics, while the latter signs of acute and massive blood loss are rare; as to signs elicited by direct abdominal examination, the palpability of any mass depends on its location and rapidity of development. Palpability is thus a most variable guide. Consequently, *local tenderness, spasm, and rebound are the most important signs*—they indicate an irritation of peritoneal surfaces by blood, enteric content, or pus, and can provide an accurate picture of the problem when all else is absent. Certainly, such irritation is not here due to pus, and only rarely due to enteric contents because a ruptured viscus would then have to be assumed, a most remote possibility. As a reflection of intraperitoneal bleeding, therefore, its localization can suggest the probable source, and, once this is established, selected abdominal x-rays, serial hemograms, and clinical progress will determine the need for surgical intervention.

**Ruptured Spleen.** The ruptured spleen can give rise to hemorrhage that can be rapidly fatal or agonizingly insidious, dependent entirely on the site and degree of rupture. But localizing signs will be present, and there is always evidence of blood loss. There will be evidence of peritoneal irritation, not only in the left upper quadrant, but often on the left diaphragmatic surface through left shoulder pain referral, and in the left lower quadrant as blood flows down the left colic gutter.

**Lacerated Liver.** The lacerated liver gives rise to tenderness in the right upper quadrant, down the right colic gutter with peritoneal irritation in that area, and possibly referred to the right shoulder (from right diaphragmatic irritation).

**Enteric Rupture.** Enteric rupture from blunt external trauma is another entity repeatedly emphasized in the surgical literature, but it must be here considered only as a very rare picture of clinical peritonitis, free intraperitoneal air, and variable signs, and not as a commonly encountered athletic injury. Forceful perforation of the transverse colon, the small bowel, or the cecum is a remote possibility and must always be kept in mind, but hemorrhage from liver or spleen is the most common and, therefore, the most likely.

In all instances, local tenderness, spasm, and rebound are uniformly present, and surgical evaluation can proceed therefrom. More important, in all instances there is a uniform, subjective feeling of internal upset that can be depended upon to focus the athletic physician's attention on potential visceral injury. As with so much in athletics, accurate diagnosis is always possible when one is looking for it, while the most frightening problem is to know when to look for it.

**Solar Plexus Blow.** To further confuse matters, there is the frequent impact to the abdomen that results in prostration, inability to breathe, an ashen pallor, and the appearance of primary shock—the picture of the athlete with his "wind knocked out." The differentiation of this clinical picture, the *wind,* or the *solar plexus,* is impossible; every aspect is classical for more serious injuries, hence treatment must be expectant, waiting for it to subside, encouraging the frightened athlete by urging him to breathe rhythmically and slowly, to relax, to stop fighting for air, to stop struggling, to let it pass spontaneously. No attempt is made to pump the legs, bounce the trunk up and down, or institute the other maneuvers familiar to sports fans, because it is our belief that the entire picture is one of diaphragmatic, abdominal, and intercostal spasm, brought on by impact to the upper abdomen. Secondary to this spasm, there is a sudden acapnea and acute air hunger, which immediately leads to panic. A quiet, commanding reassurance and a concentration on restoring normal respiration have a most remarkable effect on a writhing, terrified, acapneic young man. It makes a good deal more sense than vigorous external measures spectacularly applied. Beyond this little can be done until there is spontaneous recovery, usually in 1 or 2 minutes.

Meanwhile, close questioning of the athlete usually reveals the reassuring fact that this episode is identical to others in the past, reassuring because the question of deep abdominal trauma remains unanswered. Our experience has been that the athlete can be depended upon to complain of any symptoms more significant than those stemming from the routine "solar-plexus blow." One stalwart half-back, who experienced a splenic rupture, insisted that the splenic injury was distinctly more painful and subjectively "different" from the "solar-plexus blow" despite the identical clinical picture initially. This is small consolation to the physician, caught between the two possibilities, but it is of significance. The subjective feeling is apparently different to the experienced athlete, objective physical signs do persist and do become even more marked in the more serious instance, and the lesser of the two evils always subsides rapidly.

## URINARY TRACT INJURIES

**Contusion of the Kidney.** Contusion of the kidney, even a forceful tearing of the renal pedicle, does occur in sports; hence any complaint in the area of the 11th or 12th rib must be simultaneously evaluated for accompanying renal injury. This is simply done by examining a gross urine specimen, because renal injury is usually, though not always, accompanied by bloody urine. (In one instance, the chief complaint was inability to urinate hours after injury, directly caused by blood clots that had completely blocked the urethra.) There may be difficulty in evaluating a urine with only microscopic hematuria, since some degree of microscopic hematuria is normal after any strenuous athletic contest. The latter hematuria, however, does not persist beyond 12 hours, so observation of voided specimens beyond this period should provide an accurate diagnosis. Alertness to the possibility of renal trauma assures accurate diagnosis by immediate intravenous pyelography before secondary hemorrhagic shock or other complications supervene. Once diagnosis is established and pyelography has demonstrated a minor distortion of parenchyma, bed rest and careful observation should suffice. Cases with obvious extravasation of dye or gross calyceal distortions should be carefully evaluated by a urological surgeon, since emergency surgery may be indicated. In either instance, no further contact sport should be allowed for at least a year after injury, simply to assure maximum healing of a most vital organ. Should nephrectomy be necessary, contact sport should be barred permanently.

**Bladder Rupture.** Unlike renal contusions—seen in basketball, football, hockey, and a number of contact and non-contact sports— bladder rupture is virtually never seen despite its frequent occurrence elsewhere. This is predominantly due to a very simple expedient, yet one that should never be forgotten in any athletic program: the absolute necessity of micturition prior to any practice or contest. Such a basic rule assures that the empty bladder remains behind the bony protection of the pelvis throughout that period of activity; barring massive injury to the pelvis, virtually impossible in athletics, bladder integrity is thereby assured.

## INJURIES TO THE EXTERNAL GENITALIA

**Contusions.** Secure protection is not afforded the external genitalia, the occasionally used "cup" protector nothwithstanding. The *testes* are vulnerable, and painful contusions are routine in every sport. Needless to say, the magnitude of subjective symptoms from such contusions bears no direct relation to the extent of actual injury, but this profits the victim little. The shock-like pallor, the acute protopathic pain, the lower abdominal symptoms, and the nausea are so familiar that they need not be discussed in detail, except to emphasize that they are common to all such injuries no matter how glancing or crushing the blow. Consequently, each instance should be thoroughly examined within minutes, if the symptoms fail to subside, and later, if recovery occurs within 2 or 3 minutes as it usually does. Despite the overall frequency of these incidents a certain small number very shortly exhibit the characteristics of acute injury, with bleeding to an extent that can be incredible. Firm support to the scrotum will suffice in the vast majority, but those with continued bleeding must be placed on bed rest under urological observation and must be given adequate support and local ice packs. Local supportive treatment is imperative because of the structural nature of the tissues involved and the tremendous volume of blood that can accumulate quickly. Scrotal extravasation can take months to absorb, during which time the involved testis cannot be accurately palpated. A well padded "cup" supporter will suffice as post-injury protection as soon as local discomfort and swelling subside, but truly significant testicular injury can result in a non-functioning structure or, worse, an atrophic one.

### Testicular Rupture

Case 2, K.H.: This 20-year-old football player jumped high into the air for an end-zone pass and, while spread-eagled in the air, was hit forcibly from below and upward by the helmet crown of a defending back, receiving the full impact on his scrotal contents despite the presence of a routine athletic supporter. Pain and disability were immediate, but after a few moments of hesitation he returned to the huddle for the next offensive play. Close questioning on the sidelines after completion of that particular offensive series confirmed the nature of the problem, but he was able to continue the game without interruption. Examination at the end of the contest revealed mild scrotal edema and marked bilateral testicular tenderness more marked on the right than the left, a normal testicular outline to limited palpation in the face of exquisite tenderness, and a soft thickening in the retro-testicular area on the right side, suggestive of early bleeding. Despite the increasing local pain, recommended observation in the Infirmary was refused, and instead a dormitory regime of scrotal support, application of ice locally, and bed rest was assiduously followed by the patient. However, pain persisted, extending into the right groin, and within 48 hours there was a well established hematocele, which during the subsequent 48 hours showed no evidence of resorption. Consequently, the patient was admitted to the Urological Service at Yale-New Haven Hospital, where on the 6th day following injury an exploration of the scrotum was carried out under general anaesthetic. A traumatic disruption of the right testis was found, with gross extrusion of the testicular contents requiring meticulous debridement prior to careful reapproximation of the tunica albuginea (Dr. Bernard Lytton, Professor of Urology, Yale University School of Medicine). Postoperative course was uneventful, and the patient returned to classes on the 10th day. Followup since that time has indicated a testis that is normal in size, consistency, and, presumably, function.

In another instance, a lineman, assigned to the protective wall directly in front of the kicker in punt formation, bent forward to block an onrushing opponent, was knocked backward, his hips full flexed, just far enough to receive the full force of the punter's foot in his scrotum and perineum. The force of the blow was sufficient to lift the victim off the ground, and the result was scrotal swelling to melon-like proportions despite intensive local measures. Disability, even visible in his gait, lasted for 6 months. The rarity of his injury gave him little consolation for his truly monumental agonies, nor did it prevent the eventual outcome—a fibrotic, presumably *nonfunctioning testis* on one side. Fortunately, his remaining testis was palpable and functionally normal. Further similar cases have been reported, several from another Ivy League school, and a review of the literature reveals an incidence which, though small, cannot be ignored. And what if there is but a single testis to begin with?

**Displaced Testis.** Another rare occurrence in athletics is the displaced testis. In our only such instance the responsible forces were so minimal as to be virtually unnoticed in the midst of a football-scrimmage pileup. The athlete, however, subjectively aware that something was definitely though not too painfully amiss, discovered to his horror that there was but one where two had been before.

His apprehension brought him to examination post-haste. Examination confirmed his observation that there was but one testicle in the scrotum. The missing one was not to be found at the external ring nor just above it, nor was it in the lower inguinal canal. Instead, it had lodged just external to the internal ring with at least a portion of it pushed through the ring. Return of the gland was easily accomplished by judicious milking, but, had the causative force been greater, operative intervention would have been necessary. The incidence of such mechanical displacements is rare, and displacement to the internal ring or into the abdomen is even rarer; nonetheless, it should not be unexpected in activities of such random violence as contact sports.

**Testicular Torsion.** Testicular torsion is most frequently encountered in the age group of our athletes—the teens and early twenties—and the price of late recognition is a gangrenous testicle that must be removed surgically. This is particularly tragic because early diagnosis is so simple. Any young man with acute testicular pain and swelling will seek help, and, though the differentiation of this condition from epididymitis or orchitis is at times difficult, the finding of a rotated and mobile testis is pathognomonic. The normal epididymis is always posterior and should be sought in this position in every instance of spontaneous testicular discomfort. Even if it is posterior, hypermobility of the testis and epididymis within the tunica vaginalis should be checked carefully. It is not unusual to find a complete 180-degree torsion that on examination reverts to normal or to find nothing more than demonstrable hypermobility. Torsion with spontaneous detorsion is a recurrent problem, and a careful history usually reveals a number of brief episodes of testicular discomfort that subsided spontaneously without medical attention. Consequently, immediate urological consultation should always be sought to evaluate the desirability of surgical fixation, even if the acute torsion is no longer a problem. To temporize solves nothing, and the ultimate price may be a gangrenous, unsalvageable testicle.

# 9

# The Face and Head

As stated in our discussion of equipment, football injuries about the face and head have dropped off remarkably in recent years, but they still do occur. Furthermore, with the exception of the minimally effective helmet and cage in lacrosse, the fencer's mask, the baseball catcher's mask, and the specially made fiberglass goalie's mask in hockey, all other contact and non-contact sports provide no protection from direct impact in these areas. Consequently, the physician in athletics sees every variety of injury in and about the face and head. Their frequency and the constant need for optimal cosmetic results demand a thorough evaluation of every such injury and the application of cosmetic surgical techniques in all facial lacerations.

## THE FACIAL BONES

### Clinical Evaluation

Anatomical review of the bones of the face reveals that, despite the obscuring edema and induration that rapidly distorts injuries to this region, these bones are largely subcutaneous, hence accessible to direct palpation either from the external surface or through the mouth. Examination can therefore be meticulous and painstaking and subsequent x-ray demonstration of fractures can be correctly anticipated or suspected. Such optimism may seem misplaced to clinicians accustomed to seeing those injuries in hospital emergency rooms or in their offices, but the key difference is the time element. Examination on the field is carried out within seconds of the injury before edema and bleeding even begin, and therefore it can accurately delineate bony crepitus, irregularity, fracture-line tenderness, or displacements and angulations that within 10 to 15 minutes are completely obscured.

The maxilla can be thoroughly palpated, including the external surface of the antrum, the nasal spines, the alveolar ridge, the entire zygomatic arch, and the infraorbital rim. Crepitus, fracture-line tenderness, and displacement are immediately obvious, while their absence can be considered as good as a negative x-ray. The mandible can be thoroughly and accurately evaluated, first by checking the integrity of the gingiva overlying the alveolar ridge (rarely intact in a fracture), then by palpating the entire body, angle, and ascending

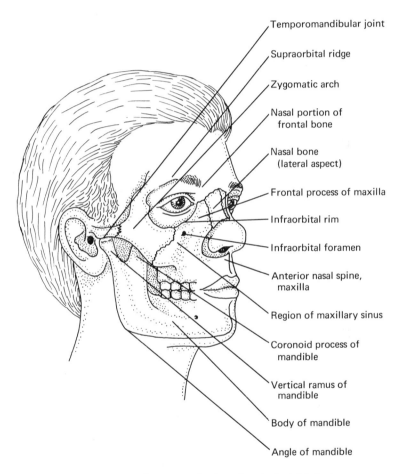

Temporomandibular joint

Supraorbital ridge

Zygomatic arch

Nasal portion of
frontal bone

Nasal bone
(lateral aspect)

Frontal process of maxilla

Infraorbital rim

Infraorbital foramen

Anterior nasal spine,
maxilla

Region of maxillary sinus

Coronoid process of
mandible

Vertical ramus of
mandible

Body of mandible

Angle of mandible

Fig. 9-1. Palpable bony check points in facial injuries.

rami, double checking the latter both by palpation and judicious rocking on the temporomandibular joint. Mandibular or maxillary continuity is further assured by having the athlete check for any subjective changes in his bite. The coronoid process is tested by direct intraoral palpation as well as by the significance of deep pain on contraction of the temporal muscle. The nasal bones can be evaluated by direct palpation and inspection, with particular attention paid to the lateral nasals (for any crepitus or fracture-line tenderness), the nasal spines of the frontal and maxillary bones, the septum, and the overall presence of any deviation of the nasal axis from the midline vertical. The latter is usually a simple observation, but it can be complicated by the athlete's inability to recall the direction of previous deviation.

At the same time related findings should be evaluated. Anesthesia or hypoaesthesia over the infraorbital nerve distribution (lateral nose, upper lip, and infraorbital) signifies damage thereto. This is most often in the area of the infraorbital foramen due to fracture, or worse, deep to the foramen under the floor of the orbit, indicating *disruption of the infraobital plate* and the ominous possibility of permanent diplopia from an accompanying inferiorward orbital displacement. Subjective aching discomfort, deep in the maxillary antrum and radiating to the canine fossa on that side, may indicate the increasing pressure of intra-antral hemorrhage, almost certainly due to a *fracture in the wall of the antrum.* A sudden steady drip of fluid from the nose following an impact suggests a *fracture of the cribiform plate* and *cerebrospinal rhinorrhea* with its dire implication of secondary meningitis; if the fluid is watery clear and continues to drip steadily, the diagnosis is virtually certain, and, x-rays or no, such a case demands immediate neurosurgical care and occasionally intracranial surgery for flap closure of the leak; if the fluid is yellow and glairy and all flow ceases within 10 minutes, it represents the commonly seen spontaneous drainage of a stopped-up sinus, and at the completion of such drainage in 5 or 10 minutes, the athlete can return to full activity feeling better than he has for days—in either case, until the diagnosis is established, nothing should be thrust into the nose to absorb the drip despite its annoying character, and the victim must be admonished to let it drip and not blow his nose for any reason whatever!

**X-Ray Diagnosis.** Such detailed emphasis on thorough clinical examination may seem superfluous to those doctors accustomed to seeing injuries only after x-rays have been evaluated and fractures thereby delineated. The simplest solution for the athletic physician would be to x-ray all facial bones in every case, but for every fracture there are a score of facial contusions without bony injury. Furthermore, the proper positioning and exposure of x-ray films for this area is technically difficult. More important, radiologists, able to read and interpret these films accurately enough to render an authoritative "no fracture" verdict, are hard to locate in the late afternoon and evening when these injuries most commonly occur. If the doctor on the field were to x-ray every such injury to assure himself of negative readings, the traffic to and fro would soon reach ridiculous proportions. X-rays would pile up waiting for the "no fracture" blessing—which is far more difficult to bestow than reading clinically obvious fractures. It would soon become obvious to the squad members that their doctor was "playing it safe," while they, in turn, were forced to leave practice or game, shower, dress, then find their way to x-ray, only to find that the entire trip and time lost were more often than not unnecessary. Their inevitable reaction would be to stop reporting injuries that they themselves do not think need x-ray, an intolerable development. This is not to say that x-rays should not be obtained in instances in which there is clinical suspicion, but it behooves the physician to exercise the most careful judgment. This demands thorough examination of each injury. With the necessary mental picture of the site and nature of any possible fracture in the locality, the doctor will be surprised how uniformly he can outline and predict the exact fracture site and at the same time pronounce the majority of these athletes fit to return to action.

Many readers will rebel at the clinical approach just outlined, since it applies equally to all athletic injuries and to all x-rays that might otherwise be obtained "to rule out fracture." However, those fractures that occur without pain or disability are rare and can be easily kept in mind. The ordering of unnecessary x-rays of pelvis and femur, for example, to rule out fracture in an obvious high contusion of the quadriceps is hardly analogous: Fractures of the femur or pelvis do not occur without pain and disability, and to obtain x-rays "just in case" is illogical. There are reported incidents in which a star athlete is rushed to the hospital for an x-ray in the midst of a game and then rushed back to resume play because the x-ray was negative. If he was well enough to return so promptly, why was the x-ray necessary in the first place?

**Fracture Management**

If meticulous examination fails to elicit any sign of facial fracture, locally applied ice will suffice to control local edema and bleeding; with adequate protective devices the athlete can return to full activity without delay. On the other hand, fractures that are suspected and then confirmed by x-ray must be treated promptly. The services of a trained maxillofacial surgeon or an otolaryngologist with special interest in this field offer the maximum medical benefit to these particular injuries, be it simple elevation of a depressed zygomatic arch, the packing of a smashed maxillary antrum, the packing and elevation of a depressed infraorbital plate, the wiring of the fractured mandible, or the correction of an over-riding fracture of a lateral nasal bone and the concomitant restoration of nasal integrity in the vertical midline. These are specialty problems and should be handled by specialists. The team physician struggling without specialist help should manage these problems to the best of his ability, aided by surgical and specialty monographs on the subject. But the obvious cosmetic evidence of a bad result may be enough to discourage such desperate efforts.

What of the ultimate disposition of the athletes with the facial fractures described above? How long are they barred from competitive athletics? Much depends on the specialist-consultant involved, but barring those major injuries that necessitate extensive surgery or internal fixation, simple linear fractures are considered adequately stabilized within 6 to 14 days, at the end of which time a return to full activity with special protection against recurrent injury can be anticipated. The birdcage face mask is usually adequate in football; in the other sports special fiberglass appliances can be devised to fit the need, always "bridging" the injury from normal bony prominences.

**Temporomandibular dislocation.** The anterior displacement of the mandibular condyle out of its temporal articulation and the subsequent masseter and temporal spasm are described in every textbook, and the classical mouth-agape helplessness of the victim need not be discussed in detail. However, it should be remedied immediately. The repeated advice to pad the thumbs well can not be too strongly emphasized, for their position on the molar and premolar surface of the mandible bilaterally, with thumbtips pressed firmly against the coronoid processes and fingers grasping the body and angle externally, places the thumbs in a most disadvantageous position when leverage is exerted to slip the condyles posteriorward. Reduction is immediately followed by the snap of both masseters and temporals in unison, and the jaw slams shut with instantaneous and painful finality.

## DENTAL INJURY

With regard to the teeth, per se, discussion must be limited to where medicine stops and dentistry begins. The overall picture of dental injury in football has changed remarkably even within the past 10 years, owing to the face mask. In addition, specific rules have been adopted in recent years on the secondary school level, requiring the use of molded dental mouthpieces, the surest way of avoiding virtually all dental injuries. It is to the credit of the dental profession that they have insisted upon this ruling. Until 1974, however, it is an optional adjunct in collegiate football. We still see an occasional chipped incisor or cracked premolar, requiring immediate dental care if the nerve is painfully exposed. Failure to adopt the mouthpiece has been due to several factors, most of them subjective on the part of the athlete. Thus, mouthpieces are difficult to breathe through in the heat of combat when air hunger is most acute; they sometimes fall out, and the replacement of a dirt-caked, saliva-muddied oral appliance is hardly pleasant. Fortunately our athletes are increasingly products of secondary schools requiring the mouthpiece and therefore consider it a routine part of their equipment. As a result, mouthpieces will soon be universal, thereby reducing dental injuries to zero.

## THE EYES AND ORBITS

**Lacerations.** The most common injury encountered in the orbital area is laceration. The frequency of these sometimes extensive and bloody integumental splits is easy to understand in football, in which the face mask virtually rules out the possibility of lacerating forces in any other region of the face, but its frequency in other sports must be due to the local characteristics of the site most commonly involved, the supraorbital ridge. This bony prominence seems to play the part of a ridged anvil to the impacting agency, thus cleaving the intervening skin and brow. In any event, these lacerations are uniformly much deeper than apparent at first, may penetrate the underlying orbicularis oculi to expose bony ridge, and may glance tangentially off the ridge to undermine one margin extensively. Since the eyebrow is most often directly contiguous or actually part of the split, the first inclination is to shave it off to assure a sterile field. This is a common practice that must be condemned. A considerable percentage of eyebrows so shaven (some say one in four) do not grow back, and an additional percentage grow back scantily! Suturing a laceration while pushing hair out of the way is not ideal, but it is preferable to leaving half an eyebrow for life. Closure of the laceration should be meticulous and up to plastic surgical standards, for the ideal linear scar is even more important in this particular area, in which vulnerability implies an increased likelihood of recurrent lacerations. Each succeeding scar must be as minimal as possible, in order to avoid the eventual accumulation of dense scar tissue so characteristic of the veteran professional pugilist, the so-called "boxer's brow."

**Lid and Conjunctival Injuries.** Almost as common in most sports, especially football, are lid and conjunctival injuries. The former are usually splits in the skin of the lid, occasionally extending down to and exposing the tarsus in the upper lid or undermining the lower lid extensively; each of these must be cleansed and sutured with 5-0 or 6-0 suture material for maximum cosmetic and functional results. Conjunctival injuries are usually abrasions either by an intruding object, such as a finger or stick, or by foreign material from the playing field. Thorough examination of the entire conjunctival surface is mandatory, but, if dirt is the cause, the gross particulate matter must be removed before anything can be seen. A thorough lavaging of the eye with copious amounts of sterile saline would seem the ideal method of cleansing. Practically speaking, however, the amount necessary to accomplish this in the presence of the incredible amount of muddy dirt often encountered renders a second method more advantageous: namely, gentle physical removal of the gross matter with a thoroughly moistened gauze sponge, followed by a limited lavage with sterile solution. Close inspection of all conjunctival surfaces can then be carried out by everting the upper lid upon itself and assuring that there is no break in the smooth integrity of the entire sac. Subjective symptoms are of exceptional importance in judging the efficacy of this ocular toilet, for any residual foreign matter or the slightest abrasion is persistently obvious to the victim. If there is abrasion without bleeding, an antibiotic ophthalmic ointment can be instilled. If the abrasion is persistently symptomatic, this treatment can be extended to include a few drops of Pontocain solution. This last is not without risk, since the resultant anesthesia could lead to further new injury to a benumbed surface. But the likelihood of this is sufficiently remote to allow consideration of its use.

**Corneal Abrasions.** The same measures apply in corneal abrasions, incurred simultaneously with the above or independently. They should be carefully sought for either with an angled slit-attachment to the usual ophthalmoscope head or with the fluorescein dye method. Such injuries are uniformly painful to the extent that hospitalization may be necessary for sedation; symptoms aside, they constitute a permanent threat to normal vision unless properly treated. Fortunately the protective reflexes surrounding and protecting the eye are maximal in the athlete; so extensive corneal abrasion is rare. This fact, however, does not alter the potential danger of these injuries, and every instance of possible abrasion should be thoroughly examined and evaluated, antibiotic ophthalmic ointment instilled, an eye pad applied, and the patient placed on bedrest in a darkened room until symptoms subside. In the meantime ophthalmological consultation should be sought, to assure added expert evaluation and authoritative clearance for a return to full activity. Uncomplicated corneal abrasions heal completely in 3 to 5 days at the most, and an experienced specialist is certainly the best qualified to assure the earliest return to play.

**Ocular Hemorrhage.** An essential in ocular evaluation is the funduscopic examination of the eyegrounds. *Anterior and posterior chamber hemorrhages* occur from *optic "concussion"* and must not be neglected simply because thorough examination failed to include an intraocular evaluation. Hemorrhage may be sufficiently gross to be detectable to the naked eye, but any athlete who complains of the slightest blurring of vision in any eye deserves a thorough visualization of the bulb contents. This is necessary to detect the more frequent type of slow bleeding that gradually obscures vision over a period of hours. The finding of any such intraocular damage demands immediate specialist attention and should not under any circumstances be handled by those unfamiliar with ophthalmology.

**Contact Lenses.** Some mention must be made of the *contact lens,* now so familiar in athletics that the sight of athletes and officials crawling about on hands and knees in search of some invisible object is an instant cause of public merriment. Contact lenses are a practical solution to the problem of the poor sighted athlete in contact sports. And they are now worn in preference to glasses by many athletes in all sports, contact or no. The original scleral type has been universally superseded by the tiny corneal type for a number of reasons. It is more economical, more easily tolerated for long periods of time, more easily adjusted-to initially, and can be inserted with ease. The scleral type required 3 to 5 minutes of concentrated effort over a mirror to insert correctly, was tolerable for only 2 to 3 hours at a time, and caused mild episcleritis with daily use. Advantages can be disadvantages, however, and the principal advantage of the tiny corneal type—its ease of insertion—is also its greatest disadvantage: namely, the ease with which it can be knocked out and lost, or knocked off center. In the latter instance, the athlete can usually milk it back into place, but occasionally it is so far off center that the physician finds himself searching frantically for it in the deepest conjunctival fornices, which may be far deeper and more inaccessible than he ever imagined. The ease of insertion has also given rise to the pernicious habit of using saliva as a surface lubricant, preparatory to insertion. The well-known bacterial content of saliva is such that its potential effect on the cornea is frightening, nor is it surprising that there have been reports of serious corneal ulcerations from these lenses.

## THE EXTERNAL EARS

The external ears are prone to injury in all sports. Even football with its all-encasing helmet provides us with the common *laceration-abrasion,* secondary to a carefully inserted enemy finger and fingernail. Or an unwary player will wedge himself into his snug helmet (with an effort unfamiliar to the non-athlete) and then forget to straighten out his ears; any pinna so folded for a 2 to 3 hour practice swells, bleeds along the artificial crease, and thus causes intense local pain; furthermore, the area will be aggravated and reaggravated each time the player dons or doffs his helmet—sometimes for the remainder of the season!

**Perichondral Hematoma.** Much more important is the perichondral hematoma, the familiar "cauliflower ear" of wrestling. It is seen in many other sports and is a reflection of the basic pattern of injury in a peculiarly constituted tissue structure, where there is little or no subcutaneous fat, the overlying skin is taut and thin, and the supporting framework is an elastic type of fibrocartilage that, nonetheless, has limits to its flexibility and can be fractured. Thus, the first result of injury, bleeding, is confined between cartilage and overlying skin. Hence, it is immediately visible to the naked eye and to the athlete. Whether the hematoma thus formed is between cartilage and perichondrium, or perichondrium and skin, is academic. It is clearly present and something must be done about it. Not surprisingly the most obvious method of dealing with such a superficial fluid collection, straightforward incision, is a common practice. This must be condemned, because to open a dead space to outside contamination, a dead space rich in nutritive blood products and debris, is to open the entire space to secondary infection, which can easily progress to *perichondritis* and *chondritis.* In the last instance, the relatively avascular cartilage possesses little if any capability to resist infection, and a sequestrating, necrotic, cartilaginous slough can supervene, with chronic drainage and permanent disfigurement, a high price to pay for a hematoma! On the other hand, careful aspiration through a

No. 25 needle under aseptic conditions can be carried out repeatedly if necessary, until the separated surfaces of dead space adhere solidly, with no visible residual and little if any pain. Admittedly, recurrent bleeding and/or serum collection is frequent, yet a patient regimen, that after aspiration splints the part with molded collodion-soaked cotton and tiny strips of adhesive tape, then controls further aggravation for 2 to 3 days—with repeated aspiration as indicated,—is safe and always successful. The wrestling ear guard minimizes this common problem both prophylactically and post-injury, but it is unpleasant to wear and most boys prefer to take their chances without it.

**Lacerations.** The danger of secondary infection in the pinna is doubly important in *lacerations of the area,* which commonly expose or involve cartilage. Meticulous débridement and cleansing are an absolute necessity, and prophylactic antibiotic therapy, not in general a surgically acceptable practice, is justified here. In the male the external ear cannot be hidden under the hair, so any deformity or ugly scarring is extremely noticeable. In spite of the risks of superinfection, drug sensitivity, and bacterial resistance every effort should be made to attain the maximum cosmetic result. This requires approximating well trimmed and débrided cartilage meticulously with the finest absorbable sutures, suturing the perichondrium as a separate layer, closing the skin with 5-0 or 6-0 cosmetic sutures, and, finally, administering adequate doses of a broad-spectrum antibiotic.

**Otitis Externa.** A condition most commonly seen in competitive swimming is otitis externa. Infection in the external auditory canal is conditioned by the nature of the tissues involved: a thin skin tautly stretched over supporting structures that are rigid or semi-rigid with no elasticity to allow for expansion within layers. Hence, a mild cellulitis rapidly matures and localizes into a tense furuncle accompanied by local symptoms that painfully outweigh the inflammatory process. Because pain rapidly becomes intolerable, local efforts should be prompt and vigorous. Moreover, additional considerations must be given to the sport responsible, most commonly swimming. Constant immersion of the skin of the external canal does not hasten resolution or foster resistance to recurrent infection. Pool work must be banned until there has been full recovery, while the athlete tries to maintain some semblance of condition by other means. At the same time measures must be taken toward the control of future episodes. This is done locally by the instillation of, for example, half-strength Burrow's solution after each workout and generally by assuring adequate chlorination, filtration, and bacterial check of the pool water. Some swimming squads routinely instill a solution such as Burrow's to minimize the incidence of these infections, and most otolaryngologists advise such routine medication in those with recurrent problems. In any case, the association of these infections with competitive swimming and their disabling effect in terms of lost practice and competition time must be recognized and appreciated by every physician in athletics.

# 10

# Skin and Soft Tissue Injuries

The body integument, covering all in a continuous envelope, is necessarily the first to suffer insult from without no matter what the nature or ultimate effect of the intruding forces. It is either contused, abraded, lacerated, or punctured. Sometimes integumental trauma is the sole result of such external insult, other times it is the least of many overwhelming problems, but it is always present.

## CONTUSIONS

Bleeding from disruption of minor vascular channels can be quite brisk, and the resulting swelling may be more directly related to the vascularity of the tissue involved than to the degree of total injury. Hence, the contusion, or bruise, of soft tissues can be a significant problem of itself. Closed soft tissue swelling from direct impact is one of the most frequent minor problems in contact sports. By early recognition and vigorous initial treatment it can and must be prevented from developing into an unnecessary difficulty.

Representing as it does an area of extravasated blood and crushed though not necessarily devitalized tissues, every gradation of swelling is seen, from the puffy subcutaneous superficial bruise, involving no more than subcutaneous fat, to huge fluctuant hematomas. The initial objective is to stop the bleeding by means of ice, compression, and elevation, until bleeding has definitely stopped. Local injections of a "spreading-factor" or systemic enzymes are not indicated (nor have we found any circumstance where they are). Because heat or activity during the first 24 to 48 hours only restarts bleeding, both are contraindicated.

Once bleeding has stopped, which may not require 48 hours in the most minor and superficial contusions, normal activity is resumed and only the amount of local heat needed to relieve local soreness is applied. Increased activity is then encouraged, first to tolerance, then to the level demanded by the sport. In the meantime, a special pad is designed to protect the area from further impact. This may be a simple piece of sponge rubber or a specially molded fiberglass bridge over the area. In any case the pad must be sufficient to avoid recurrent damage to resolving local absorptive and healing processes.

**Bone Bruise.** Of special significance is the *"bone bruise,"* which may present in certain specific sites, as a "heel bruise," affecting the plantar surface of the os calcis, the "stone bruise," affecting the second or third metatarsal head, or the "bruised hamate," deep in the proximal hypothenar eminence. These are simple contusions that involve a subcutaneous surface of bone and hence the periosteum thereof with its extraordinarily rich vascular supply and sensory nerve endings. Consequently, immediate examination after impact will rule out any palpable fracture-line tenderness; the mechanics of the injury will rule out other skeletal trauma; yet the area impacted will become progressively tender, to a degree out of proportion to the initial damage. This tenderness will persist long after true soft tissue tenderness has since subsided. X-rays are invariably normal, but this extraordinary sensitivity of the area to the slightest blow will remain for months.

In the case of the *"heel bruise,"* the injury is the result of impact through the athletic shoe, which may be heelless as in track, and hence offer no protection other than a single thickness of thin, flexible leather. The *"stone bruise"* is the result of striding full weight onto some hard irregularity with the ultra-thin and flexible running shoe, painfully bruising the metatarsal heads and transverse arch. The *"hamate bruise,"* seen in the stick, racquet, and bat sports, is the result of impact on the hamate prominence either by falling on outstretched hand or by force transmitted thereto through stick, racquet, or bat. In each of these instances, even more than other bone bruises from flying hockey pucks, baseballs, elbows, walls, and goal posts in areas where bone is comparably superficial, there is an added difficulty owing to the nature of the site. The runner with a "stone bruise" is virtually disabled as long as the prolonged tenderness persists, as is the batter or hockey player suffering from the "hamate bruise," special padding notwithstanding. Some "tough" athletes can perform successfully in spite of these handicaps, but in top-level competition significant deleterious effect on performance must be anticipated. Accordingly, intensive local therapy must be instituted without delay to stop initial bleeding, following which special padding should be designed to be worn at all times, padding that may be commercially available (such as the routine and effective "heel cup" for the heel bruise) or that may tax the ingenuity of trainer, equipment man, and doctor alike. Once the proper padding is obtained, a modicum of local heat to relieve initial soreness plus the pad should suffice for a return to active athletic participation, regardless of persistent local tenderness that may last for months.

**Hematomas.** The ultimate contusion, the *hematoma,* in which extravasation is so rapid as to collect in one fluctuant fluid mass, can form anywhere and at any depth. Symptoms are uniformly minimal and directly related to associated tissue injury, unless the inflammatory stage of tissue response involves a directly contiguous joint surface. Hematomas trigger a marked inflammatory response to better absorb the large blood collection, which in turn causes a marked increase in local tenderness and heat to a degree that cellulitis is often simulated. These last effects around or beside a joint surface may lead to much frantic x-raying and searching for chip-fractures, occult fractures, septic arthritis, and similar dire conditions. Yet the entire process will disappear spontaneously within the 2 or 3 days that the hematoma requires to pass through this stage.

The mature, fluctuant hematoma is characteristically non-tender and singularly unalarming. Surrounding ecchymosis may be striking or absent, depending on the age of the lesion. The degree of fluctuation will vary from an early "doughiness," indicating a more-or-less solid clot, to a classical fluctuation, indicating liquefaction of the initial clot and the admixture of serum and tissue fluid. In any event, initial treatment consists of local cold and local pressure by elastic bandages and, where possible, the application of a molded sponge rubber pad cut to size. Results from such treatment can be impressive, with many large hematomas being completely obliterated in 24 to 48 hours. After disappearance local compression and/or padding should be continued for 8 to 10 days, to assure lasting resolution.

Some large hematomas will not respond to this treatment (though this can never be predicted) and require further attention. If fluctuation is already well established, aspiration through a No. 19 gauge needle can be easily done under careful aseptic precautions, followed by thorough compression. Occasionally a semi-firm clot will effectively resist aspiration except from needles much too large in gauge to assure adequate external sealing after withdrawal, thereby increasing the possibility of secondary infection. Continued compression and padding should then be resorted to, until such time as the clot liquefies secondarily, usually in 2 to 5 days, after which aspiration can be accomplished in the usual manner. Under no circumstances has open incision and drainage been necessary, nor can we imagine an instance where it would be. We have cared for enough hematomas so drained by others; the foul, mixed infection that inevitably supervenes, the prolonged drainage, and the prolonged disability can last for weeks or months. Ten or even twenty needle aspirations are far more preferable!

### ABRASIONS, LACERATIONS, AND PUNCTURE WOUNDS

With regard to more extensive integumental trauma, the basic concern is the control of secondary infection: There is never a circumstance in athletics in which any abrasion, laceration, or puncture wound can be considered clean in the surgical sense. This is particularly true of the turf sports such as football, but prophylactic precautions should apply to all athletes and to all sports. Personal cleanliness can be safely presumed for what it may be worth, since athletes are the most thoroughly and frequently washed group in an average student body, nor are they as likely to allow dressings or bandages to become filthy through neglect. (Those who deal with both athletes and non-athletes are repeatedly reminded of this difference, due undoubtedly to the fact that daily strenuous exercise makes showering a necessity rather than a choice.)

More important, by the exercise of centralized control and authority over the athlete through each coach and squad roster, a completed tetanus toxoid immunization series can be insisted upon and followed through to completion (without entering into futile arguments with unwilling students and parents over freedom of choice, overpaternalism, and therapeutic nihilism). The importance of this immunization program cannot be overemphasized. Despite control of one's own facilities to assure that horse manure is not a routine fertilizer, such control cannot be exerted over foreign fields. (This is illustrated by the annual use by the Yale Rugby team, which includes a number of football players, of a horse armory for certain out-of town games.) The value of toxoid immunization has been so well proven by the military that nothing more need be said here.

Decisions concerning a return to action following any of these injuries must be tempered by a knowledge of the stresses of the sport involved. One must remember that once useful exercise has been resumed there is no practical way that the wound, be it an abrasion, laceration, or puncture, can be kept dry. It is unreasonable to expect an athlete to "work up a sweat" and then prevent him from showering by the admonition to keep the dressing dry (it will be thoroughly sweat soaked anyway). Any wound that cannot be safely immersed daily in water must necessarily keep an athlete totally disabled until it *can* be immersed. Waterproof dressings of collodion or plastic are helpful but not totally protective; they are of greatest value in protecting the cleanest types of sutured lacerations, not the borderline closures. Careful thought, including thorough consideration of the local circumstances of each wound, must be given to each case before permission is granted to return to activity.

**Abrasions.** Of the specific varieties of direct integumental trauma the least worrisome and most frequent is *abrasion,* seen in every sport, from the *"floor burn"* of the basketball player to the *"strawberry"* so familiar to the sliding base runner. In each instance, the superficial layers of skin have been abrasively removed so that a weeping, hypersensitive base, prone to secondary infection, is left. Initial treatment is directed toward a gentle but thorough cleansing despite local discomfort. Abrasions from the turf sports or from falls on a cinder track can be incredibly contaminated with foreign material, all of which must be removed. We have found that a surgical soap with detergent, hence with penetrating qualities, is by far the most effective, whether or not the accompanying bactericidal effect is largely valueless. Following this gross toilet we apply an unguent providing local antibiotic effect. We purposefully avoid any ointment that might produce sensitization to future systemic needs, such as tetracycline or penicillin, and limit our choice to those of purely topical value, such as polymyxin B. With such a preparation the abraded surface is covered by an oily vehicle that is locally soothing, facilitates future dressing changes, and prevents the formation of an eschar, beneath which infection might proceed apace. Since local warm compresses are routine for infected abrasions, we see no reason to bar an immediate return to full athletic activity; a daily workout and shower followed by a daily dressing and ointment application comprise much the best treatment in any case.

**Lacerations.** With *lacerations* the general rule should be that, if subcutaneous fat is exposed, the wound should be sutured. Preliminary cleansing and débridement should be thorough, technique should be meticulous, and, if any sutures must be buried or vessels ligated, absorbable catgut should be used (reserving nonabsorbable material for skin closure only). Heavy suture material is unnecessary. The 4-0 to 5-0 is adequate in all instances, and the deep-bite vertical mattress suture is the best by far, assuring edge-to-edge approximation as well as deep apposition and obliteration of dead space. Use of this suture technique often eliminates the need for deep buried sutures, always a source of concern in a potentially dirty wound.

In addition to the above, there must be thorough exploration of the wound in every direction (an elementary injunction, yet one occasionally forgotten by capable surgeons). If early return to full activity is contemplated, the closure must be a solid one, not a flimsy edge-to-edge skin apposition. Finally, every effort should be made to secure primary, cosmetically adequate wound healing regardless of site. None of these essentials can be successfully fulfilled on a squirming, wincing patient, no matter how "tough" he may be. It is mandatory, therefore, that local anesthesia be used whenever suture is indicated. The anesthesia of choice is usually the direct infiltration type, since field blocks are not practical in a crowded locker room. The sole exception is the tiny slit, requiring no more than one quickly placed stitch, since here the pain of infiltration outweighs that of suture placement. Because no athlete welcomes a needle, all of them will try to "gut it out." But, once one squad member experiences the advantage of local anesthesia, it soon becomes general squad knowledge and objections will be overcome.

**Bursal Lacerations**. Two common sites of lacerations are frequently mishandled due to a failure to explore the wound thoroughly prior to suture because it is acutely painful in the unanesthetized patient. The first is the area overlying the *olecranon bursa;* the second, the area overlying the *prepatellar bursa*. Both areas absorb the greatest punishment, and in both the elbows and knees the bursa is directly subcutaneous, its deep surface directly contiguous to and grossly indistinguishable from the underlying periosteum. A *penetrating laceration,* therefore, can carry contamination into a natural dead space that possesses the propensity to secrete large amounts of fluid when irritated. A remarkable degree of swelling can be anticipated, swelling that can be pure blood from disruption of vascular subserosal surfaces or a mixture of blood and bursal effusion. In either case, it is an ideal culture medium for secondary infection that can rapidly spread to involve the contiguous bone. Consequently, lacerations in these areas can never be viewed as routine, until the possibility of bursal penetration has been positively eliminated by direct visualization of all corners of the wound. Should such a penetration be demonstrated, immobilization of the knee or elbow is mandatory, together with daily inspection of the wound to assure that initial local measures—namely, thorough irrigation, careful débridement, separate layer closure of the disrupted serous surface, meticulous hemostasis, and local pressure dressing without drainage—have succeeded in attaining rapid primary healing. Additional systemic antibiotic therapy is desirable because of the dire implications of secondary infection, and we have employed it without hesitation. If infection does develop, open drainage is necessary. By and large, however, initial recognition and intensive measures as outlined should suffice except in cases of gross contamination and extensive bursal disruption. In any event, prolonged immobilization of at least 8 to 10 days must be anticipated to assure optimum results, and the athlete and coach must be apprised of this necessary ruling.

**Puncture Wounds.** The third variety of major integumental trauma, the *puncture wound,* can vary from minor penetration, of little or no clinical significance, to rare, major penetrating wounds from misdirected javelins or buttonless fencing foils. In the latter instances, hospital admission and special surgical care is of course necessary. This must include thorough evaluation of the possibility of deep damage by appraisal of the angle and site of the entrance wound, evaluation of x-rays, assessment of the degree and rapidity of blood loss, and exploration on the basis of these and other clinical indications. Details of the studies required, the indications for exploration, and its technical performance are part of the surgeon's trade and do not concern us here. On the other hand, the common puncture wounds of the plantar surfaces of the feet as well as other areas are part of the athletic physician's trade and must not be ignored. Tetanus toxoid boosters must be insisted upon regardless of the type of contamination. The wound must be thoroughly inspected. Probing a puncture wound to its depths is not a necessity; careful evaluation of the deeper structures by palpation and by appropriate functional tests indicates much more without deepening the contamination. The entrance wound should be inspected and its adequacy as a drainage point determined, since under no circumstances should the wound be closed to entrap an unknown degree of contamination within the tract. Should the wound appear too small, it should be further opened under local anesthesia to assure proper drainage. Daily dressings, thorough inspection, palpation for deep infection, and daily saline soaks can then assure that no pocketed abscesses develop. Under this regimen rapid secondary healing without residual tenderness may be anticipated within three to five days.

**Foreign Body.** If a foreign body is implicated, it should be searched for immediately, under local anesthesia if necessary: it should be teased out of its tract with a sterile needle until enough is exposed to grasp securely; following removal the residual tract should be treated for what it is, an open puncture-wound.

## BLISTERS

Despite their benign appearance, blisters are truly the athlete's bane. An intradermal reflection of local irritation, they inevitably accompany every athletic endeavor, afflicting the feet in the running sports, the hands in crew and stick sports, even specific fingers in sports that require specialized finger grips, such as fencing. Because they afflict the part that is the most used, they are acutely disabling. The basketball player with blisters on the soles of his feet cannot perform effectively, nor can the baseball pitcher with blisters on his throwing fingers.

**Prevention.** More important, therefore, than the treatment of blisters is their *prevention*. An area of irritation, the "hot spot," can be detected subjectively prior to the actual formation of a blister, and every athlete should be trained to recognize the symptoms. Caught at this early stage, a protective dressing of vaseline and gauze effectively prevents further irritation. Of course, measures should be taken to anticipate the areas of irritation in each sport, and steps taken to circumvent blister formation. Thus, in basketball a thin moleskin can be adopted, applied to the plantar surfaces at each early practice; alternatively, there can be a thorough "greasing" of the entire foot with liberal dollops of lanolin ointment, which seems to eliminate blisters but also devours athletic socks. Similarly, the football squad can be issued a pair of shoes to "break in" and practice in through the summer months, thereby assuring that they will return for pre-season practice with feet well toughened by shoes that they can continue to wear.

**Treatment.** Once a blister is established, *relief* is an absolute necessity, and it must be prompt. The painful distention must be eased somehow, yet nothing should be done that will transform an intradermal sterile reaction into an infected open wound. Some have routinely employed sterile aspiration of the blister contents followed by local pressure with good result. Others routinely open the blister, release the fluid, and excise the external flap of skin, leaving the blister base exposed. Although initially effective, the first method almost always results in a rapid reaccumulation of fluid, necessitating early reaspiration (sometimes twice in a single workout). The second method removes the thick outer-layer of blister and exposes the very thin inner layer, which can then be abraded easily; thereby the area is converted into the equivalent of a third degree, full-thickness burn, with the strong likelihood of secondary infection of the raw surface. We have used a compromise method that has been most satisfactory. The blister is opened widely, but the outer skin left as the natural deep-dressing; thereby a continuing drainage is accomplished yet at the same time the thin inner layer of skin is protected from abrasion by gauze or other coverings. The inner layer rapidly thickens in two to four days, the excess skin falls off, and the athlete has not lost a day of competition. Secondary infection remains a threat until resolution is complete, and an unguent containing polymyxin B is utilized—to "grease" the surface, so to speak—to maintain drainage by inhibiting crust formation and prevent infection for the two to four days that the deep layer needs to thicken up.

**Blisters Under the Callus.** Unlike the straightforward blisters seen in the first 2 to 3 weeks of any sport season is the *blister under the callus* that develops in mid-season. The mechanics of this phenomenon are quite simple and avoidable. Callus is built up in an area of chronic irritation. If untreated, it soon creates a thick keratinized plaque, that of itself gives rise to acute irritation in the deepest layers resulting in a painful fluid-taut blister. This may be largely invisible under the callus. Treatment is the same: opening the area widely but leaving the overlying skin in place until the inner-layer thickens up, and trimming off the excess keratin either by excision or, preferably, by abrasion with a piece of fine emery board, the familiar "callus-file" of the training room. The file when properly used prevents these incidents by planing off the excess keratin as it forms. (Such regular foot care is usually neglected until one acute episode has occurred, after which the victim needs no further urging.)

## FURUNCLES

Of minor significance in normal clinical practice, the furuncle assumes considerable stature in athletics. Despite the fact that personal hygiene is above average in the athlete, his peculiar needs can ofttimes transform a simple, uncomplicated furuncle into a major problem. This is chiefly due to two factors: the local and systemic effects of any particular sport on the condition itself and the effect of any such superficial infection on others.

The ideal *local treatment* of any furuncle involves proper localization of the purulent process without breaking down the natural barrier of fibrin, acute inflammatory cells, and debris that the body normally establishes around it. Basic requirements are protection of the external aspect of the inflamed area, elimination of any local pressure factors, and prevention of overzealous motion of the affected part. At the same time local erythema (hence blood flow to the area) should be gently stimulated to increase the effectiveness of the inflammatory process already under way. This requires frequent warm soaks to encourage "pointing," after which the area is opened and external drainage established to assure that pressures within the abscess do not cause a deep penetration instead. These requirements can effectively limit continued competition, for the usual furuncle sites cannot be protected effectively against external pressure or impacts nor can the part be kept at rest. This is particularly true with the multiple furuncles that commonly afflict football squads between the 1st and 3rd week of pre-season practice in and around the knee areas—the combination of perspiration, the twice-daily exposure to dirt and abrasion from the lower end of the pant and the knee pad, and the overall high temperatures characteristic of pre-season practice combine to create a perennial problem. Athletic demands notwithstanding, the treatment of furuncles should be as outlined without compromise. The result of a single impact on a benign furuncle can be a deep, burrowing cellulitis that requires intensive treatment and results in many days lost.

The effect of superficial infection on others is also a factor, particularly after drainage has been established and the furuncle is largely under control. The close association and the body contact of any athletic squad assures that virulent organisms in the drainage are rapidly disseminated unless strict precautions are taken to isolate the victim together with his clothing, dressings, and personal equipment.

## WARTS AND CALLOSITIES

The callosity, particularly the plantar callosity, can be the source of acute disability through its role in the formation of acute deep-lying blisters. To circumvent this, it has been recommended that the callus file be used regularly. Of even more unique significance is the effect of repeated immersion on callosities, as seen in competitive divers from time to time. Their incessantly intermittent immersion leaches out all natural oils from the keratinized plaque, which then cracks and splits by progressively penetrating degrees until dermis is reached, bleeding ensues, and secondary infection disables the athlete. Treatment is simple: the liberal use of lanolin ointment on the keratinized area after it has been planed down with a callus file. No further difficulties need be anticipated, but, until secondary infection has completely subsided, all pool work must be banned regardless of the effect on athletic performance.

Unlike the simplicity of the above, *the plantar wart* presents a persistent problem. Although never totally disabling, its annoying chronicity can hamper performance in any of the running sports. As a specific variant of the common everyday wart (verruca vulgaris), differing only in those characteristics secondary to its site on a weight-bearing surface (i.e., pressure inversion and local hyperkeratinization), it is caused by a virus that is said to be neurotropic. It seems to spread at times by local "seeding," and it appears and disappears without apparent reason. Treatment varies from total surgical excision and primary closure to pressure injections with saline, novocaine, xylocaine, or distilled water and to "dry ice," liquid nitrogen, high-frequency coagulation, and radiation treatments. No one method has proved entirely satisfactory; in fact, it has been demonstrated that a form of psychotherapy can banish a plantar wart, and one remarkable report mentions successful utilization of "x-ray treatments" that were comprised of exposure to the audible whirring of the rotating anode without any x-rays at all.

No treatment is worth considering, that replaces a temporary wart with a permanent structural change in the area, such as a surgical scar or a scar from overenthusiastic electrocoagulation. The immediate results of such radical treatment are painful. Weight bearing must be limited for the first few days, and secondary infection is always a risk. All this for a condition that may disappear without a trace next week or next month! Consequently, the least traumatic treatment seems best: A gentle keratolytic such as 5 per cent salicylic acid in a collodion base has proved ideal. The horny surface of the wart is softened and steadily reduced in thickness. The lesion has every opportunity to resolve spontaneously under the influence of whatever psychosomatic factors may be implicated in the regular daily application of medication. By these means the local situation has always improved, and no athlete has lost a single day of practice or competition.

## UNGUAL INJURIES AND SUBUNGUAL HEMATOMATA

Direct injury to nail and nail bed of either fingers or toes is extremely common and ranges from a subtotal avulsion of the nail to its very base to splits and tears into the distal bed. Pain and disability need not be described, since the penetrating magnitude of symptoms is familiar to all. However, the nature of the affected tissues must be kept in mind. The nail bed is directly contiguous to the underlying periosteum of the bony phalanx. Bleeding, therefore, may be from a fracture of that phalanx through the disrupted nailbed. Consequently, the mechanics of the injury must be reviewed and careful differentiation made between the forceful avulsion without bony injury and the crush injury which may involve bone. Initial treatment may be necessarily identical in either instance, but the dangers of secondary infection are different.

*The avulsed nail* can be painlessly removed if hanging by a few shreds. If it is still firmly attached at the base, it should be replaced and bandaged in place. The athlete is then cautioned to keep it taped down thereafter to avoid catching it on clothing and the like, until such time as it painlessly separates off with the growth of new nail (3 to 6 weeks). Either way, the open distalward drainage effectively circumvents closed-space hemorrhage or infection.

In *the subungual hematoma* such fortunate drainage does not evolve, and immediate relief is mandatory. The best and simplest method has been the "red-hot paper clip" method, crude but effective, wherein the end of a paper clip is heated over an alcohol lamp to incandescence and then thrust through the intervening nail. On striking the entrapped blood it immediately cools; thus, it causes little if any discomfort and affords immediate relief. There is one disadvantage to the technique: the channel established not only affords welcome drainage to the outside but also provides an ideal entry-way for secondary contamination. In such a closed space full of blood products a foul purulent infection may readily supervene. This can be easily remedied by excising the overlying nail, but it must nevertheless be anticipated, particularly if there is an accompanying bony injury. Hence, some type of dressing must be kept over the drainage point until the danger of infection is past. Contrariwise, if there is no pressing need for pain relief, such drainage should be best avoided, especially if bony injury has been demonstrated—a secondary osteomyelitis of the distal bony phalanx is a high price to pay for local pain relief, the more so if the accumulated blood and the associated symptoms have already begun to grade off.

# 11

# *Cervical Injuries*

Within this short segment of anatomy passes every essential to a functioning existence. Injuries of magnitude can be catastrophic. In no other area will the doctor on the field feel his responsibility more, for the dire possibility of skeletal injury and subsequent medullary or cord damage can happen at any time.

It is no consolation that the most minor rotary subluxation of the upper cervical vertebrae can lead to quadriplegia or even death without a single warning symptom to differentiate it from the most minor muscle strain. Should the doctor transport every athlete with a stiff neck to the hospital, his neck immobilized with sand bags, for a multiple series of cervical-spine films that are always difficult to interpret accurately? Should he hospitalize in cervical traction every athlete with a stiff neck until certain that no possibility of subluxation remains? Or should he reserve such measures for those with clinical evidence of deep skeletal injury or significant neurological dysfunction? If he chooses the last course, sooner or later he will encounter a serious neck injury with little or no symptoms that will pass unrecognized until obvious and disastrous symptoms develop, and he will then be accused of deplorable negligence. If he chooses the former, however, he will be overtreating hundreds of cases for the sake of the one possibility in 10 or 20 years, which even then may proceed to serious complications without being recognized. The physician on the spot will find himself condemned one way or the other!

There is no easy solution to the physician's dilemma, and we can only advise that, if he remains constantly on the alert for the slightest indication of deep cervical injury, if he analyzes every cervical injury in terms of the mechanics involved, the symptoms elicited, and the findings of thorough examination, if he remains alert to the slightest clue that does not ring true for the more minor injury, if he looks for deep injury first and last—in short, if he always "runs scared"—he will at least have done his best.

**Clinical Evaluation**

What does an adequate examination consist of? An analysis of the mechanism of injury comes first. Was it hyperflexion, hyperextension, lateral flexion, or hyper-rotation? One is usually forced to depend on the athlete's own recollection of the circumstances of injury, which may not be dependable or even recollected. If a true picture can be reconstructed, the next step is inspection. Is there spasm and rotation, deviation from the usual position, pain that prevents any motion? If so, where is the pain and where does it radiate? Most important, is there sensory or motor change in any of the four extremities? Only after every item has been checked and found in order can direct examination of the neck begin: first, palpating for spasm of any muscle group, then gently testing for any pain and/or limitation on flexion, extension, lateral flexion, and rotation. As a last check, the lateral masses of the palpable third through seventh cervical vertebrae, lateral and deep to the glottic and laryngeal compartments, should be palpated thoroughly and inspected for any deep tenderness or swelling.

**Strains and Contusions.** Such examination will reveal particular tenderness and particular spasm of specific muscle groups, pinpoint the problem, and eliminate concern over deep injury. It is even possible to palpate soreness and slight swelling in the scalenes, deep to the sterno-cleidomastoid, in rare instances of *acute scelene strain. Trapezius and longissimus capitis strains* stand out like steel cords, easing the doctor's primary concern over deeper injury. *Contusions,* as revealed by history or observation, are identified with ease by careful examination since they appear as localized tender swellings that are unmistakable.

**The "Hot Shot."** If the injury is not a simple strain or contusion, rapidly amenable to a cervical collar for 1 or 2 days, what is it? First of all, there is the very common *"hot shot,"* the familiar *"pinched nerve"* of the sportswriter, characterized by a sharp, burning pain along the course of one or more of the branches of the cervical plexus and radiating into the posterior scalp (greater and lesser occipital) up to and behind the ear (greater and lesser auricular), around the neck (cutaneous colli), or down the top of the clavicles and shoulder (suparclavicular). (Figure 11-1.) The most important thing to determine in the presence of such symptoms is the position in which they arose. If the neck was forcibly bent laterally *away from the affected side,* there is little cause for concern, because this is the classical "pinched nerve," catching the involved branch somewhere in the powerful musculature behind the sternocleidomastoid around whose posterior aspect these nerves normally emerge. As such, the symptoms subside within 2 or 3 minutes, leaving a brief residual soreness and a paresthetic area. The athlete can return directly to full activity.

**Deep Skeletal Injury.** What if these radiating neurological symptoms arise on lateral flexion *toward the affected side?* This is an entirely different matter. In this position the muscles are relaxed, while the invertebral foramina are compressed to their narrowest. Signs of

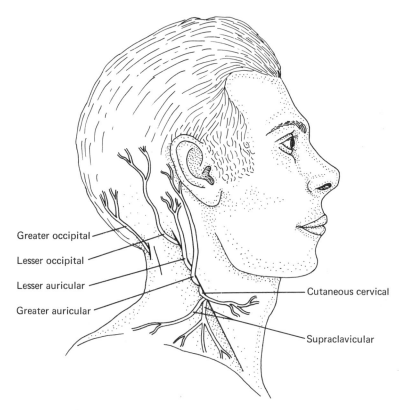

Greater occipital

Lesser occipital

Lesser auricular

Greater auricular

Cutaneous cervical

Supraclavicular

Fig. 11-1. The cervical plexus and the "hot shot."

nerve compression here suggest but one thing, *deep skeletal injury,* either fracture or rotary subluxation, in any case a serious question that must be answered without delay by immediate neck support, transportation to the hospital, and detailed cervical-spine studies. Similarly, if straight *axial compression* on the top of the head elicits radiating cervical root pain, either unilateral or bilateral, deep injury must be considered and immediate action taken.

**Brachial Plexus Traction.** What of the nerve pain that radiates down into the arm and possibly into the hand, sometimes following root dermatomes, sometimes following peripheral nerve distributions from *the brachial plexus?* These are rare, and the usual signs are sufficiently peripheral to absolve bony pathology. The mechanism is one of forceful depression of the shoulder girdle on the affected side, stretching the plexus in its supraclavicular position. However, unlike in clinics where reports indicate a certain percentage incidence of plexus traction injuries that tear the posterior cervical roots at the foramina (even causing dural-cuff leaks of cerebrospinal fluid), in athletics injuries of this magnitude are not encountered. This is perhaps due to the protective muscularity of the athlete. It is something to be kept in mind, but not a source of great concern.

## Mechanism of Injury

More important are the mechanism of these injuries, the reason why they occur, and the measures that can be taken to avoid them, temporary though most may be. It has been our experience that a boy who gets one "hot shot" is certain to get many more, to the extent that he may become "gun shy" and therefore ineffective. Equally important, these injuries are becoming more commonplace as the years pass. The reason for this may be the efficiency of the helmet-face-mask combination, which encourages football players to hurl themselves headlong into situations that would in earlier days have knocked out all their front teeth in one impact. A second possibility is that coaching techniques have taken advantage of the protection offered by the helmet-face-mask combination to alter blocking and tackling mechanics so as to utilize the head as a battering ram. A tackler, for instance, facing an elusive ball carrier, stands a much better chance of stopping his opponent if he aims at the numbers or just below with his face and head, for this effectively neutralizes the ball carrier's head fakes, hip fakes, and fancy footwork and, if the impact does not knock the latter off his feet, it does hold him up until pursuit-help arrives. Even with the head up and "neck bowed" the torsion and flexion forces on the cervical spine are greatly increased by this "spearing" technique and we can only join the growing numbers of doctors who have criticized its development.

## Prevention of Cervical Injury

Control of cervical injury requires a careful appraisal of every football candidate. If he is thin, poorly developed, and has a long neck and observation of his performance reveals only a minimal coordination, he should be discouraged from further play. Secondly, build-up of the cervical musculature should be an integral part of a football conditioning program. "Bridging" exercises are best and require no special equipment; some authorities have characterized these exercises as harmful, as indeed they are for the average non-athlete, but the dire risk of serious injury from cervical under-development would appear to overbalance possible injury from the exercises themselves—and these exercises are indeed effective as witnessed by the heavy cervical musculature that so characterizes most football players! Thirdly, all candidates must be reminded incessantly that they must keep their head up and their neck bowed. In this position, they can see what is coming and prepare for it. Employing the muscles they have developed, they can fix the cervical spine in its most stable position—particularly against a lethal hyperflexion, but against lateral flexion, hyperextension, and torsion as well.

**Athletic Equipment.** Aside from measures directed toward the athlete, his physical abilities, and the techniques he must employ there is little that can be done. The possible role of certain types of shoulder pads has been touched upon. The low-profile pad of increasing popularity has been indicted by some as responsible for the growing frequency of "hot shots" because of the minimal support afforded the cervical region in contrast to that by the bulkier models. However, we have never adopted the low-profile model (for precisely this reason), yet we have noted a rise in "hot shots" and similar neck problems parallel to the rise reported elsewhere. Regardless of the explanation the victim of one or more of these painful incidents has no particular desire to experience more, and arguments about the style of shoulder pad or repeated admonitions that his technique is faulty do not solve his problem. Instead, some means must be employed to minimize the characteristic lateral flexion phenomenon, yet allow rotation, extension, and some degree of flexion.

**Cervical Collars.** Obviously, a rigid collar of the Thomas type only succeeds in either throttling the wearer or so limiting his cervical mobility that he is unable to perform at all. Nevertheless, any really effective support demands rigidity, which is in direct proportion to its effectiveness. Searching for a compromise solution, one that would allow effective performance yet provide support, we began to use a felt collar enclosed in stockinette, to be tied around the neck after pads and jersey were put on, thus adjustable to tolerance by the wearer while limiting lateral flexion somewhat. Results with this appliance surpassed the most optimistic expectations. It or the alternative semi-rigid rubber tubing of large caliber that is similarly adjustable and no more rigid, has become standard in all instances of recurrent "hot shots." Some experts have scoffed, pointing to the fact that these appliances cannot provide adequate support to the neck against the impacting forces. We agree that as simple support mechanisms there is no reason why they should have any value; nonetheless, they do!

The answer lies in a very simple mechanism, yet one that became apparent only after many conversations over the years with the only sources of accurate information: the wearers themselves. It became clear that the collars do not provide support of value, but they do capitalize on a combination of sensory and motor coordination that is maximal in the trained athlete. In essence, the collar appliances trigger a protective twisting of the entire upper body and shoulder girdle the moment that lateral flexion proceeds beyond tolerable limits. The mechanism of injury is immediately altered thereby; the depressed shoulder is swung forward and brought up, and the angle between cervical axis and shoulder is reduced. Viewed in this manner, the efficacy of the cervical support is understandable.

## A Case Report

The following case illustrates some of the problems discussed in this chapter.

Case 3, L. H.: A sophomore halfback of impressive agility but dangerously small stature combined cat-like mobility with a total disregard for his own anatomical integrity (to the extent that he had missed freshman football, recovering from a second fracture of his left clavicle sustained in high school football). He was noted for a habitual preference for his own headlong, suicidal version of blocking and tackling. Despite our fears of what might happen to a 145 pound frame flung about with such utter abandon, he performed remarkably well as a regular until a major out-of-town conference game. On a kick return in the open field he launched himself into a typical flying, full-body block. At the conclusion of the play he was prone and motionless. Examination within 10 to 15 seconds revealed him to be gathering his faculties, aware only that he had received an unexpected blow on the head. (Subsequent study of movie films revealed a violent unexpected impact to the right temporal area, slamming the head into a momentary leftward lateral hyperflexion.) There was no other complaint; he moved all limbs equally and within a minute was fully oriented, though he had obviously suffered a brief but definite cerebral concussion. Consequently, he was helped to his feet and walked to the sidelines under his own power, his gait steady, his sensorium clear. Immediate sideline examination subsequently confirmed this rapid recovery; his cranial nerves were normal, his ocular movements coordinated and steady, his vision acute, his orientation normal.

The diagnosis seemed clear and recovery was excellent, hence the only conclusion was that, having lost consciousness, he would not be able to return to the game. However, in 2 to 3 minutes the subject noted that his neck was becoming stiff and called the examiner back. Further examination of the neck revealed beginning spasm of the muscles on the left, a slight tilt of the head to that side, and a progressive limitation of extension, though active flexion remained free and painless. Rotation was becoming more limited as spasm increased and, most important, any passive extension or rotation of chin to left, no matter how gentle, caused acute radiating pain behind and above the ear on the left, as did lateral flexion *toward the affected side*. There was, then, evidence of deep injury, along with the ominous sign of pain increased by any narrowing of the intervertebral foramina on that side.

Any attempt to assume the supine position became immediately painful, the only comfortable position being bolt upright with the head held rigidly on the neck in a fixed position, slightly tilted to the left, chin slightly raised but midline —a position only the victim could control. Therefore, despite the now-certain evidence of some deep-lying skeletal injury, it was decided that the best method of transport to the dressing room would be that controlled by the patient himself. He was walked in, a distance of about 100 yards. Immediate orthopedic help was summoned, and immediate hospitalization undertaken, with the victim still sitting bolt-upright in the ambulance, maintaining his own head position.

Multiple x-ray studies under the vigorous direction of the orthopedist himself revealed a suspicious suggestion of compression of the left lateral mass of C-1, which was further confirmed by more studies. Within the hour, tongs were inserted and traction established, still without further neurological signs, other than a hint of sensory paresthesia in the T-2 dermatome that appeared during the x-ray examinations and just as promptly disappeared.

Recovery, following tongs, minerva jacket, and, lastly, fitted collar, was without incident and was considered complete at the end of 6 to 8 months. But the possibility of further football was categorically ruled out. The final diagnosis by x-rays of subsequent bony healing pattern was

1. Fracture of ring, C-1, in two places (Jacksonian).
2. Fracture, with impaction, lateral mass, C-1.
3. Fracture (?) of odontoid process, C-2.

The reader cannot doubt the role of pure luck in this case. There was no reason to suspect neck injury when the boy was walked to the sidelines. Even after a significant neck injury was suspected, though its nature remained unknown, it was impossible to move him in any other way in spite of the unknown risks. The injury fortunately took place at the one field in the Ivy League that is within one-half block of a modern, fully equipped medical center. Thanks to the expert specialist help that is alway available there, the suspicion of serious injury was sufficient to assure maximum medical care in the shortest possible time.

But the fact remains that a boy with multiple fractures of C-1 (an ominously lethal combination) was walked off the field and transported to the hospital bolt upright in spite of the clinical suspicion of skeletal injury. Criticisms from medical onlookers after the diagnosis was publicized were more than a little unsympathetic. Yet the symptoms were such that, despite suspicions, there was no other way to move him without risking possible cord or medullary damage that so far was not evident. It was a beggar's choice, and the choice had to be made alone. X-rays confirmed suspicions but even then failed to demonstrate the true gravity of the situation until much later. Who can say what might have happened had traction and the prone position been insisted upon at the outset?

# 12

# *Injuries to the Shoulder Girdle*

As the principal fulcrum for all upper extremity action as well as the portion of the anatomy best suited for forcible ramming, the shoulder is the most common site of minor, disabling injuries. These range from local contusions, ligament strains, and muscle strains to irritative bursitis and to neurological deficits of long-standing significance. Moreover, as the central attachment for the upper extremity, it is the focus of all abnormal forces that may primarily affect the arm and through the arm the shoulder—culminating in subluxations, complete dislocations, fracture dislocations, and grossly displaced and angulated fractures. Shoulder problems can afflict and disable athletes in all sports. Next to the knee, it is the area that is most often a chronic source of persistent disability, from year to year as well as from sport to sport.

A review of the regional anatomy (see Fig. 12-1) reveals that the superior aspect of the shoulder girdle is not nearly so well supplied with supporting musculature and is largely subcutaneous, in contrast to the inferior aspect buried deep within layers of heavy muscle. Consequently, muscular action is preponderantly one of fixation of the girdle in an inferiorward position, the better to provide a stable fulcrum for arm movement. Aside from the trapezius and strap-like levator scapulae there is nothing comparable to elevate the girdle of itself or to resist actively violent depression of the girdle by impact from above downward. It is no wonder then that football, with its incessant demand on this last mechanism is the most common cause of injuries in this region (inside and outside cantilever shoulder pads notwithstanding).

Because of the anatomical characteristics of the area a thorough sequential examination can be carried out, followed by a progressive series of functional tests. If carried out properly, these provide an accurate diagnosis without added x-rays "for the record." The first step is a careful review of the history of injury, the manner in which it was incurred, the angle of impact, and the position of the upper extremity at the time. Next is a careful inspection of the area, combined with a thorough palpation of the entire subcutaneous length of the clavicle, the acromioclavicular joint, the coracoclavicular area deep thereto, the glenohumeral area, and the acromion, passing thence posteriorward to the scapular spine. Only after this thorough an appraisal should functional tests be undertaken. These are done first

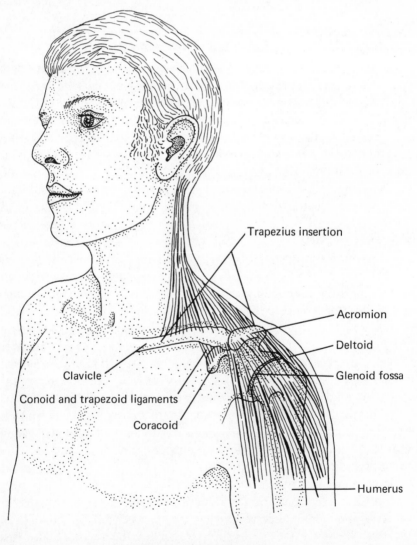

Fig. 12-1. The shoulder.

without resistance then with resistance: testing abduction and adduction in the forward and in the lateral plane for any limitation or pain, then testing rotation at the glenohumeral joint. Lastly, a check should be made for serratus anterior fixation of the scapular body by "wall-walking" the hands, looking for the slightest "winging."

By means of these principles of examination major orthopedic injuries are clearly demonstrated, and proper disposition and treatment are facilitated. Such an examination also pinpoints lesser problems that are no less disabling in athletic terms, but that, properly recognized and treated, can be assured the earliest possible return to activity.

No matter the injury the most important therapy in shoulder problems is an early return to active motion. Prolonged immobilization and the "frozen shoulder" must be kept in mind whenever a plan of treatment is implemented. Any immobilization not based upon the necessity for a solid restoration of significant tissue disruption (as in a glenohumeral dislocation or demonstrable acromioclavicular separation) should be avoided assiduously!

## Trapezius Strains and Contusions

Because of its broad origin and insertion the trapezius is one of the most prominent of the subcutaneous muscles, particularly so in the athlete. Its distal portion—that is, that which is distal to the spine of the scapula—is rarely the source of acute disability in athletics. In contrast, the proximal portion, running from the occipital protuberance and the ligamentum nuchae to the posterior aspect of the distal clavicle, the acromion, and the spine of the scapula, is the only muscle of significant size that can prevent forcible depression of the shoulder girdle or forcible deviation of the neck. Accordingly, the proximal portion is subject to strains of varying severity in addition to contusions from blows over the superior aspect of the entire shoulder.

**Strains.** Trapezius strains can be severe enough to fix the neck in spasm, with the entire proximal half of muscle taut and tender. They can, on the other hand, simply prevent effective use of both the shoulder and the ipsilateral upper extremity because of soreness and intermittent spasm. In either case, the findings are easy to demonstrate, ofttimes even the exact area of strain, and the area of hemorrhage in rare instances can be palpated. Disability can be crippling—in a basketball player, for example—yet it can start for no reason at all, with no history of acute onset. The problem here is spasm, as it is with all back strains, and the spasm must be overcome one way or another. Heat is indicated, directed toward relief of spasm and restoration of motion, without concern for bleeding as with the usual soft tissue injury. Any modality is effective, but some are more so than others. Radiant heat applied directly twice a day is best. This should be combined with three to four hot showers, since the latter allows a certain amount of gentle motion that facilitates resolution. If available, skilled massage of the taut musculature is also beneficial in hastening eventual resolution of the process. Without predictable pattern, resolution can be incredibly rapid or disappointingly persistent, with or without treatment.

**Contusions.** Contusions of the trapezius occur most often in the contact sports from direct impact just medial to the lateral end of the clavicle. Such contusions can be surprisingly painful, with acute tenderness and swelling easily outlined by inspection and palpation, with voluntary depression of the entire shoulder girdle, and with disability that because of pain effectively prevents abduction of the ipsilateral upper extremity despite the absence of any injury to the latter. Just as in the "shoulder pointer," cursory examination and observation of the gross disability can easily mislead the examiner into the diagnosis of acromioclavicular separation. However, a sling to the affected arm, ice to the exact area for 24 hours, and hot showers and active motion thereafter restore full strength and function in a matter of 3 to 4 days, in contrast to the course of a true acromioclavicular separation.

### The Shoulder Pointer

Though the term "shoulder pointer" has been discarded by the Committee on Nomenclature of the A.M.A. as inexact, it succinctly describes a particular injury so well that we prefer to retain it for both descriptive and therapeutic purposes. It is a contusion of a very specific area of the shoulder, and carries with it a consistent picture of acute disability that is at first glance indistinguishable from a true acromioclavicular separation. For this reason some feel that it is actually a Grade I separation—a strain of the acromioclavicular fibers overlying the joint without demonstrable laxity or motion. However, local findings in the "shoulder pointer" are not limited to the area of the acromioclavicular ligament, and treatment of the injury as if it were a separation always results in greatly increased discomfort.

Essentially, the mechanism of injury is a blow received on the top of the shoulder in the acromioclavicular area, which receives the brunt of the impact because of its prominence. Because of the increased musculature of the trained athlete (Fig. 12-2), there is a simultaneous contusion of the deltoid laterally and the trapezius medially, both of which in the athlete encroach closely on the A-C area. Caught thus between the impacting force and unyielding bone, these muscles are severely bruised. Acute tenderness and swelling are always demonstra-

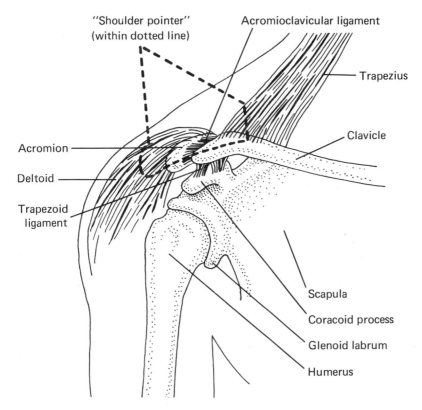

Fig. 12-2. The acromioclavicular area.

ble in these areas, at times much more remarkable than directly over the A-C joint. Hence, differentiation is not difficult; there is no laxity of the A-C joint, there is no demonstrable tenderness in the coraco-clavicular, trapezoid, or conoid ligament areas, while there is obvious tenderness and swelling of the trapezius, and/or deltoid.

Treatment is simply a sling, a shoulder-cap strapping, and ice to the area, continued for 2 days and followed by hot showers and active motion until full strength and mobility are restored, usually a matter of another three to four days. At the end of this 5- to 6-day period, a special pad can be applied to prevent recurrent impact. The athlete, sore but fully functional, is then returned to complete activity.

## Acromio-Clavicular Strains and Separations

As a disability seen almost exclusively in athletics, acromioclavicular pathology, particularly the "shoulder separation," has become a routine part of every sports journalist's working vocabulary and is routinely included in team "medical reports" all over the country. Nevertheless, as a review of the regional anatomy demonstrates (Figs. 12-1 and 12-3), the area is a complex one, with one true joint, the acromioclavicular joint, and three ligaments. One of these ligaments, the acromioclavicular, might also be considered part of the proper acromioclavicular joint capsule, hence subject to the usual stretching and tearing of any joint capsule. The remaining two, the conoid and trapezoid ligaments, fix the clavicle to yet another part of the scapula, the coracoid process. The simple fact that the acromion and coracoid are integral parts of the same bone is of particular significance, since any injury in this area can be then viewed in its proper light; that is, as the result of abnormal disruptive mechanisms that force the clavicle up from its attachment to the scapula, to which it is firmly held inferiorly by the trapezoid and conoid ligaments, and laterally by the acromioclavicular ligament-joint capsule. Given the far greater holding power of the heavy conoid and trapezoid ligaments, any significant injury in the area must be accompanied by a tearing of these particular ligaments, unless the lateral portion of the clavicle fractures at the same time, which of course does happen at times. Conversely, if the conoid and trapezoid maintain their integrity, hence their holding power of clavicle to coracoid, very little of significance can happen to the acromioclavicular joint or joint capsule.

**Symptoms and Signs.** Viewed in this manner, the myriad variations in symptoms and signs in this area fall into a logical pattern. The least injury, and one that can often be ignored, is a minimal stretch to the joint capsule, a *Grade I strain* by standard nomenclature. This could be likened to a synovitis from a simple sprain and responds very rapidly to local ice, shoulder-cap strapping, sling overnight, and a rapidly graduated rehabilitation. Findings are limited to minimal swelling over the joint line and local tenderness, some pain on motion, but no demonstrable abnormal mobility whatever. Identical thereto is *the chronic A-C strain,* more a reactive synovitis to incessantly repeated joint stress, as is occasionally seen in hard working swimmers. It is responsive to equally simple measures: a reorganization of workout requirements to minimize overhead resistive work for a short period and then building back up to it over a period of 10 days to 2 weeks.

Beyond this very limited and easily managed degree of injury are the *infinite gradations of separation and elevation,* all requiring some element of stretching and/or tearing of the dense coracoclavicular attachments. Differential signs in each and all of these injuries are an abnormal mobility of the clavicle in relation to the acromion and, related thereto, varying degrees of tenderness *inferior to the clavicle* in the coracoclavicular ligament area. Tenderness here is most significant, as it may be present in spite of minimal false motion at the acromioclavicular joint and thus the sole indication of a disabling degree of injury, one that may take up to 2 weeks for recovery. In confirmation of this initial finding, it is not unusual to note the subsequent appearance of subcutaneous discoloration 7 to 10 days later as a reflection of the deepest injury. At other times tenderness may be accompanied by visible and palpable swelling in the same area, still lacking a remarkable degree of false motion at the joint above yet consistent with the subsequent disability. Another reason for this emphasis on palpation of the coracoid area for evidence of conoid or trapezoid injury is the not infrequently encountered laxity of the acromioclavicular joint, that is an asymptomatic residual of long past injuries and is of no contemporary significance. These, obviously, exhibit no such localized tenderness despite unquestionable A-C motion, hence can be discounted.

Nonetheless, the *demonstration of significant false motion remains the essential part of the diagnosis in any acute separation,* since any separation worthy of the name must exhibit demonstrable laxity in the acute stage. A dependable method of evaluating such laxity is pivotal. X-rays with weights in the hand and like maneuvers notwithstanding, special equipment is not actually necessary, just so long as two prerequisites are met. The first is *examination within minutes of the injury* because swelling within and around the area completely obscures significant false motion within one or two hours; the swelling creates the illusion of a tender but stable joint. The second prerequisite is *proper and controlled stabilization of the scapula during examination.* Thus, the best method of examination is quite simple. Done early enough after injury to fulfill the first requirement above, it is surprisingly painless. The body of the scapula is grasped in the fingers of one hand, thereby fixing it in place, while the examining hand measures the degree of laxity by fingertip. By this simple maneuver the usual pitfall of examining a supine patient is obviated, since he must be upright in order to provide a firm grasp on the scapular body. At the same time, the controlled scapula can be displaced in different directions, the better to demonstrate the true extent of displacement.

Using this method, it has been our experience that x-rays are seldom successful in demonstrating any greater laxity or separation, routine weights or no. Not infrequently, objective and significant motion fails to show up on x-ray as demonstrable separation. X-rays should of course be taken if there is any suspicion of accompanying bony damage. Fracture can and does occur and may be missed, particularly as it involves the distal clavicle, is without displacement, and frequently incomplete. Hence, careful palpation of this virtually subcutaneous segment of bone should be an integral part of every routine shoulder examination—if it is, the physician is unlikely to miss the bony tenderness that inevitably accompanies such fractures.

Finally, it must be pointed out that many athletes without history of previous injury have demonstrably loose A-C joints and quite remarkable prominence of the distal clavicles above the smooth level of the shoulder-line. Whether this is due to chronic insult or heredity is difficult to say, though its frequency among wrestlers suggests some correlation with long-standing strain to the area. In any event, the apparent abnormality is always bilateral and does not seem to be of functional significance; yet it behooves any examiner to look at both shoulders first, before deciding that the one side with a prominent distal clavicle is a significant finding.

**Treatment.** Passing now to *treatment* of these injuries, it is important to remember the variability of degree in separations, from the barely demonstrable but definite finding of 1 to 2 millimeters of false motion to complete disruption of all ligaments and a distal clavicle that points upward at a 45 degree angle, threatening at any moment to perforate the skin. All these varieties will be encountered in any active athletic program over the years, and they should serve to underline the obvious error of those who acclaim one or another universal treatment for any and all A-C injuries, regardless of degree. Certainly the least of them can be handled by *sling alone* with restoration of motion as soon as local reaction will allow.

Those with elevations of 4 millimeters or more should be placed in a *Watson-Jones strapping,* carefully applied to exert axial pressure upward along the length of the humerus (not toward flexion of the forearm) and downward over the errant clavicular end. If a Watson-Jones strapping is considered necessary in the first place, however, it must be because the ligamentous disruption is sufficiently extensive to require such immobilization. It should, therefore, be rigidly maintained for at least 3 to 6 weeks. To apply it for any shorter period of time, then remove it, and allow what little healing that may have occurred to redisrupt under the weight of scapula and arm is illogical, and to point to subsequent laxity as proof of the superiority of open reduction is a further absurdity.

*Open reduction,* with fixation by screw, pin, wire, fascia lata, kangaroo tendon, silkworm gut, and all the other appurtenances favored by orthopedic surgeons, is certainly much the best treatment in gross displacements. This is the orthopedist's province, and it remains only for the field physician to evaluate the injury correctly. If there are demonstrable ligamentous damage and significant false motion that require at the least a Watson-Jones strapping for the requisite period mentioned, he should call in the orthopedist and leave the method to him, whatever it may be.

It is only when the athlete recovers that he again becomes a problem. No matter what the method of treatment a residual of disability remains that requires a prolonged period of *vigorous rehabilitation.* Also, there is the ultimate moment of truth when he returns to full combat: We have seen pins break, screws break, pins bend, screws work out of holes, wires snap, and even completely stable joints disrupt again under the stress of the more violent contact sports. In a majority of instances, no difficulties are encountered, but one can never be sure.

### The Sternoclavicular Subluxation

By and large, the impacting forces responsible for these injuries have a common pattern. They are violent and drive the shoulder forward and medialward usually through an uncontrolled fall. These same forces have been indicted in the common "greenstick" midshaft fracture of childhood and adolescence. In fact, the injury may be another version of the same thing, altered by the fact that in the athlete of college years the clavicle is more mature, is more sturdy, and, hence, transmits the same disruptive forces medialward along its intact length to the sternoclavicular articulation. Pain is immediate, as is disability, while examination of the clavicle is completely negative until the medial sternal end is approached, at which point there is acute swelling and tenderness of the joint. Sometimes there is demonstrable false motion. If there is crepitus, x-rays should be taken to determine the presence of chips or articular comminution. However, neither has ever been encountered. The problem has always been one of a joint subluxation of limited degree with some capsular disruption secondary thereto. The intracapsular swelling, the edema and soreness about the joint, and the pain on motion are the same as encountered in any "sprain." The treatment is the same; namely, ice to the area, compression with a felt pad, strapping directly thereover, and rest by means of sling to that side.

Disability for all sports is prolonged, as might be expected in a joint of such key importance for all shoulder girdle movement, and it is rare that an athlete can return to full activity much before 10 to 14 days regardless of the severity of initial symptoms or findings. This arbitrary period is directly related more to the subjective discomfort that even the least of these injuries produces than to the actual anatomical damage, but, regardless, stable healing in the area is better assured thereby. Local pressure with pad and tape should be maintained throughout this period and beyond, totalling about 4 weeks. However, once full-scale workouts have been resumed in the 2nd week (trunk and leg work are resumed much earlier), pressure is necessary only during the exercise periods. Good stabilization has always accompanied healing under this regime, yet it may prove difficult to justify keeping an athlete out of contact work for so long. Nonetheless, any attempt to shorten the period of disability inevitably results in a recrudescence of symptoms and signs that simply prolongs convalescence. In short, "sprain" of the sternoclavicular joint is one of a certain few injuries seen in athletics that, regardless of initial severity or the intensity of local treatment, requires a fixed period of time to stabilize to the degree mandatory for contact sports. This period cannot be rationalized, and the athlete and coach must be aware of this from the start.

**Deltoid Strains and Subdeltoid Bursitis**

As the most powerful abductor muscle for the upper extremity as well as the most extensive in total area, the deltoid muscle is the most frequent source of both acute and chronic disability in the glenohumeral area. With the underlying bursa, whose broad extent encompasses the acromion, the coracoid, and the greater tuberosity of the humerus, the deltoid and subdeltoid area can give rise to myriad problems. These problems tend to merge into one another, as contiguous structures become involved either in the acute injury or in the basic stages of healing. Initial evaluation must therefore be painstakingly accurate before these confusing developments make their appearance. Treatment may be strikingly similar regardless of this initial evaluation. Nevertheless, the anticipated period of disability in terms of athletics, always an important factor, can be accurately predicted only upon correct evaluation of each separate condition.

**Acute Deltoid Strain.** Thus, we have the very common acute deltoid strain, which can be divided into three separate entities: the anterior, the middle, and posterior deltoid strains, each secondary to acute muscular effort in differing directions.

*Anterior deltoid strain,* the most common of the group, occurs most frequently in football as the result of the "arm tackle," a deplorable technique of desperation, in which a frustrated tackler finds himself grasping laterally for a ball carrier with a single outstretched arm that is totally inadequate to even slow the progress of a determined young man of 170 to 225 pounds. Symptoms may not be immediate. More typically they become more and more disabling over the ensuing 6 to 8 hours, with palpable and occasionally visible swelling in the anterior third of the muscle, pain and weakness on abduction in the forward plane, and clearly defined tenderness in the anterior third of the muscle. Ice, shoulder-cap strapping, and sling comprise the initial treatment. This is followed by active motion under a hot shower in 1 to 2 days and a return to full activity immediately thereafter on the 3rd or 4th day and for the remainder of the convalescence.

*Middle Deltoid Strain.* Middle deltoid strain, in contrast, occurs with over-enthusiastic abduction against resistance in the lateral plane and is encountered in all sports without predictable pattern. It is characterized by a similar slow onset. There is tenderness in the middle third of the muscle, and pain and weakness on abduction in the lateral plane serve to differentiate it. Treatment consists of ice, shoulder-cap strapping and sling, active motion under a hot shower in one or two days, and a return to full activity thereafter.

*Posterior Deltoid Strain.* Posterior deltoid strain is encountered in any and all sports. It is not directly related to any specific action, but is usually a result of some strain exerted in a posteriorward direction, such as the butterfly stroke in competitive swimming. Tenderness is clearly defined in the posterior third of the deltoid, a portion of the muscle that in the non-athlete is the most poorly defined. Disability and treatment are identical to that above.

**Acute Subdeltoid Bursitis.** In each of the above conditions, the signs and symptoms are quite clear, the treatment is the same, and the disability is predictably brief. However, any of the motions that give rise to them can cause instead an acute subdeltoid bursitis, which presents an entirely different picture. Tenderness is diffuse and deep-seated, pain and weakness accompany any and all shoulder motion, and there is often a palpable swelling of the entire bursa. More important, there will be signs that reflect the diffuse nature of the process, hence signs pointing to the short and long tendons that pass through the bursa, the bicipital, the rotators, and the subscapularis.

Disability is acute, but never to the degree usually encountered in clinical practice. This is true for several reasons. Firstly, even the slightest sign of irritation is immediately detected by the athlete, for he is noticeably disabled thereby and seeks help far earlier than the average patient. Secondly, these are young men in their teens and twenties, and the exertions that have given rise to the irritation are usually far beyond the capability of an average human being; hence, the process is clearly related to abnormal strain. Thirdly, the symptoms are usually minimal in the true clinical sense, in that ordinary activity can be carried on normally without discomfort.

Treatment is not simply "inject and be done with it." Unquestionably, needle aspiration and instillation of steroids offer an adequate answer to the usual chronic, calcified, recurrently acute bursitis of middle age, and in these cases it is clearly superior to x-ray therapy, ultrasonic treatment, infra-red lamps, diathermy, aspiration and irrigation, and all the other more or less painful or ineffective procedures. Because of the reasons that were enumerated above, however, subdeltoid bursitis differs markedly in the competitive athlete and in comparison to the average case is truly subclinical. Steroid injection, which is distinctly uncomfortable initially and for the ensuing 8 to 10 hours, provides relief mainly in relation to the acute pain that has gone before. It offers the complaining athlete very little. In fact, he often feels much worse afterward than before; firstly, because his was a minimal complaint to begin with, and, secondly, needles are always anathema to young men of this type.

It has been our experience that a careful analysis of the strains involved, initial rest with sling, then a logically graduated program of active rehabilitation return a happy athlete to his labors within 5 to 7 days at the most, sometimes less. Such a program must provide for complete rest of the part for at least 24 hours. A daily check is then made, as shoulder motion is gradually resumed. Continued exercise to all other body parts is encouraged the while. Each increment of shoulder activity is checked carefully by direct palpation and functional strength tests; activity is never pushed if local symptoms increase. So treated, the rapidity with which the most demanding exertions can be resumed is most gratifying, and is in distinct contrast to the results of immediate injection that have been carried out elsewhere. The treatment is fitted to the complaint and not the reverse.

## Rotator Cuff and Supraspinatus Injuries

The subscapularis, supraspinatus, infraspinatus, teres major, and teres minor muscles comprise the deeper muscles around the glenohumeral joint and for functional purposes can be separated into three groups.

The subscapularis passes in front of the joint and together with the powerful teres major (the latissimus dorsi is an even more powerful component of this motion, though not usually considered a short rotator) rotates the humerus inward. The supraspinatus pulls the humerus into the glenoid and initiates abduction for the first 10 to 15 degrees, before the deltoid can operate effectively. Lastly, the teres minor and infraspinatus, acting through the rotator cuff, work together as external rotators of the humerus.

**Functional Rehabilitation.** Viewed in this manner, these muscle groups can be practically evaluated by certain functional tests illustrated in Figure 12-3. With the degree of injury clearly indicated either by weakness or pain on passive motion, active motion, or active motion versus resistance, the problem can be accurately delineated, and a program designed to progressively restore strength without undue aggravation. In a swimmer this means elimination of all arm work until acute symptoms subside, followed by a graduated series of pulley exercises and light stroking, then by a gradual speeding of distance work, leaving the violent sprints to the last. A baseball player must be cautioned to discontinue all throwing until soreness completely subsides, following which easy tosses in "pepper games" can be started and working up to full motion throwing undertaken in a graduated manner. In baseball more difficulty than in any other sport may be anticipated. If the arm "feels good," both athlete and coach are likely to consider a few minutes of hard throwing a good thing, ignoring the fact that even one hard throw too early can undo all the healing that has gone before. Patience is the byword, checking the situation daily, rigidly controlling all activity, and measuring increasing tolerance and

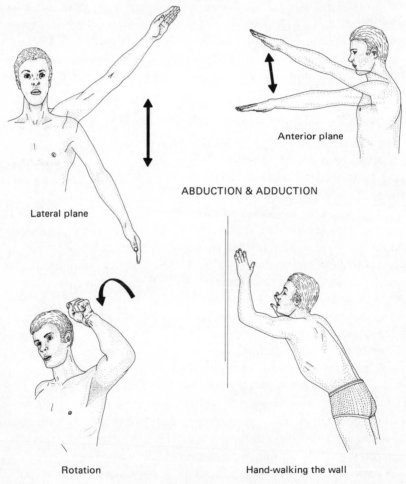

Anterior plane

ABDUCTION & ADDUCTION

Lateral plane

Rotation                                    Hand-walking the wall

Fig. 12-3. Functional shoulder tests.

strength against the ultimate demands expected. The total period of close observation may last 2 to 3 weeks—even longer in an uncooperative case—but the end result will be a fully functioning athlete, unhampered by chronic difficulties.

**Muscle Tears.** Aside from the gratifying results, another possible advantage of so closely controlled a rehabilitation program may be the rarity of permanently disabling tears of these key muscles, tears that have been reported by many and are well known in the professional sports. With the exception of a few athletes with permanent disability, dating back to secondary school injuries, there have been no instances among our athletes of the classical functional loss seen with *complete or even partial tears of the supraspinatus or rotator cuff.* We have never seen a total loss of initial abduction, said to be a sign of supraspinatus rupture, nor have we seen an example of the rotation loss in the throwing motion, said to be a result of actual avulsion of the rotator cuff. Finally, we have not seen the disability ascribed to demonstrable avulsion-fracture of the glenoid rim by the triceps. It could be that our athletes do not throw as hard as others, but this is hardly likely. Instead, the uniform historical pattern with those who have such permanent disability dating back to pre-college days is significant; their initial pain and disability were either ignored or at the most treated with local heat for no more than 3 to 5 days, after which hard throwing was not only encouraged but actually demanded as a sign of "guts." Under such circumstances it is not surprising that a muscle strain, still edematous and friable, could be converted into a complete tear. To confirm this impression, we have been unable to find a single instance in which such complete functional loss arose de novo.

A controlled program assures that any instance of "sore arm" is immediately referred to medical care either by the athlete or his coach, without the risk of subsequent aggravation under uncontrolled self-treatment or coach demands. This may be the answer to the striking difference in our incidence of these serious injuries. Be that as it may, the functional loss that reflects these serious and permanent injuries should be kept in mind at all times, should be actively sought out, and orthopedic assistance or surgery requested before dense and disabling scarring occur. Most important, if extensive damage to this degree is even suspected, the athlete should not be allowed to return to activity until that suspicion is laid to rest.

## Scapular "Winging" and the Long Thoracic Nerve

Paralysis of the serratus anterior muscle through injury to the long thoracic nerve of Bell is another condition that must be considered whenever an athlete reports with vague symptoms referable to his shoulder. Rare in clinical practice, it is not uncommon in athletics, averaging one or two a year in our program. As with so many athletic-medical problems, it is protean in its earliest manifestations yet can be diagnosed relatively promptly. This is true because the disability associated therewith (noticeable to the average patient only after advanced atrophy of the serratus anterior has occurred) is quite obvious to the athlete as a subjective weakness he cannot define. Therefore, he will report the problem quite promptly.

**Clinical Evaluation.** Examination may not be remarkable except for a weakness of abduction in the lateral plane inconsistent with the usual muscular power seen in these active young men. Abduction in the lateral plane, against resistance, may nearly lift the examiner off the floor, yet there is visible rotation of the scapula with the effort. The visible and well-defined serratus digitations on the ribs will appear normal and certainly far better defined than on the average patient. "Walking the wall" (see Fig. 12-3) may be so distorted by heavy latissimus, trapezius, and rhomboid muscles that the classical and dramatic winging of the scapular body is not immediately apparent. Nonetheless, if symptoms of vague weakness on abduction continue to suggest long thoracic nerve injury, repeated examinations should be carried out. When all else fails, the athlete during examination should do a series of pushups, which quite often demonstrates the lateral rotation and "winging" of the scapular body (provided that the number of pushups is sufficient to constitute a real challenge to the athlete's normal strength and endurance).

**Treatment.** Once the diagnosis is established, treatment and disability are uniform; namely, a repeated faradic electrostimulation of the nerve on a daily or thrice-weekly schedule, and a total discontinuation of all athletic activity for the duration of the symptoms. Though harsh, this policy is based on consideration of the various factors involved. The injury is never completely explicable, hence no program can be designed to avoid the specific cause. As a pure motor nerve, the long thoracic has no sensory fibers to reflect the presence of regeneration, hence progress cannot be accurately determined at any one time. The prolonged winding course of the injured nerve, so familiar to surgeons during a radical mastectomy, makes accurate localization of the actual nerve lesion impossible. Nor can any mechanism be pinpointed, for we have seen it in swimmers, high jumpers, football players, and basketball players. We must, therefore, be content to continue stimulation of the muscle, in hopes of preventing irreversible atrophy while regeneration proceeds undisturbed, and at no time risking re-injury to the nerve, however it may have occurred.

Case 4, R. G.: A champion backstroker reported with a vague complaint of weakness in his left shoulder, which was completely negative to routine examination except for a suggestive rotation of the scapula on resisted lateral abduction. Muscular development, as with all competitive swimmers, was such that the scapula was buried under layers of overlying musculature and the anterior serratus stood out as firm, distinct digitations on the anterolateral rib cage. The athlete volunteered that in high school he had suffered a "nerve injury" for which he received electrical stimulation, with prompt recovery within 3 months, and that his present complaint was somewhat similar subjectively. With this very helpful item, further search was made for the slightest evidence of scapular "winging," and additional pushups at last revealed a definite suggestion thereof despite the heavy trapezius and rhomboid development. Electrostimulation was immediately started and all swimming discontinued.

Further attempts to analyze the basic injury with this exceptionally alert young man (who subsequently went on to medical school) failed to pinpoint any specific factor other than the "backstroke flip." This is a very complex motion that combines an extreme of abduction at the shoulder with extreme external rotation of the humerus, and in that position, an explosive muscular effort that pushes off the pool wall, turns the flexed body around, and partially somersaults it, all at the same time. However, the countless times that this particular maneuver had been repeated in 1 week, much less in a month or year, fails to explain why injury should have taken place this once or whether there was any real connection with the previous episode. At any rate a gradual return to function was noted over the ensuing 6 months, with treatment and improvement continuing into medical school.

This case illustrates two additional facets of diagnosis and treatment, that are unique. First, the diagnosis would have been delayed had it not been for the unusual medical interest of the athlete himself, and this saving in time must certainly be viewed as a valuable dividend—treatment is the same, regardless of the stage at which diagnosis is made, but there is clear advantage in treatment before significant serratus atrophy has supervened. Second, the effect of a stringent ban on swimming, in this case limiting post-season national competition as well, was less traumatic emotionally because of the extraordinary insight and experience of this particular young man. (One can imagine the problems that might have been encountered had he been a "gung-ho hard-head.")

## Injury to the Axillary Nerve

Of interest is another nerve injury, reportedly much more common than the foregoing, but, in our experience, of less long-term significance—axillary nerve trauma. As a branch of the posterior cord of the brachial plexus, it swings posteriorward out of the axilla by way of the same anatomical space as the circumflex vessels. This is a space bounded by the teres minor above, the teres major below, the humerus laterally, and the long head of the triceps medially. Thereby the axillary nerve reaches its destination to supply the deltoid. Contusions have been described, impacting the nerve in its course between the coracoid and the head of the humerus, with scarring and neuroma formation necessitating surgery. Loss of abduction through loss of deltoid function is the obvious result of such injury, and operative treatment is clearly mandatory.

However, the only instance of significant axillary nerve involvement in our experience was more notable as a demonstration of anatomy, while serious injury has not been encountered. Thus, a quarterback reported that he noted some minor weakness of abduction after "straining" his arm, but was most disturbed by a numbness and tingling over the sensory distribution of the axillary nerve, along the upper lateral arm and shoulder, on the motion of "handing-off." On examination there was little weakness demonstrable. Instead, there was soreness and swelling of the teres major and teres minor, high up in the posterior axilla. Rest of the arm in a sling, followed by graduated rehabilitation, resulted in prompt resolution of spasm and swelling in the involved muscles and therewith prompt subsidence of the paraesthesias. Anatomical analysis of the neurological signs could only lead to the conclusion that the space through which the nerve normally passes had been impinged upon by the intrinsic muscle swelling, which swelling appeared to be related partially to throwing as well as to the jerky motion of turning, faking a belly-handoff, then cocking the arm to throw. Intriguing as this case was, with the mechanism so clearly demonstrated, we have searched in vain for another yet feel that it must be more common!

**Glenohumeral Dislocations**

Complete dislocation of the glenohumeral joint is a relatively common injury in athletics, occurring with uniform frequency in the contact sports and less so in the non-contact sports. *Recognition is not difficult, simple palpation and inspection suffice* to demonstrate an empty glenoid fossa, with humeral head position depending entirely on the type of displacement, be it subglenoid, subcoracoid, or posterior. Often the athlete himself volunteers the diagnosis. Examination then proves him right. Occasionally, a posterior dislocation in a heavily muscled young man may cause some difficulty in diagnosis, since it allows internal rotation and adduction; tests depending on this particular limitation then reveal nothing. However, acute disability is unquestionable, and simple, thorough examination cannot fail to make the diagnosis.

*Treatment should be immediate reduction,* as soon as possible but without panic. As with everything else in medicine, blanket rules cannot be made. Every effort should be made to effect reduction in the brief period of 5 to 10 minutes post injury when local numbness and shock are present. This does not mean that dogged persistence, attempt after attempt, should be insisted upon, especially when under the lightest anesthesia a gentle, atraumatic reduction can be obtained. Furthermore, many feel that no reduction should be attempted without preliminary x-ray, to circumvent the medico-legal problem of fracture of the glenoid rim and its temporal relation to manipulation. Be that as it may, to leave a dislocation untended for the time required to get x-rays, study them, and decide upon treatment, when one forceful attempt may effect immediate reduction and relief of pain, is not reasonable, legal problems notwithstanding. Instead, *one* vigorous try should be made, using the familiar "foot in the axilla" method of straight traction. If distraction does not occur in the first few seconds of pull, failure is likely, for the musculature of the trained athlete may balance the pull of the average-sized doctor. Regardless of that no levering type of reduction should be attempted—in particular, the Kocher maneuver—because the athlete's powerful musculature surrounding the dislocated shoulder will almost surely crack the rib cage, the fulcrum of this particular maneuver! Once reduction has been accomplished, there is immediate relief of pain. *A sling with controlling swath around the chest will suffice thereafter.* Local discomfort subsides as rapidly as the extent of soft tissue damage allows, rarely lasting more than 3 or 4 days, at which point differentiation and decision must be made between the divergent treatment for primary dislocation and for the recurrent dislocation.

**Primary Dislocation.** In the case of primary dislocation, local symptoms are severe in view of the extensive capsular damage and soft tissue trauma. However, within the usual period mentioned above, the athlete feels much like himself again and wishes the sling removed. A decision has to be made at this early date concerning the routine period of immobilization in primary dislocations. Some orthopedists feel that all primary dislocations are simply the first of many, that is, are more directly related to shallow fossa, deficient glenoid labrum, and the like, hence brief or prolonged immobilization means little. Others feel that it is impossible to predict which case will prove to be the recurrent type, hence immobilize the primary dislocation for at least 6 weeks in hopes of avoiding recurrent problems except in those with anatomical disposition thereto. Having seen the violence involved in many primary dislocations, we find it hard to believe that any shoulder, no matter how normal, could withstand such disruptive forces. We feel, therefore, that any treatment that affords a damaged but basically normal shoulder the best chance to heal solidly is the more sensible.

**Recurrent Dislocation.** On the other hand, recurrent dislocation is an entirely different problem in that the history is usually quite clear-cut, the impacting or dislocating force is at times minimal (e.g., turning over in bed), reduction is usually simply accomplished, and the local problems subside within 36 to 48 hours. Here there is no question that prolonged immobilization will gain anything of value, hence early active motion can be resumed as soon as local symptoms allow, without fear for an already determined future. Instead, some decision is necessary concerning *surgical fixation* of the permanently loose joint. This is an orthopedist's decision. The type of repair depends on the decision of the orthopedist. The Putti-Platt, Magnussen-Stack, and Bankhart fixations, all have been observed at one time or another, all with equally satisfactory stability in athletic competition.

The added value of the *cuff and chain,* an appliance that effectively prevents or limits abduction beyond 45 degrees, remains a question. It is quite hampering to useful motion of the involved arm yet does have some prophylactic effect, though we have seen dislocations with the device still firmly in place. It is the orthopedist who must decide whether he wishes to protect an operative result with a cuff-and-chain or if he cares to risk it at all. Most return our athletes to action without the cuff and chain, though this is by no means uniform.

More important in our opinion is the *proper timing of corrective surgical procedures.* Should they be done simply to allow a boy to return to football or to assure the boy of a trouble-free life after contact sports and after college? Should a postoperative shoulder be exposed to the risk of another massive injury in contact sports? And is it sensible to bar football postoperatively, while allowing basketball where all strains and violence "under the boards" occur with the arms outstretched and abducted?

Our personal feelings reflect those of our late staff orthopedist at Yale and follow his conservative bent: Thus, surgical fixation of the recurrent shoulder dislocation should be done primarily to assure the patient of a trouble-free future life, not as a direct expedient to return him to football; postoperatively, the shoulder should be protected from the possibility of extensive recurrent damage by cuff-and-chain regardless of its bulk and inconvenience. Lastly, all sports must be individually evaluated in terms of a shoulder that has had one major operation already, and therefore deserves protection. Athletics are certainly important, but education and a trouble-free life after college are much more so. A professional athletic career changes all, but the difference and the reasons for the difference are clear and should be so recognized.

Case 5, D. H.: A highly rated schoolboy offensive end had a history of multiple recurrent dislocations of both shoulders, the right more often than the left. At his position as a potentially stellar pass receiver, any limitation of abduction by cuff-and-chain would have been virtually disabling. Moreover, with bilateral problems, which side deserved limitation? Because of the history of more numerous episodes on the right and another recurrent episode on that side during his freshman football season, a cuff-and-chain was finally ordered for the right shoulder upon his return to pre-season football as a sophomore despite his lamentations. The effect of this ruling on his pass-receiving was then awaited with great interest, but, before any valid observations could be made, he suffered another right shoulder injury with the applicance still firmly in place.

The mechanism of this latest injury was impossible to reconstruct accurately, but the victim adamantly insisted that his shoulder was "out." Examination revealed no loss of deltoid contour, and palpation of the glenoid area was next to useless because of overlying deltoid spasm. But the humerus could be palpated along its axis toward the glenoid fossa and did not appear grossly out of line. Internal and external rotation were painful but without limitation, adduction was painful but without limitation, and the combination of internal rotation and adduction was sufficiently free to allow him to touch his opposite shoulder without difficulty. Abduction was even more painful but could be passively demonstrated to above 90 degrees.

Nonetheless, the injured boy insisted that the shoulder was "out." And so indeed it was posteriorly, and locked over the posterior glenoid rim by spasm, requiring general anesthesia and considerable manipulation to obtain reduction. Post-reduction discomfort was more severe than usual, since this was his first posterior dislocation in contrast to the countless anterior ones, but full motion was eventually restored in 6 to 8 weeks.

Surgery, repeatedly deferred over the years for numerous reasons, was now inevitable and was carried out at home during the ensuing winter. The procedure was reportedly a difficult one, as might be anticipated with such chronicity and with a fresh posterior capsular disruption as well, but recovery was excellent. His orthopedist, true to his surgical convictions, did not bar football nor did he insist upon external support. Nonetheless, it seemed reasonable that any protection was better than none in this much abused shoulder, and we explained our feelings to the athlete. He in turn was not at all anxious to risk further injury to the operative shoulder, nor did he wish further trouble with his untreated and occasionally symptomatic left shoulder. Any further surgery, no matter what the reason, was definitely not a part of his plans. Fortunately for everyone concerned, after a few days of badly needed pre-season conditioning and much "agonizing reappraisal," he decided that football was not that important. We are convinced that his was the proper decision.

**The "Loose" Shoulder.** As if such problems were not enough, there is still the "loose shoulder" that has never dislocated. A clear-cut history of *repeated subluxations without a single accompanying episode of clinical dislocation* is not infrequently encountered. The mechanism by history alone is one of violent force and a pre-existing capsular laxity, which combine to ride the head of the humerus up on the rim of the glenoid, where for a brief moment of pain and limited motion it remains, only to slip back into the fossa with an audible and painful click. Such a disconcerting incident may occur but once or several times in a week or a day, yet repeated examination reveals only some residual soreness and an unquestionable laxity in the capsule. This last is best demonstrated by placing the subject's hands behind his neck with elbows abducted in the lateral plane, testing glenohumeral stability by forcing the elbow posteriorward with one hand while palpating high in the axillary dome over the glenohumeral capsule with the other. (This test always demonstrates significant anterior capsule laxity, but it can also accomplish complete dislocation. It must be done with care.)

The question must then be answered: Is this shoulder loose enough to warrant external support to protect it, or should it be exposed to whatever forces its owner chooses to inflict upon it with the fatalistic attitude that dislocation is inevitable? And how often is "too often" for subluxation to occur before something must be done?

There are no simple answers to this problem. If episodes are recurring with increasing frequency to the extent that performance and dependability are jeopardized, some type of external support is necessary. By the same measure, if the discomfort of each incident is more than the sport is worth to the boy, he should be so advised. If he or his parents wish some guarantee that these episodes can be controlled and clinical dislocation thereby avoided, the unhappy facts and the risks must be clearly outlined. Beyond full knowledge of the incidents and the underlying anatomical factors, the physician can bring little of worth to any discussion of the future and what should be done. Surgery is certainly indicated, should the condition proceed to one of recurrent clinical dislocations, but few orthopedists would recommend internal fixation for a history of episodic subluxations. If the use of external support, such as the cuff-and-chain, effectively prevents further aggravation, does it not still leave the athlete neither here nor there, with a shoulder bad enough to be somewhat undependable yet too good for surgical fixation?

Shoulders such as these are subjectively bothersome only in the more stressful contact sports, such as football and wrestling, which by and large end after graduation, to be replaced by sports equally active yet less damaging to specific joints. Consequently, if significant aggravation of a loose shoulder can be controlled by cuff-and-chain until the more violent sports are voluntarily abandoned, the patient is, so-to-speak, "home free" and is unlikely to have similar problems thereafter. Unless of course he goes on to a professional athletic career. But this puts an entirely different light on the problem, with surgical indications that are solely determined by performance requirements and criteria that are based on saleable athletic capabilities for today and tomorrow, not at future age 40. As an entirely different framework of reference, within which otherwise unacceptable standards have a special validity, professional athletics should be recognized for what they are and not the standard by which the overwhelming preponderance of permanently amateur college and secondary school athletes should be treated.

# 13

# *Injuries to the Upper Extremity*

Examination for upper extremity injuries must include some method for accurate appraisal of skeletal integrity, because fractures and dislocations must be identified and treated before anything else. Inspection and palpation, in the course of obtaining an accurate history of how and why the injury occurred, are the keystone of any such examination.

Despite the greater muscularity of the competitive athlete, the skeletal framework of the upper extremity is easily palpated. The entire length of the humerus, up to the surgical neck and glenohumeral area, is essentially subcutaneous along its medial aspect, as are the medial and lateral epicondyles. The ulna, from styloid to olecranon, is similarly palpable along its entire length. The radius, despite the heavy overlying brachio-radialis and supinator muscles, can be palpated from radial head to broad distal end, including the dorsal articulating rim. The carpals present a more difficult problem but careful localized pressure over the scaphoid (dorsally) and the lunate, pisiform, and hamate (ventrally) provides significant information about the four carpals most likely to present problems. Finally, each metacarpophalangeal ray is largely subcutaneous on one or another aspect, so can be inspected and palpated accurately.

By this means fracture-line tenderness and swelling, crepitus, angulation, and actual bony deformity can be detected before anything more vigorous is attempted. In the presence of any of the above signs there is little need to demonstrate false motion. Forceful manipulation of any single bone to demonstrate axial integrity should be reserved as a final check of structural continuity, not as further proof of that which already clearly requires x-ray. Should there be no other signs to indicate fracture, then and only then should more vigorous pressures be applied to rule out impacted or greenstick fractures. A forceful levering, cross-wise and axially, must then be performed before pronouncing any such injury free of fracture. The examining physician must maintain a high index of suspicion and must never allow an athlete to return to action with an injury that suggests fracture. Similarly, he must not decide without x-ray that any suspected fracture is safe from aggravation by continued sport participation. If a fracture is suspected, it should be x-rayed and then judged on its own indications, not by any special athletic considerations. If treatment might be altered to particular needs, it can then be done deliberately with the x-ray indicated fracture line before one.

## Strains and Tears of the Proximal Biceps

Having examined the upper extremity and satisfied himself that there is no fracture or dislocation, what then should the doctor look for? Beginning at the shoulder, he must consider the bicipital muscle and its problems, some of which are within the shoulder. The biceps, as the most powerful flexor of the elbow as well as one of the most powerful supinators, is properly respected by athletes and other laymen as an indicator of overall strength. Less well recognized is the fact that, because of its involvement in virtually all complex upper extremity functions, strains of this large muscle can appear entirely within its proximal portion, hence within the shoulder area, as often as in the more obvious tendinous area on the flexor aspect of the elbow. *Strains,* even *tears,* of the long head of the biceps along its course up the bicipital groove to the glenoid rim are not infrequent and can be a persistent, even crippling problem (to a baseball pitcher, for example). Such strains are often accompanied by a *tenosynovitis* along the tendon sheath, rendering all motions of the shoulder painful. With the typical increase in pain on forceful flexion of the biceps against resistance and the typically acute tenderness over the bicipital groove along the upper anterior humerus, they present a striking picture that is distinctly separable from true shoulder problems. Similarly, *tears of the long head* typically exhibit a classical disalward motion of the contracting muscle belly despite an intact short head and are therefore unlikely to be confused with any true shoulder problem.

**Treatment.** Treatment of the complete tear is surgical and need not concern us here, the difficulties being one of adequate exposure and then approximation of the frayed and "rolled-up" tendon ends in a hopefully secure manner. But the strain and/or tenosynovitis of the long head of the biceps presents a less clear-cut problem, hence one for which treatment is even less clear cut. Rest with sling is the first step and should be continued until local tenderness and pain on motion subside completely. In the vast majority of cases this will suffice and can be followed by a judicious resumption of activity in graduated steps. With a pitcher, this may take an additional 2 to 3 weeks, just as would any similar injury within the shoulder area. Refractory cases should be assessed as to whether advice has been followed closely; more often than not, it is soon apparent that the impatient pitcher has been "testing" the shoulder by throwing "a few hard ones," thus negating the entire effort. If conservative measures are clearly inadequate, injection of the tendon sheath with cortical steroid has been reported as quite effective; however, in our one such instance, it failed to restore pitching effectiveness.

## Distal Bicipital Strains

Strains of less long term significance occur at the other musculotendinous end of the biceps, along the thick and powerful distal tendon from the junction of muscle with tendon to its insertion on the ulna, and are usually secondary to either an overenthusiastic effort at weightlifting (particularly the "curling" exercise) or, even more often, to an accompanying hyperextension of the elbow. Tenderness is easily elicited along the course of the tendon to its insertion, commonly extending distally and medially to the insertion along the exact course of the associated lacertus fibrosus. Rest with sling for one or two days and a little common sense suffice for the weight lifter; the hyperextended elbow (in the football player) is more of a problem, and will be discussed later as part of the discussion of the elbow.

## The Brachialis Contusion and Calcification

One of the more common contusions in contact sports, particularly in football, is that involving the bulk of the brachialis muscle. In the athlete this is quite highly developed and is visible as a firm belly on the antero-lateral aspect of the upper arm. It is distinctly separable from the lateral head of the triceps posteriorly and the deltoid proximally. In this exposed position, just below the football shoulder-pad epaulettes, it is subject to multiple impacts, is easily contused initially, and is doubly prone to recurrent contusions and bleeding thereafter.

**Treatment.** Immediate application of ice and compression usually controls the first episode. Because of the peculiar local circumstances, however, secure padding of the area against recurrent impact is difficult without a locking of the pad up against the epaulette, which thereby limits abduction unreasonably. Consequently, *recurrent contusion* is almost inevitable.

### Calcification of the Brachialis

Recurrent trauma and bleeding in an area directly contiguous to the intermuscular septum that runs distal to the deltoid tubercle along the shaft of the humerus must have significant long-term effect, and it is not surprising that *calcification and bony spurs* develop, emerging from this area of the humerus and penetrating into the muscle belly itself. Serial x-rays and direct palpation reveal this to be a true bony spurring that matures progressively to a point where excision may be a temptation. The likelihood of recurrence, however, and the technical difficulties of dissecting a calcification that penetrates between and through muscle fibers (which then rebleed in turn) are factors to be seriously considered.

With proper padding we have not found such radical treatment to be necessary. Others have recommended ultrasonic treatments, but these have succeeded only in making an asymptomatic, though calcific, area sore and swollen without altering the degree of calcification. In the long run we have found it to be a condition best inspected, then padded, and looked upon as a permanent and harmless souvenir from football.

### Injuries About the Radial Head

The radial head and neck, together with the annular ligament, present an anatomical and functional unit that can be quite easily palpated and accurately evaluated. As the key articulation for the indispensable pronation and supination of the forearm, the least symptom referrable to this area is noticed as a hampering disability by the competitive athlete; hence it is reported promptly. Direct treatment, however, is never completely encouraging or satisfying.

**Fractures.** If there is an acute onset attributable to some distinct trauma, the first diagnostic consideration should be of a possible impaction or infraction-fracture of the radial head. This is characterized by acute swelling in the joint, acute tenderness of the radial head, and pain on pronation and supination—these same findings are present in all instances of radio-humeral pathology and are too general for accurate differential diagnosis. Hence, *x-rays are absolutely essential whenever radial head trauma is suspected.* If the suspicion is strong enough, a negative initial film should be discounted and followed by repeat films in a week. During this interim rest with sling should be instituted, because fractures of this area may not show up until a week of bone absorption has taken place along the originally invisible fracture line. The intervening week of full athletic disability serves to quiet local symptoms and signs unrelated to a fracture, eliminating thereby the need for follow-up x-rays should the signs and symptoms disappear entirely.

**Acute Sprains.** More common are the acute sprains involving radio-humeral joint capsule and annular ligament, which present acute signs identical to those above and of similar acute onset. They necessitate identical diagnostic and therapeutic measures until spontaneous resolution eliminates the possibility of more significant skeletal trauma. Injection of local anesthetic or cortical steroid has been recommended for the relief of local pain. This can be simply done, should acute symptoms so warrant; however, simple rest with sling has proved adequate for our needs, with the added advantage that spontaneous resolution of symptoms and signs can then be used as an accurate guideline, not only to the probable period of athletic disability, but to the diagnosis itself.

**Radio-Humeral Bursitis.** Even more difficult to deal with is the chronic radio humeral bursitis, the familiar *"tennis elbow,"* that plagues athletes in those sports that demand a repeated elbow extension combined with a snapping supination or pronation. Since it is this last motion that gives a "twist" to the tennis service or puts the "break" in the pitcher's curve, it is not a motion that can be dispensed with or advised against. Radio-humeral bursitis is, therefore, a totally crippling athletic problem during each acute episode. Since it is characteristically recurrent, its effect on the competitive athlete can be disastrous.

In essence, it is no more than an acute exacerbation of chronic synovitis, with swelling, heat, and acute pain in the radio-humeral area, and is exacerbated by flexion and extension of the elbow (but most by pronation and supination). Intensive treatment of each such episode can shorten severity and duration, but has little effect on the likelihood of recurrence. *If pain is the principal problem,* injection of local anesthetic or cortical steroid brings rapid relief, but this is purely symptomatic and does not guarantee a prompt return to full athletic proficiency. In fact, too rapid a return to full activity, simply because the area has been rendered painless, assures that the process will become even more aggravated and more injections will be required. Rest with sling is still a very necessary part of the total treatment, even after injection has relieved the local pain, and the overall saving in time lost from competition is more apparent than real.

It must be pointed out that with most competitive athletes mild discomfort and associated weakness of vigorous function is the usual complaint, not pain of itself. *Primary relief of pain is not as important as with the usual clinical case;* restoration to full and completely painless function under competitive conditions is the more important consideration. In view of these factors it is not our policy to inject these bursae; rather, we place the part at *rest in a sling* until the local findings subside, usually 2 to 4 days. A *graduated and controlled program of activity* can be then outlined, that gradually restores motion and function as rapidly as tolerated, the while maintaining overall general physical condition. The athlete thus remains active, the injury is remobilized according to criteria that he himself can observe and feel, and there is no argument that he can go full speed because of an artificially benumbed, hence subjectively healed injury. Such a regimen would be a total failure in the middle aged tennis player, whose throbbing pain has prevented sleep for days before help is sought. But there is a distinct difference between these two examples, a difference that should be recognized as significant, and the treatment varied accordingly.

## Humeral Epicondylitis

As the proximal anchor-points for the extensors and supinators laterally, and the flexors and pronators medially, the humeral epicondyles can become the seat of acute and chronic strains that by their effect on these precise muscle actions can seriously hamper athletic performance. Strength of grip is affected as well as supination and pronation; and these are functions that with the exception of soccer and track are an integral part of all athletic performance on a competitive level.

**Acute Epicondylitis.** Significant acute epicondylitis is not a frequent problem. Furthermore, all instances of either medial or lateral acute strain respond rapidly to sling and rest, without the need for injection, special strapping, or physical therapy. More important than the specific treatment, therefore, is a careful analysis of the cause of the acute strain. In accordance with the overall rarity of these acute probems it is virtually certain that the causative factor will be an abnormal one, hence easily correctible. Thus, a baseball pitcher who decides on his own to develop a new breaking pitch may devote hour after hour in a furor of youthful enthusiasm—with predictable results. A modicum of sensible control, after a respectable period of rest to the abused elbow, will suffice and will prevent future chronic epicondylitis.

**Chronic Epicondylitis.** Chronic humeral epicondylitis, usually associated with veteran professional baseball pitchers after years of service, had not been encountered on the college level until recently, when a few cases began to show up on our entrance medical screening. History and findings were strikingly similar; the process palpably and roentgenographically involved the medial epicondyle, all cases were former Little League pitchers who had shown great potential until they developed "sore arms," and all cases are pitchers no longer!

The significance of these common factors is impossible to assess accurately in view of the very small number involved, but there are several implications. Chronic degenerative changes were present in all and were permanent, so could not be altered by treatment. Further, the more frequent involvement of the medial epicondyle indicates a greater likelihood of chronic strain in the pronators rather than the supinators, which is confirmed by the fact that the "slider," a pitch that requires a snapping pronation on delivery, was the original cause of the "sore arm" in each of our few instances, rather than the commonly indicted "curve" which requires a snapping supination on delivery and is a basic part of every pitcher's arsenal. A discussion of the worth of Little League baseball is not relevant here, nor can any conclusions be drawn from so few cases out of such a vast program. However, are these few cases merely the first of many to come? Should some attempt be made to outlaw the "breaking pitch," or should the "slider" be outlawed in the lower age-groups?

### Contusion of the Musculospiral (Radial) Nerve

Because of its dramatic nature direct contusion to the radial nerve deserves special mention, though it is of limited long-term significance. In its course in the musculospiral groove along the lateral aspect of the lower third of the humerus the radial nerve is relatively superficial, between brachialis proximally and brachioradialis distally. Contusions over this portion of the arm result in a sudden radiating pain distalward along the radial sensory distribution and a simultaneous paralysis of the extensors, over and above the acute local discomfort from what is at the same time a painful contusion of bony humerus.

This is the so-called *"dead arm."* Yet, despite this acute and widespread symptomatology, surely a frightening experience for the victim, there is rarely permanent damage. The vast majority of these incidents subside spontaneously in a matter of minutes. Local ice, reassurance, and adequate padding thereafter usually suffice. The remote possibility remains that more permanent injury to the radial nerve may occur, but this has not been encountered, nor is it likely to be missed either by the doctor or the athlete. Any persistent symptoms clearly warrant further investigation, x-rays, and neurosurgical consultation, but such gross disability is rare.

### The Hyperextension Strain of the Elbow

Of significance because of its frequency in football as well as its disabling chronicity, the hyperextended elbow is a familiar sight to all trainers and team physicians. The mechanism of injury is one of hyperextension and is closely akin to the posterior dislocation of the elbow. By the same measure those structures that subsequently exhibit tenderness and swelling—namely, the bicipital tendon and the associated lacertus fibrosus, the collateral ligaments both medial and lateral, and the pronators and flexors from the medial epicondyle—are precisely the same structures that by their presence and their functional strength probably prevented the dislocation in the first place. Depending on the degree of force involved, there is a varying degree of local reaction, ranging from the least limitation of extension to 180 degrees and a minimal soreness of the structures named, to a limitation of extension to 150 to 160 degrees, acute tenderness and swelling of all structures, palpable swelling of the joint capsule posteriorly, and palpable tenderness deep in the olecranon fossa of the humerus from forceful impaction by the olecranon.

**Treatment.** Treatment is rest of the part in a sling, with elastic support and ice to minimize initial swelling. If there is a subjective history of actual subluxation and there is an accompanying acute tenderness and swelling over the coronoid process deep in the antecubital fossa, x-rays should be obtained to rule out fracture. Response to the conservative local measures is quite dramatic, with subsidence of swelling and limitation in 2 to 4 days. Full extension, however, remains limited by 5 to 10 degrees and should only be regained by the most gentle means over the ensuing 2 to 3 days. Any vigorous manipulation negates previous progress in short order. By passive restoration of extension progressive improvement proceeds uninterrupted, while an early return to full activity is anticipated by the usual general conditioning program. When 180 degrees of extension has been regained, weight work with the small bar and 20 pounds will rapidly restore functional strength. Full activity can then be resumed.

**External Support.** The principle difficulty encountered in this early a return to full competition is the likelihood of recurrent injury, since the mechanism of injury is quite common to all athletic activity. If extension can be artificially limited short of 180 degrees, there will be little if any aggravation of the resolving process no matter how vigorous the sport. However, a single episode of hyperextension immediately reproduces the entire injury. Some type of external support is therefore essential to assure continued resolution of the original injury while strength and function return. For this purpose the "elbow-cinch-strapping" (Fig. 22-2) is invaluable as a daily adjunct to full activity, not only for the first few days but for 2 to 4 weeks thereafter. The athlete can be advised to avoid hyperextension in the future by abandoning "arm-tackling," but, since this is usually a desperation maneuver at best, the "cinch strap" is likely to prove of more value than any such advice.

### Olecranon Bursitis

Because of its exposed anatomical site the olecranon bursa is subject to laceration, puncture, abrasion, and direct contusion. All require intensive local treatment to avoid unnecessary complication. Once direct or indirect involvement is recognized and the proper measures taken, no problems should arise. However, possible bursal injury must be recognized before it can be treated. It behooves the physician to keep the anatomical limits of this troublesome sac before him at all times, mindful of the unusual volume and total area thereof in those athletes with a past history of previous trouble. It is not unusual to see bursae that extend midway to the ulnar styloid and up over the olecranon to the triceps area, all secondary to an acute contusion and traumatic bursitis years previously.

**Acute Olecranon Bursitis.** Acute olecranon bursitis with tense, fluctuant swelling of the bursa and surrounding redness and tenderness can occasionally develop *de novo,* but far more frequent is a combination of intrabursal hemorrhage from impact, superimposed on this acute reaction, culminating in a huge fluctuant swelling that can reach impressive proportions. *Treatment is by aspiration, not by open incision.* Aspiration of up to 50 or 75 cubic centimeters of sanguinous fluid is not unusual, and should be immediately followed by firm elastic compression and ice for at least 24 to 48 hours. Recurrent swelling may or may not develop; so it is our policy to withhold local cortical steroid injection until the initial aspiration has proved futile. *If reaspiration is necessary, a long-acting steroid* or some similar instillation has been strikingly successful in ending the problem. In either case, *elastic compression, heavy protective padding, and controlled activity* for 1 or 2 days are indispensable.

Furthermore, certain *chronic changes* in the serous surfaces within the bursa must be expected following such an initial episode. Regardless of therapy some thickening and an increased tendency toward recurrent swelling upon the least impact must be anticipated. Therefore, each acute episode will need padding for a prolonged period, probably for the remainder of the season, to avoid that which is reasonably certain to otherwise develop. Elbow pads are a nuisance, and the need for them may require considerable direct reinforcement by the doctor and trainer to keep the athlete from discarding the pad as soon as his acute problems have subsided. Fortunately, logical explanation and repeated reminders usually suffice.

**Chronic Olecranon Bursitis.** If a chronically thickened and swollen olecranon bursa recalcitrant to steroid injection then evolves, operative excision may be necessary, but the surgeon should be cautioned that operation in such an exposed area must be timed to assure a solid scar long before any contact sport season begins—otherwise, local symptoms about the scar will cause as much discomfort as the original condition. Meticulous operative technique is mandatory, since the periosteum of the olecranon forms the deep limit of dissection and secondary infection and chronic osteomyelitis are possible complications. Whether the introduction of the long acting steroids over the past few years has had any role is difficult to prove, but it has been our impression that the thickened, edematous, chronic bursae have disappeared, and with them the indication for operation. More intensive treatment of the acute episodes and more rigid control of subsequent protective padding may have also played a part. Whatever the reason, the last such bursal excision in our direct experience was over 15 years ago.

### Contusions and Strains of the Forearm

As any football enthusiast knows, the forearms are the lineman's favorite weapon whether applied legally or illegally. They absorb the brunt of impact from other helmets, face masks, cleated shoes, an occasional soft part, and the ground itself which in late autumn may have the resiliency of reinforced concrete. Every kind of contusion, abrasion, puncture wound, and laceration is seen, as well as painful bone bruises of the ulnar shaft from olecranon to the lower third, even an occasional angulated fracture. Thorough examination, particularly palpation of each such injury, tells the story in most instances, though an occasional direct bruise of the ulna may prove so painful that x-rays must be obtained to rule out direct fracture. Fortunately, fractures are rare, although as always they must be treated on their own indications, athletics and continued participation being secondary. The innumerable *contusions* require a faithful adherence to *routine ice, compression, and elevation with sling,* regardless of how minor they may appear in the first few minutes—swelling can be quite hampering once established in the taut muscularity of the forearm. These contusions, even early hematomas, disappear upon proper treatment with gratifying rapidity and without lingering disability. It only remains then to assure that adequate protective padding is applied and maintained for 2 to 3 weeks thereafter, keeping in mind any specific rules, for example, those covering rigid appliances below the elbow.

Much less routine in character and quite difficult to handle are the *strains of the forearm,* usually in the flexor group. Aside from minor acute strains, secondary to overenthusiastic weight training (rapidly responsive to routine measures of rest and reappraisal of training techniques), the persistently recurrent strain of the flexor muscles constitutes a real problem in competitive athletics. These cases are always related to strain that is an integral part of the sport involved, hence they cannot be as easily dealt with as the usual minor strain. The medical solution is obvious, namely that the sport is injurious, is forcing inordinate strain on the forearm flexors, and must be barred. At times this is the only answer. Crew, for instance, is a sport that most varsity-level competitors take up in secondary school and never leave, so great is their enthusiasm. No other sport devotes as much of the year, from September to June, to such purely mechanical drudgery, yet this drudgery is indispensable to the machine like precision of a successful eight-oared shell. To inform such an enthusiast that his forearm muscles are just not up to the strain and that he must give up the sport is a most difficult task. Instead, every effort should be made to find out why he has such a problem. Often a word with the coach to check closely on the oarsman's technique provides the answer, with rapid resolution thereafter of the spasm, thickening, induration, and tenderness in the flexor groups. At other times a simple rest for 1 week, followed by a self-paced stroking in a single shell before undertaking the incessant demands for coordinated and continuous effort in the "eight," solves the problem. But what of the young man who after such a program tolerates all his two-mile and shorter sprint distances, but cannot manage the final four-mile distance without recurrent acute spasm and pain? Should one then advise abandonment of that one final race? Or should one undertake multiple injections of steroids, even surgery, just to get that second two miles out of him? The answer is obvious and is consistent with our original thesis. Every effort should be made to allow a competitor to succeed in his chosen sport, using those abilities and strengths with which he is naturally endowed; however, when the demand is clearly more than he is able to meet, he must be advised to face facts, not grasp at desperate medical "straws."

## Wrist Sprains and the Carpal Scaphoid

Examination of the flexor aspect of the wrist is the least satisfactory of any appraisal in the upper extremity because of the bulk of tendons, nerves, and vessels that crowd through the carpal tunnel between the pisiform and hamate hook, ulnarward, and the navicular and greater multangular, radially. Nonetheless, the pisiform and hamate hook can be palpated by firm pressure thereover, and deep pressure over the lunate can be of diagnostic value. Dorsally, palpation is much more satisfactory, particularly over the carpal scaphoid (or navicular) in the anatomical snuff-box. At the same time the ulnar styloid and the dorsal articulating rim of the distal radius, can be thoroughly tested for bony tenderness or crepitus.

**Wrist Sprains.** These anatomical points scarcely need emphasis, so well known are they, but they must always be surveyed without fail, for the *"jammed wrist"* or *"sprain"* is one of the most common complaints in sports ranging from football to tennis. Examination is virtually useless after swelling has become general in the wrist; in fact, if it is delayed more than 8 hours it should be accompanied by an x-ray. On the field, however, detailed examination will be possible within minutes of the injury, and thorough palpation can then be strikingly accurate, to the extent that the majority of cases can be pronounced clear of fracture, strapped immediately, and the athlete returned to action.

Of equal importance in such a field appraisal, aside from the careful palpation mentioned, is an accurate reconstruction of the precise mechanism of injury, the direction of deviation of the wrist, and the subjective sensation at the moment of injury. Acute dorsiflexion strain, for example, is accompanied by tenderness along the volar aspect of the wrist and occasional tenderness along the dorsal articulating rim of the radius, without crepitus and of a degree short of fracture-line bone pain. Acute radial deviation is accompanied by corresponding tenderness in the ulnar-metacarpal collateral ligament.

**Wrist Dislocations.** These will be quite obvious after such a detailed examination. As with other dislocations, a single attempt should be made to attain reduction during the brief period of post-traumatic numbness. Increasing the deformity with a levering manipulation has been more successful than straight traction in our few such instances. Regardless of method, reduction under anesthesia should be the only method of choice after the first attempt. With the complexities of dislocation classifications, each with its own unique complications, early orthopedic assistance should be the team physician's first consideration.

**The Carpal Scaphoid.** A warning about *the carpal scaphoid* is in order: If there is the slightest suspicion of scaphoid tenderness on pressure in the anatomical snuffbox, x-rays must be obtained and scrutinized carefully. Even then, despite a clearly negative film, the wrist should be splinted, and activity controlled for the ensuing week, after which a second set of films should be taken. Bone absorption along the fracture line usually will have progressed by this time to a point where the fracture will be plainly visible. However, if symptoms remain well localized in the face of a second negative set of films, splint and inactivity should be continued until a third set has been obtained. It is not unknown for such fractures to show up later than two weeks after injury despite repeated x-rays that are completely negative. If symptoms disappear entirely during this same period, activity can be safely resumed, using the latest films as a matter of final record. But, regardless of earlier x-rays, if the symptoms are there, if the localization of pain is there, one must continue to look for fracture.

Once the diagnosis is made, treatment should be the classical cock-up cast, and both athlete and coach should be warned of the possible long-term disability so common with this fracture (e.g., nonunion and osteonecrosis). As with all fractures and major dislocations, orthopedic supervision and treatment is essential.

### Injuries to the Hand

Discussion of hand injuries will be limited to those commonly encountered in athletics, leaving the more extensive problems to the orthopedist, general surgeon, and/or hand-surgeon.

Examination of acute hand injuries should include careful palpation of all bony points. Axial and levering pressures should be exerted on all bones. Bone length should be checked by comparison with the opposite hand. The physician should remain aware of the common incomplete fractures, impacted fractures, and occult fractures. For aside from bony injury which, if suspected, must be confirmed or denied by x-ray, serious injuries such as tendon, nerve, or vascular trauma are virtually never seen in competitive athletics.

**Contusions.** Contusions of every description are seen, ranging from the common palmar bruise, overlying the metacarpal heads in the "glove hand" of the baseball player or hockey goalie, to multiple contusions of the dorsum (e.g., when a pinned-down football player is forced to watch his helpless hand disappear beneath the rigid cleats of friend or foe; under such circumstances, occasional compound fractures of the metacarpals can result, though they are rare). Each hand injury should be thoroughly evaluated for fracture, although aside from the classical fifth metacarpal break from blunt impact to the bony axis skeletal injury is not frequently encountered. Nevertheless, even the lesser contusions, particularly on the dorsum, can swell to arresting proportions unless ice is applied from the first, with elevation and elastic support immediately thereafter. They can therefore be acutely disabling. Most contusions upon prompt treatment subside rapidly with minimal disability, but they must still be treated intensively.

**Hamate Bruise.** One exception to the usually benign course of a properly treated contusion is the "hamate bruise," mentioned heretofore as a particular variety of bone bruise in the pisiform-hamate area deep in the hypothenar eminence. It is of particular significance in the stick sports, in which its chronicity and repeated aggravation may result in deep swelling, distal neuralgia, and vascular effects identical to a true "carpal tunnel syndrome." However, even in this last simple rest and careful padding after resumption of activity suffice, and surgery is unlikely to ever be necessary.

### Injuries to the Fingers

Injuries to the fingers are seldom of the magnitude seen by the average industrial surgeon. They follow a predictable pattern with sprains of varying severity, occasional dislocations, and rarely encountered fractures. Abrasions of the "knuckles," minor lacerations, ungual injuries of agonizing but minor character, and blisters form the overwhelming bulk of cases. Despite the prompt response of these common injuries to early treatment, nothing can render these abused appendages totally painless after injury, and a sprained thumb in a first-team quarterback may constitute more of a problem for everyone than three fractured fingers in a soccer player. Clinically there can be no comparison between the gravity of the two, yet in football the sore thumb may cripple the entire team offense for the 10 days to 2 weeks that it remains symptomatic, while the soccer player can continue to play without the slightest difficulty.

**Finger Sprains.** Finger sprains or "jammed fingers" require careful examination for excess mobility, either counterjoint or in the lateral plane; complete tear of collateral ligaments is not unusual. If normal range of motion is present without limitation and there is no detectible crepitus on palpation of the joint line, a simple strapping of the finger to its adjacent fellow will usually suffice. By this means lateral mobility is limited, overall flexor strength increased, and hyperextension prevented. For the 1st week thereafter a molded splint in the partially flexed anatomical position should be applied after each workout and worn until the following workout, at which time the finger-to-finger strapping is reapplied. After the 1st week no particular reinforcement is necessary except in instances of complete collateral laxity; splint and strapping are then best continued for at least four weeks. One might assume that under this admittedly Spartan regimen local pain and swelling would be a considerable disadvantage. However, possibly because of the early motion engendered exactly the opposite has been true: Usually the injured joint is indistinguishably normal in 2 to 3 weeks despite daily violence.

**Traumatic Dislocations.** Traumatic dislocations of every description may be encountered. These can be easily reduced immediately, usually by increasing the deformity and levering the distal articulating surface back into position (rather than by straight traction). The usual post-reduction treatment would then be a splint for the routine 4 to 6 weeks, ending with a stiff and painfully swollen joint for at least 3 weeks thereafter. After immediate reduction, on the other hand, provided motion is then without limitation and the joint surfaces are not crepitant, treatment can be identical to that for sprains of the finger: finger-to-finger strapping for uninterrupted workouts and a molded splint between (prolonged for 4 to 6 weeks). Pain and swelling have always been minimal under this regimen, a stable and freely mobile joint has been readily apparent from the 2nd week onward, and no late problems have developed. If there is a suspicion of articular comminution, it should be confirmed by x-ray, for such results cannot then be reasonably expected. However, prompt reduction is neither as likely under these circumstances nor will motion thereafter be free of limitation, so differentiation should be clear from the beginning.

**Avulsion of the Extensor Tendon.** A problem common to all sports is the *"mallet-finger," the "baseball-finger,"* or the *"dropped finger"*— the familiar avulsion of the extensor tendon from the distal phalanx. If upon x-ray there is no accompanying fracture (the rule rather than the exception), those methods of treatment directed toward fracture seem somewhat radical (e.g., Kirschner wires passing in various directions and the finger immobilized in extension at the distal and flexion at the middle joint for 6 to 8 weeks). Alternatively, when bony avulsion is not a prominent feature, prolonged splinting has been recommended, with the distal joint in hyperextension and the middle joint in 90 degree flexion, anatomically relaxing the extensor hood, hence relaxing tension on the torn tendon margins. This latter position and treatment may be fine theoretically, but will bar almost all competitive sports for a minimum of 6 to 8 weeks, a price no athlete will pay to rectify a painless droop of one fingertip. Consequently, a *compromise* has been necessary to assure even a modicum of cooperation. Much to our surprise, *simple hyperextension* of the distal phalanx for 8 weeks of uninterrupted athletic competition, with no regard for the proximal joints, has proved uniformly successful, even in a varsity basketball player.

We have not discussed *"the split finger,"* which certainly qualifies as an athletic injury because of its association with baseball catchers and errant foul tips. However, the omission is deliberate, because it can run the entire gamut of finger injuries, from painful but simple ungual avulsions to compound comminuted fractures and fracture-dislocations of any of the three phalanges of the finger with accompanying integumental splits, capsular disruptions, tendon avulsions, and soft-tissue tears of every description and variety. Each injury must be thoroughly evaluated of itself and treatment initiated that will assure maximum functional recovery, just as with any such injury regardless of the cause, and said treatment should be carried through to maximum benefit regardless of the time required. There should be no compromise whatever for the sake of an early return to athletics. A functioning digit is far more important than a season of baseball no matter the anguished protests of the injured athlete. This is not to say that there will not be an occasional instance of bizarre soft tissue splitting that will best be served by a simple molded splint dressing without suture, but such treatment can only be applied after thorough appraisal of the total injury has eliminated the possibility of skeletal, capsular, or tendon injury, not as a routine measure for all "split fingers."

# 14

# *Injuries to the Trunk*

## THE CHEST WALL

The chest wall with its supporting rib cage is readily accessible to thorough inspection and palpation anteriorly, laterally, and posteriorly. The covering muscles are extremely well developed and defined in the competitive athlete, particularly in the pectoral region anteriorly and even more so in the rhomboid and paraspinal areas posteriorly. The upper rib cage is obscured laterally by the shoulder girdle and its own heavy musculature. Nevertheless, a combination of careful palpation for swelling, tenderness, crepitus, or deformity with a judicious springing of the resilient rib cage should provide the examining physician with all that is necessary for a reasonably accurate diagnosis.

### Fractures

*Fractures of the ribs* can be detected by such means, even in the face of negative x-rays. By the same means *fractures of the costal cartilage,* invisible by x-rays in this young age group, can be detected and directly evaluated. Likewise, *sternal injuries,* often impossible to demonstrate roentgenographically except with the most elaborate laminographic technique, are immediately apparent, as are minor dislocations and displacements at the angle or xiphisternal junction.

*Treatment* of all these and other injuries of the chest wall is largely uniform. Some type of splinting support must be provided for so long as symptoms last. This is complicated in athletics by the fact that for any truly competitive sport deep and labored respiration is mandatory. Hence, these injuries might be termed "self-limiting," that is to say, while the least symptom persists, the athlete cannot exert himself to any useful degree. Local pain from rib fractures or costal cartilage fractures and separations can be quite severe but becomes rapidly controllable with adequate splinting support. The more serious problems of paradoxical motion from multiple rib fractures remain a remote possibility, but such massive trauma is not often seen, even in our most violent contact sports. Consequently, the need for external traction devices has never been a factor despite the theoretical possibility.

The tried-and-true canvas rib belt with adjustable buckles and one over-the-shoulder supporting strap has proved ideal, providing the support necessary to control both initial and subsequent discomfort yet constantly adjustable for the prone position in bed or the increase in upper abdominal girth that follows the usual athlete's meal. Rib injuries of every variety, involving the fourth in the mid-axillary line and downward, have proved amenable to this supportive treatment. However, injuries above this level, more directly subject to stress from muscles of the shoulder girdle, require a more indirect sling immobilization of the ipsilateral shoulder and arm to control discomfort. Barring internal visceral injuries, discomfort in either instance is usually controllable by these simple measures without resorting to paravertebral injection. It remains only to wait patiently until all symptoms subside.

### Injuries Involving the Pectorals

**Pectoral Strain.** With regard to the specific injuries that are more or less unique to athletics, one of the most common is the pectoral strain, a result of overenthusiastic exertion of the pectoralis major, sometimes bilaterally (too many pushups, for example), other times unilaterally (occasionally seen in shot putters). As with most muscle strains, the aching pain and tenderness are maximal at the origin or insertion on the skeleton, hence are found either along the digitations overlying the costal cartilages of ribs II to V and the intervening lateral sternal border or along the anterior axillary fold formed by the arching fibers of the pectoralis major as they merge into the humeral tendon. Soreness is usually the complaint as well as the finding, indicating a mild strain. Swelling is also present, occasionally indicating an actual disruption of muscle fibers with bleeding.

In both instances, rest of the muscle is indicated, best attained by a sling to the ipsilateral arm and shoulder in unilateral cases or an elimination of pushups and the like in bilateral cases. By and large such simple treatment will suffice. Symptoms and signs clear within 2 to 3 days, and full activity can be resumed.

In instances of actual swelling local ice should be applied for the first 24 to 48 hours, following which motion should be started only to tolerance and without resistance. A gradual controlled resistance after full painless motion has been regained restores functional strength rapidly over the ensuing 5 to 7 days. If it takes longer, so be it! To become impatient with the time lost in these cases, to succumb to the temptation of injecting the pectoralis with local anesthetic and/or steroid, may render the athlete free of disabling pain and determined to resume full activity with or without medical approval. The outcome inevitably is a torn pectoralis major muscle of permanent significance, a high price to pay for a few days "saved."

**Tears of the Pectoralis Major.** Such tears are rare, but they are always the result of some such ill advised enthusiasm. The visible and palpable defect usually appears in the anterior axillary fold area, is occasionally amenable to surgical repair (though the postoperative result may be worse than the injury), and is rarely disabling whether repaired or not.

**Tears of the Pectoralis Minor.** A similar injury occurs deep under the pectoralis major in the pectoralis minor area, seen as the result of falling heavily on the elbows with most of the body weight, effectively "breaking" the fall but producing a constant, increasing ache deep under the pectoralis major and a palpable swelling high up and medial beneath the anterior axillary fold. The swelling can reach lemon size without detectable change in the smooth external contour of the overlying pectoralis major. Aspiration has never been attempted, simply because disability despite the swelling has never been sufficient to warrant such an undertaking. Disability persists as a deep-seated ache, that is aggravated only by falling in precisely the same manner. Falling thusly is not good technique at best, hence it should be discouraged, but in this particular situation it should be avoided entirely. If such is impossible, all contact work must be barred until the swelling completely disappears; otherwise, since the swelling may take several weeks to disappear completely, a cautious, graduated return to supervised action within 8 to 10 days would seem reasonable.

## Contusions of the Lower Rib Cage

Of much greater frequency and much more of a problem are the contusions of the lower rib cage. A review of the skeletal anatomy reveals the basis for these injuries as well as the problems presented. In addition to being subcutaneous, the entire costal margin and anterior chest wall is largely cartilaginous, hence invisible by x-ray. Moreover, in the competitive athlete the lower anterior rib cage is considerably more prominent than usual owing to the flat muscularity of the abdomen below. It is thus more prone to injury from blunt impact. A further review of anatomy also demonstrates the digitations of the external and internal obliques and, toward the midline, the rectus muscles, all of which attach on this protuberant area, all of which are highly developed in the athlete, and consequently become involved in the most minor contusions as well as the more significant major fractures and separations.

### Costochondral Involvement

A whole series of related injuries is seen as a result of abnormal forces impacting upon the anterior chest wall, not to mention the possibility of those deeper visceral effects discussed in a previous chapter. For instance, blunt sternal injuries rarely cause bony disruption in a controlled athletic program, but over and above the direct "bone bruise" tenderness, which may last for some time, there are additional problems associated with the anatomical factors enumerated above. The natural springiness of this particular area will conduct and focus impacting forces upon those particular points of maximum stress, the articulations between bone and cartilage, the costochondral junctions. Direct conduction of the forces causes tenderness to appear at the *sternal angle,* over the adjacent *costosternal junctions,* as well as over the more remote yet anatomically contiguous *costochondral junctions,* all as a direct reflection of the area's "springiness." Similarly, blows on the tip of the xiphoid distally "sprain" *the xiphisternal junction,* giving rise to subsequent disabling and annoyingly persistent symptoms because of the constant association of the attached and contiguous rectus muscles with every normal body movement and every change of position.

**Treatment.** *Costochondral "sprains,"* with local tenderness but without palpable discontinuity, as well as the more severe *costochondral separations,* with palpable discontinuity and occasional false motion, inevitably limit any return to activity until local symptoms subside. *External support by rib belt* provides maximum initial pain relief as well as long-term healing in all instances, but recovery of athletic efficiency depends entirely on the individual's pain threshold. Some rare boys return to action without visible problems in 2 to 5 days; others require 2 weeks of patient rehabilitation and reassurance before they can resume competition.

The problem, therefore, is essentially "self-limiting," with effective competition possible only after all necessary athletic functions have become painless, no matter how long such recovery may take.

**Fracture of the Costal Margin.** This cannot be "gutted out." It is disabling from the moment of impact, it is palpably evident by local deformity or palpable crepitus on respiration, and it is as painful as a broken rib. Because it is cartilage, it does not heal rapidly or kindly. This unfortunate characteristic is attested to by the persistent post-operative difficulties encountered by patients who have undergone abdominothoracic procedures, persistent despite a direct visual apposition of the divided costal-margin ends and internal skeletal fixation. Hence, regardless of the rapid subsidence of acute discomfort in 3 to 5 days with the help of a rib belt, disability must be measured in weeks to months. A solid union or a demonstrable nonunion is an absolute necessity before any athletic activity, even solo running, can be approved. Some authors have suggested local injections to relieve pain and speed recovery, but nothing has as yet offered a means of assuring rapid and solid cartilaginous healing, and this is the disabling factor, not the local discomfort.

## The "Floating Ribs"

Attention should be directed to the "floating ribs," the eleventh and twelfth. In the athlete as well as in others of their age these ribs are truly "floating," moving with certain limitations with every movement of the trunk. The serratus anterior, the external and internal obliques, the intercostals, and the transversalis muscle, all attach on these ribs to a greater or lesser extent. Direct impact, particularly to the free ends of these ribs, can result in local swelling and pain, that may involve all of these muscles to a point where even normal walking is difficult. It should not be surprising, therefore, that immediate application of ice, continued for 48 hours, will barely suffice to control the discomfort. The concomitant bruising of the bony tip of the rib further complicates matters and delays recovery, while every movement utilizing the muscles above, which can scarcely be avoided even by strict bed rest, inevitably aggravates and prolongs disability. And it must be remembered that with each injury there is a serious possibility of even more dangerous and disabling renal injury. Hence, patience and close follow-up are mandatory. Initial cold application to control bleeding must be followed by a very deliberate exercise regimen, specifically designed to use in a graduated program just those muscles named, culminating in a running and twisting pattern of increasing vigor and violence. Only then can any thought of full competition activity be entertained. Such a program takes upwards of a week to 10 days, but even the most careful daily check and supervision does not effectively shorten this period.

### "Stitches"

Discussion of the *"stitch in the side"* is in order. The acute unilateral pain on inspiration, more often seen on the right side, the unique localization of pain in lower rib cage and adjacent upper abdominal quadrant, and the crippling yet temporary nature of the disability are familiar to all. The severity of the pain, its direct association with deep inspiration, hence the impossibility of deep respiration in spite of acute air hunger, all combine to stop the affected athlete as efficiently as would a broken leg. Fortunately, these attacks are always short-lived, lasting no more than 3 to 5 minutes, and they are not characteristically recurrent. There is a direct association with extreme respiratory exertion—in other words, with any activity that builds up significant oxygen debt and with it extreme respiratory exertion—and it can strike the well-conditioned athlete as indiscriminately as the novice.

There have been theories that these attacks are secondary to gas in the colon on the right or gas in the stomach on the left; others that attribute the picture to a momentary swelling of the liver in its taut capsule by a brief passive congestion secondary to a temporary left heart inefficiency. Be that as it may, the supine position with arms upraised seems to have an empirical effect in shortening the duration of these episodes. A rest of 10 to 15 minutes thereafter, followed by resumption of activity, does not cause a recurrent episode, nor are recurrences likely in the weeks that follow.

The efficacy of this empirical measure, which must owe its value to the operculum effect of the intercostals on inspiration and some mechanical alteration thereof, suggests a possible explanation of the basic symptomatic picture. A spasm or cramp of the intercostal muscles of the lower chest could give rise to the precise picture, one of pain that typically occurs when the operculum effect is at its inspiratory height. Accordingly, it should be relieved by mechanical assistance to that same inspiratory operculum effect, and, right or wrong, this particular maneuver does work uniformly.

## THE ABDOMINAL WALL

Excluding internal abdominal injuries, always one of the most difficult and important tasks of the physician in athletics, there remains a large number of muscle strains, contusions, postoperative scars, and herniae to plague the athlete.

### Muscle Strains

Strains are common, usually the result of overenthusiastic conditioning work after a long layoff but sometimes secondary to the enthusiasms so characteristic of this particular age group. Thus, the most severe *rectus muscle strain* encountered occurred in a young man who tried to break the Yale record for consecutive situps. This was attempted in an all-day effort with planned feedings "on the fly," an effort that culminated in acutely painful and swollen recti, maximally tender not only at the attachments on the costal cage and the pubic arch and at each tendinous inscription but also at the exact anatomical fusion of the semicircular line of Douglas on the lateral borders of the recti! (His chief complaint was of painfully excoriated blisters of both buttocks.)

Of more reasonable origin and of less severity, *other acute strains* are seen involving *the external oblique muscle,* usually in its digitations on the costal margin and ribs, where swelling and acute pain can be accurately localized.

All instances of acute abdominal strain, regardless of the cause or initial severity, are disabling because of the universal function of these muscles in every-day life. Hence, they fall into the category of "self-limiting" injuries in that no athletic efforts are possible until pain subsides completely after adequate rest, which may necessitate a total layoff for up to 10 days.

### Contusions of the Iliac Crest

Contusions are not usually encountered in an area that does not provide some rigid background upon which external forces can impact, so are rare in the abdominal wall except overlying the costal cage proximally or the pelvis distally. The former area has already been discussed with regard to the lower ribs and costal margin. The latter is the site of a most significant and distressingly common injury, *the so-called "iliac crest" or "hip pointer,"* of painful memory to scores of athletes in both contact and non-contact sports.

To understand the striking disability caused by this particular injury, one must return to the regional anatomy, a review of which demonstrates a firm attachment of external oblique muscle fibers to the external lip of the iliac crest, internal oblique fibers to the intermediate line of the crest, and transversalis fibers to the internal lip. In the area of the anterior superior spine these attachments become loose and areolar, as the muscle layers sweep medialward toward the inguinal area. Any blow that rides up and over this bony prominence cannot avoid tearing some or all these fibers or, short of that, crushing the overlapping bulge of muscle along the crest, a bulge characteristic of the muscular, trained athlete. Even worse, a blow that impacts the anterior spine area of loose areolar attachment can shear along the crest, stripping all the layers from their attachments as it goes. The result is acute and immediate pain, steadily increasing in severity, progressively hampering every movement, and ofttimes requiring hospitalization for sedation and narcosis to control local pain, that is agonizingly aggravated by laughing, sneezing, coughing, turning over in bed, or even emptying bladder or bowels.

So striking is the pain engendered by this injury that a search for occult avulsions, incomplete fractures, or fractures without displacement of the crest or iliac wing will at times be carried out by those unfamiliar with this classical picture. Bedrest for prolonged periods, season long athletic prohibition, and other stringent measures will also occasionally be seen as a direct result of this clinical unfamiliarity. In essence, however, the mechanisms involved are simple—the impacting blow is uniformly less than remarkable vis-à-vis the dramatic disability, and in the contact sports specific local padding is provided to further minimize the impact. Characteristically, therefore, the athlete continues for several minutes after the injury before the increasing discomfort causes him to seek help, at which time a careful history will quickly yield the diagnosis.

**Examination.** More important than the history is a painstaking examination of the injury itself. Maximal tenderness and initial swelling must be precisely and immediately located for a number of reasons.

Firstly, localization rapidly demonstrates the extent of injury despite the diffuse and increasing disability. Thus, tenderness on the iliac wing below the crest, together with tenderness in the overlapping bulge but without tenderness on the crest itself, indicates a contusion that is essentially a bone-bruise and muscle-pinch, a lesser injury with shorter disability. At the other extreme, maximum tenderness up and over the crest must mean a significant tearing of muscular attachments, hence a maximum injury and disability.

Secondly, such careful localization is possible only at the outset, for bleeding soon obscures all findings and once established creates enough local irritation and spasm to further obscure an adequate treatment program.

Thirdly, with such localization a preliminary prediction can be made as to total length of athletic disability, of vital interest to everyone. Although daily examinations must be carried through regardless, they merely serve to confirm the initial examination findings and thereby provide a guideline for a logical treatment program.

**Treatment.** Initial treatment is the same regardless of the severity or acute localization of pain, because bleeding and subsequent spasm and swelling cause a similar degree of discomfort in all of these injuries unless adequate steps are taken. An adhesive strapping is employed that tilts the trunk toward the pelvis on that side, to prevent aggravation of the growing spasm (See Fig. 22-2). Ice is then applied directly over the area and kept there for at least 48 hours (sometimes 72 hours). Local swelling and tenderness are checked daily, progress thereby ascertained, and this progress correlated with the initial findings.

In the lesser direct iliac bruise and overlying muscle pinch, swelling usually remains minimal, and symptoms are well under control by the second day. Ice can then be discontinued, and active motion begun without using local heat that may restart bleeding. At the other extreme, true crest injury will present persistent discomfort on every motion, swelling is maximal, and the full 3-day ice treatment will be necessary with few exceptions; heat should be avoided and active motion progressively resumed at a slower pace than in the lesser instances.

In all cases, each graduated step in rehabilitation must be checked daily for recurrent swelling. As motion is steadily restored, a minimum of preliminary local heat, followed by jogging and running to tolerance, can be started, culminating in sprinting, twisting exercises of increasing violence, explosive efforts such as coming out of stance and "hitting the bucker," and, finally, a return to full action with a special bulky pad over the injured area.

Such a regime returns athletes with the lesser injuries to full activity in 3 to 4 days and those with more extensive injuries in 6 to 10 days. Although these results may be viewed askance by those accustomed to total disability for 2 and 3 weeks or longer, of all the injuries commonly seen in athletics, the *"hip pointer"* provides the greatest reward to a careful day-to-day evaluation and re-evaluation of progress and a deliberately correlated rehabilitation program.

## THE DORSAL AND LUMBOSACRAL AREAS

Consistent with the limits of this volume, no attempt will be made to cover all traumas, except as they occur within the framework of competitive athletics. This limitation applies particularly to any discussion of back injuries in competitive sports. Fractures, fracture-dislocations, and major spinal cord and cauda equina injuries do occur, but their rarity is a tribute to sensible and organized athletic control. The diagnosis of these major injuries is hardly a problem, and their necessary disposition for maximum benefit of medical care is even more clear cut. It will be assumed that the reader will have had sufficient training and experience to render superfluous any brief summary of diagnosis and treatment of these injuries.

Accurate diagnosis is essential in order to differentiate between the major clinical injury, requiring immediate hospitalization and intensive specialist care, and the type of injury to be discussed more fully in this section. Examination and an accurate on-the-spot history are the primary requisites, and every physician with direct responsibility must be prepared to evaluate his findings unerringly.

In terms of history: What happened? Was it a kick, a knee, a helmet, a stick? Was it a twist or a fall? Did it happen just now or has it been building up from an incident in the past? Is there any previous history of similar episodes? If so, what diagnostic and therapeutic measures were undertaken at that time? All of these questions must be answered. Before any decision can be made about moving the injured athlete, a rapid preliminary survey must determine whether he can move his lower extremities normally, whether there are any paresthesias or other significant sensory changes, where the pain is, and how bad it is.

Unlike the frightening neck injury, certain anatomical characteristics play a pivotal role in the rarity of truly significant dorsolumbar skeletal injury. As can be seen in any review of the region, the paravertebral musculature runs alongside the spine from neck to pelvis. If one has never examined a typical competitive athlete, he cannot appreciate the potential strength and bulk of these massive muscle groups. Characteristically the dorsolumbar spine appears as a deep valley, surrounded in the dorsal area by dense rhomboids, trapezius, as well as bulging paravertebrals. In the lumbar area it is even more securely walled in by a steadily thickening mass of paravertebrals on each side. Torsions and flexions, as well as direct blows, any one of which would seriously damage and possibly cripple the non-athlete, are absorbed and dissipated by this surrounding musculature, a factor that is not only well recognized within the athletic world but is deliberately reinforced in the contact sports by a series of "back-breaker" exercises. It is for this reason that we view askance any athlete who tries to avoid the painful drudgery of strenuous back-conditioning work or obtains some vague medical excuse to avoid it. Demanding though such exercises may be, they are expressly designed to build muscle that may prevent a permanently crippling injury!

## Fractures

Despite these local factors significant skeletal injuries do occur and must be identified immediately, without the advantage of a preliminary x-ray. The initial impact is of key importance in alerting the examiner to the possibility of serious injury. If there is forcible impact, particularly if it is by some rigid, unexpected object, and impact is immediately followed by an unusual degree of pain, the possibility of a *fractured spinous process* or, if the site of maximal impact is to the side of the midline, the possibility of a *fractured transverse process* must be seriously entertained: x-rays must be obtained and necessary treatment initiated. If there is a sudden hyperflexion and examination reveals a suspicious gibbus in the area, a *compression fracture* must be suspected until x-rays rule otherwise. Most important of all, if there is any trace of sensory change, subjective or objective, *spinal cord or cauda equina injury* must never be forgotten and must be followed up immediately.

## Contusions

The incidence of potentially crippling injuries is extremely low, hence, having looked for them from the first and having found no evidence of them, with what should the physician concern himself? The overwhelming preponderance of impacts results only in *contusions,* which, if they do not involve neighboring ribs, are usually of little consequence despite their extent.

They can range from visible imprints of entire helmet tops to clearly outlined cleat prints, more painful in appearance than they actually are. As long as there is no underlying bony structure that is acutely tender at the same time (hence possibly fractured), there is neither cause for concern nor significant disability.

The sole exception is *contusion over the lumbodorsal fascia,* which owes its unique character to the anatomy of the area, in which a dense layer of fascia extends as a thick sheetlike structure over the entire lumbosacral area, passing external to the paraspinal muscles. The potential dead space beneath this layer extends from flank to flank, with only the regularly spaced spinous processes to mark the midline. A contusion in this area may give rise to a hematoma of arresting proportions. So extensive can this accumulation be that aspiration is often necessary, not just to relieve pain, which will be minimal, but to relieve the peculiar pressure effects on all trunk movements. Unfortunately, aspiration of this area will seldom suffice unless repeated a number of times, because pressure obliteration of this dead space is virtually impossible and the smooth fascia overlying the space will persist in ballooning up. Incision for drainage is far too radical, while stringent athletic disability remains difficult to justify in the face of an absolute minimum of truly disabling symptoms. Patiently repeated aspirations usually prove the most practical solution in these instances and ultimately prove permanently successful.

**Back Strains**

Much more common and even more of a problem are *acute and chronic back strains,* ranging from the usual "trade-mark" backache of the oarsman to the sudden and crippling spasm that can seize the long distance runner. In all instances the common denominator is spasm, visible and palpable. Hence, a thorough sequential examination of all backs much be performed to assure adequate differentiation and identification of the myriad varieties of backaches, spasms, "pulls," "bad back," and the like, that will always plague the athletic physician.

**Examination.** Every back should be inspected under good light and in the standing position to begin with, checking any list, scoliosis, or kyphosis. Then forward bending, lateral bending, and rotation must be tested, and any limitation carefully noted—these initial steps alone will often quickly outline a spastic paravertebral muscle group that can be both seen and felt. In the supine position, straight leg raising should be tested on both sides, lumbar flexion tested by flexing thighs on hips and rolling the hips cephalad up off the table, and any sacro-iliac pathology localized by the heel-to-knee test. In the prone position, direct search should be made for areas of discrete spasm and "trigger points."

Using these maneuvers, the whole gamut of back strains common to athletics will fall into some logical order, with, for example, clearly localized areas of spasm and strain, or tender areas of fibrosis and scarring, which can then be correlated with the causative factors and necessary adjustments made. The weight-lifter frequently reports with an acute strain of both lumbar paravertebral groups, as evidenced by bilateral spasm and acute tenderness at their insertions on the pelvis. On closer questioning he may admit to "dead-lifting" some astronomical total of weights. The lordotic distance-runner suffers spasms of low back pain toward the end of two miles, purely as a result of his peculiar posture, about which nothing can be done. The hammer or discus thrower exhibits acute spasm in the left paravertebral area, a result of the inordinate strain placed on this muscle in the effort of throwing. Not to be forgotten, the unfortunate oarsman can strain his lumbar paravertebrals acutely, not by his rowing, but by the motion of heaving the 1250 pound shell out of the water—this must be done each day, and must be done by all eight men together, for, if any one of the eight is ahead of his colleagues in the concerted effort, his back suffers without the shell having been moved an inch out of the water. Once such a strain has been established, how can the oarsman avoid persistent trouble each time he tries to row?

**Treatment.** In all these instances of strain the immediate treatment is heat, either by infra-red lamp in the prone position or, better yet, active motion under a hot shower which always relieves the spasm and pain for as long as it is applied. But the principal problem is the steady return of pain thereafter, which must be met by repeated treatments or by massage with a counter-irritant.

During the acute phase nothing whatever can be done athletically, and the victim is effectively shelved until all spasm and discomfort subside, no matter how long this may take. Even then he must undertake a graduated series of steps prior to a return to full activity, each step designed to restore strength and function without reaggravation of the original strain. This is the area in which careful coordination with the coaching staff is essential, because workouts must be carefully designed to correct whatever faults might have led to the initial episode as well as to restore the athlete to action. No attempt will be made to detail such specific arrangements, since they differ not only from sport to sport but from athlete to athlete, but the guiding principle should be a gradual restoration of activity and strength in those motions essential to the sport, without at any time placing the athlete in circumstances in which he cannot immediately desist from all effort should he suffer the slightest recurrent twinge. In the case of the track man this means a modicum of weight work and jogging, then a lot of over distance jogging and short sprints, carefully building back to all the requirements of his event before competition is allowed. With the oarsman this means working out alone in the "tubs" and single scull prior to re-entering the big shell.

**Chronic Sacro-iliac Strain**

What of *the chronic "sacro-iliac," the "bad back"?* By definition the problem is not acute, and careful examination usually reveals little if anything. X-rays will have to be taken and reviewed, though in the usual case five or ten sets may already be available. By and large no opinion should be given by the team physician unless he is an orthopedist, in which case he will be well equipped to dispose of these cases. If he is not, an orthopedic evaluation should be sought for a clear-cut diagnosis of the true disability. If there is true orthopedic disability, preventing full-scale competition, this should be made clear to the boy and further participation barred. In no instance should a back condition be allowed to modify participation in the everyday drudgery of practice while permitting full-scale game competition. If one orthopedic consultant cannot appreciate the need for these admittedly stringent standards—necessary for squad morale and for the well-being of the athlete concerned—another opinion should be sought. Nothing can be more discouraging than trying to take care of an athlete who, with a medical "blessing" so-to-speak, has back aches at his own convenience, whenever he fails or fears he will fail some competitive demand or when an unpleasant practice session does not meet with his approval. He soon destroys any confidence that coach or fellow squad-members may have once held for him; much worse, he eventually undermines his own self-confidence—a high price to pay for oversympathetic medical recommendations.

**Sciatica**

What of the occasional case of *"sciatica"?* As part of the routine back examination outlined above, tests are included that should provide the examiner with most of the usual signs that indicate a *herni-*

*ated intervertebral disc*. With symptomatic "sciatica" a complete neurosurgical or orthopedic work-up is a primary necessity, all athletic competition aside. Whether myelography should be part of this work-up is up to the consultant involved, but under no circumstances can a truly suspicious case be allowed to continue in any type of stressful competition at the risk of further herniation and possible irreversible nerve damage. Negative findings must remain negative findings in the face of the most stressful weight work and conditioning before any thought can be given to a return to full competition regardless of the circumstances. Disc surgery is neither innocuous enough nor curative enough to warrant any other decision.

## Chronic Back Conditions

The same can be said for any *chronic back condition* of clinical significance, be it congenital, such as spondylolisthesis with spondyloschisis, or a residual of past injury. None of the contact or non-contact sports, with the possible exception of swimming, can be said to deal kindly with the chronic back ailment, whatever it may be. If the ailment is already symptomatic, how can one judge the degree of aggravation or its permanent effect?

The most careful judgment is necessary in handling these cases. If, for example, the problem has been or can be completely worked up, the diagnosis agreed upon by all consultants concerned, and there is no disability that prevents a full-scale competition in all aspects of the sport in question, there can be no reason to bar such competition. However, if any of the routine conditioning and practice schedules must be permanently altered or if special appliances must be worn at all times simply to allow a limited and borderline competition, such a case must be diverted into less demanding areas of activity. In the contact sports there can be no question of the validity of this position, but serious opposition can be expected in certain of the non-contact sports. The doctor with the primary responsibility must be the one to make the final decision, and to do so he must know the varying demands of each of these many sports. For example, rowing is a non-contact sport but is clearly unkind to the low back despite the niceties of modern technique that depend as much on leg drive for power, whereas rifle shooting is quite undemanding. As another example, swimming would seem innocuous and healthful, as indeed it is on a non-competitive basis, but the flip turn, free style or backstroke, repeated incessantly throughout every competitive workout, will put even the healthiest back to a severe test. All these are factors that must be taken into serious consideration before any final decision can be reached. The broad statement of principle outlined above still holds in the non-contact sports as well: Competition and all the drudgery such competition entails must be tolerated without symptoms; otherwise, temporary or even permanent aggravation of the back problem may result. No sport is worth such a crippling outcome.

# 15

# Injuries to the Pelvic Girdle Area

The pelvic girdle will for convenience be defined to include not only the pelvic girdle itself but the hip joint and the musculature principally concerned with its movement and stabilization. Our discussion will include problems involving such muscles as the pectineus, sartorius, gracilis, and adductors, that are more a part of the thigh, because problems pertaining to them lead to disability referable to hipjoint mobility.

A review of anatomy reveals that the pubic arch, the iliac wings, the sacrococcygeal area behind, and the ischial tuberosity deep below are all bony points that are both easily palpated and tested by direct pressure. The hip joint and the neck of the femur, naturally, cannot be felt or directly tested, but the greater trochanter is virtually subcutaneous, even in the most heavily muscled athlete, hence constitutes an important check point. Because direct skeletal injury to the pelvic girdle is practically unknown in controlled competitive athletics, these structures should be checked and tested only preliminary to a more thorough examination. The attached muscles in and around the girdle are the real source of disability in athletics, and a series of functional tests is of the utmost importance in evaluating any complaint referable to the pelvic girdle.

Every such complaint must be subjected to a *simple series of tests,* all quite simply and rapidly done, with the athlete in the supine position. He is asked to raise his foot off the ground with knee straight, then, keeping his foot just clear of the ground, he is asked to abduct his leg against resistance and then adduct against resistance. Lastly, he is asked to raise the entire leg against resistance. By this means the tensor fascia lata, the gluteus maximus, and the short rotators and stabilizers of the hip joint are tested by abduction, the adductor magnus, minimus, longus, and brevis, the pectineus, the gracilis, and even the obturator are tested by adduction, and the sartorius, iliopsoas, and quadriceps by extension. By testing against resistance the precise point of discomfort can be simultaneously determined with accuracy, allowing one muscle group to be differentiated from another.

## "GROIN STRAINS"

Of all the problems encountered in and around the pelvic girdle, the most frequent and the most difficult to handle are *"groin strains."* Not very often seen outside of athletics, these are among the most common athletic complaints, characteristically seen in early season hockey and in any of the running sports after a practice or game on a muddy field. The mechanism is one of a sudden, unexpected hyperextension or hyperabduction on slippery footing. So predictable is this mechanism that we fully expect to see these problems after a rainy day in the fall or spring or after hockey practice commences in late fall. We are never disappointed. Because the muscles involved are quite sizable and because the mechanism is more a sudden "stretch" than a snap during contraction, the uniform picture is one of a slowly increasing soreness and tightness characteristic of a strain, rather than a sudden pain and acute disability characteristic of a complete tearing of muscle fibers. Because these muscles are so essential to every type of hip motion, the disability steadily becomes so hampering to all movement that further self-aggravation is very nearly impossible. These injuries, therefore, are reported relatively promptly, at times so promptly that without the functional tests mentioned above the temptation would be to ignore the complaint entirely. However, to ignore even the most minor complaint of "tightness in the groin" and to send the athlete back to "push it," as it were, can result in a true muscle tear and a disability that will last three to five weeks!

**Treatment.** Treatment should be prompt and thorough, with ice and compression by an elastic-bandage figure-of-eight "spica," flexing the thigh on the hip by 5 or 10 degrees and thereby preventing hyperextension. All athletic endeavor should be discontinued, and all effort turned toward the control of swelling (that is, bleeding) in the involved muscle group. Once bleeding becomes established to any extent whatever, the subsequent absorptive inflammatory reaction effectively increases local spasm and pain and thereby prolongs the period of enforced inactivity. And this last is the most important, not so much in terms of early return to competition but because any scarring, hence contracture, of these essential muscles will result in recurrent, chronic difficulties that can be season long, even career long.

**Rehabilitation.** Active rehabilitation must be resumed as early as possible, as soon as bleeding has definitely subsided, yet not a moment too soon. Hence, careful daily evaluation is an absolute necessity, gauging the degree of activity against the degree of local reaction in a continuing program of readjustment. "Spica" support should be continued throughout rehabilitation, sometimes for weeks, but the most important factor is controlled motion in a series of graduated steps, using local heat only in the form of a counter-irritant during these workouts, rather than as a penetrating external source that may stir up recurrent bleeding. Under this management athletes with these strains can be returned to full scale activity in 4 to 7 days without recurrent problems and without the necessity of local injections, whirlpools, massages, and other modalities. Without such direct supervision and, in particular, without early and increasing motion the resulting scar tissue will not only be permanently palpable but will hamper the athlete for weeks and months.

### Iliopsoas Strain

As to the more specific characteristics exhibited by particular muscle groups so involved, the "ilio psoas strain" warrants further discussion. Some have grouped all groin strains as ilio psoas strains, but we have been unable to confirm this opinion because it is frequently possible to pinpoint involved muscles far removed from this specific group. This is not to say that it does not occur as a real entity, for one does occasionally see instances where the pain and swelling pinpoint high up, lateral to the adductor and pectineus and medial to the sartorius, yet palpably extending up under the inguinal ligament. There can be no question that such cases represent the classical iliopsoas strain. Routine treatment, however, has always resulted in rapid recovery, possibly before the development of more chronic symptoms extending up along the psoas into the pelvis and low back.

### Sartorius Strain

A persistent minor difficulty has been uniformly encountered with sartorius strain because of its proximal insertion on the anterior iliac spine. The actual muscular disability responds in a manner consistent with the course outlined above, but with football players the squatting "ready" position may continue for weeks to give annoying symptoms either on the iliac spine or immediately contiguous thereto.

## Sartorius Tear

Case 6, R. B.: An experienced varsity oarsman, he had noted some mild "tightness" in his left groin for 3 or 4 days, never significant enough for him to report or remember but noticeable on climbing out of the shell after each practice session thereafter. The area always "loosened up" after walking around for a few minutes, was localizable in retrospect to the upper third of the sartorius, and hardly seemed worthy of his notice.

In the midst of a 2-mile sprint trial pain in the area became acute and agonizing, yet as part of an eight-oared crew and long inured to all degrees of muscular pain, he continued on, grimly working his seat slide and sweep in unison with the others. At the conclusion of the sprint he had to be helped from the shell. There was a visible swelling of his entire medial thigh and a complete loss of extension and adduction. Examination shortly thereafter revealed a massive hemorrhage of the anterior and medial thigh with a total inability or disinclination to use any adductor or extensor. Bedrest, ice, and compression were immediately instituted, with prompt cessation of further bleeding. There was slow resorption of the massive extravasation. By the 4th to 5th day the mass had localized over and in the sartorius; in another 10 days a firm and unquestionable fibrous scar could be outlined at the junction of upper and middle third of the muscle. Because of the necessary inactivity during the prolonged hemorrhagic phase scarring was extensive. A prolonged period of active rehabilitation was required, lasting 3 to 4 weeks. At the end of this period, however, functional recovery was excellent. Aside from the permanent scarred mass in his sartorius he was as well as ever.

This case demonstrates a number of unique factors that might serve to underline the preceding discussion. It is the only instance of tear in a "groin" muscle that we have encountered in 18 intercollegiate sports over a 17-year period. Despite its rarity it brings out the precise causative mechanism, namely an enforced demand on a previously strained muscle group by circumstances beyond the athlete's control, circumstances, therefore, that every physician must keep in mind when devising a rehabilitation program, circumstances that must never be allowed to overwhelm an injury before full recovery. Also it typifies the difficulties in deciding upon primary suture of a torn muscle. Here a major muscle tear was unquestionably the only possible cause of such massive bleeding, but, with diffuse hemorrhage that spread from groin to knee, where was the tear?

It must be emphasized that the clear cut history of previous strain, localizable to the sartorius, was obtained only after repeated, specific interrogation day after day and even then only after the mass had become localized. There are undoubtedly some orthopedists who would have extracted an accurate history at the very beginning and that night would have proceeded unerringly to the exact site of tear, restored continuity in a solid, end-to-end fusion of fibers, and returned the athlete to his place in the shell in 10 days rather than four weeks. Be that as it may, the subsequent scar in this case, though permanent, was not of functional significance; so we do not view the results in this case as too far short of ideal.

## Avulsion Fractures

The avulsion fracture of the adductor tubercle of the pubis by the adductor magnus and the avulsion-fracture of the lesser trochanter by the ilio-psoas tendon should be mentioned, though both are accompanied by such acute and severe disability that they can hardly be ignored by athlete, coach, or doctor. These particular injuries do occur, clearly require a complete diagnostic work up with x-rays, and demand specific surgical attention. They are rare enough to be remarkably obvious when they do occur.

## GLUTEAL STRAINS AND CONTUSIONS

**Strains.** Muscles in this region range from the massive gluteus maximus to the lesser medius, the thick but short gemelli and pyriformis, and the sheet-like quadratus femoris. All act in a similar manner, rotating the thigh on the hip and stabilizing the hip joint. Because they are indispensable for weight bearing, dysfunction of any of them is totally disabling to the athlete. Fortunately, strains of these heavy muscles are not frequently seen and are usually the result of some unusual combination of circumstances, such as a shot putter slipping just as he pivots on his back foot or the long jumper landing off balance. Hence, symptomatic local treatment will control the episode, and activity can then be resumed to tolerance, in the secure knowledge that local circumstances will probably not again combine in such an injurious manner.

**Contusions.** Contusions of the area are not as easily dismissed. Contusions can and do occur anywhere around the pelvic girdle even through padding expressly designed to minimize them. One would suppose that contusions of the sacrum and coccyx might be the only problem. This is not the case, in part because of the specific padding mentioned but also because of the heavy development of the buttocks in the competitive athlete, creating a deep valley in which the painfully vulnerable coccyx lies protected. But the ischial tuberosity and gluteals remain exposed, and contusions thereof are not only frequent but are of real significance, not because of local pain, which is usually not great, but because of the anatomical characteristics of the area. As can be seen from inspection, let alone review of the local anatomy, the buttock can swell. Because of the presence of major vessels, the superior and inferior gluteals and their branches, it swells after blunt impact to most impressive proportions. The normal concavity of the lateral buttock sometimes disappears entirely, and a mass the size of a football accumulates therein.

Local ice must be instituted forthwith even in the least of these. But how can one apply external pressure and still allow for biological function? And how can one avoid milking the area with each and every step? The answer is total bedrest and local ice despite the athlete's loud cries of protest. The tendency toward rebleeding is greater in this contusion than in any other encountered, hence bedrest and ice must be continued from 3 to 5 days with limited walking permissible only thereafter. With very little pain to remind him of his problem, the beleaguered athlete soon fills the air with his lamentations, but the physician must remain adamant, for over and beyond this uniform rebleeding tendency is the greater problem of how to prevent idential injury as soon as athletic competition is resumed. Hockey players and football players spend much of their time landing on their fundaments, and, if the athlete is from one of these two sports, as he usually is, how can one pad the area adequately? Thick sponge rubber under extra-tight girdle pads may help, but nothing has really worked out well. Time is the best of healers; if further aggravation can be avoided for about 4 weeks after injury, one can stop worrying; until then these contusions remain a problem.

## THE TROCHANTERIC BURSA AND THE "SNAPPING HIP"

The trochanteric bursa, as the subcutaneous "cushion," so-to-speak, overlying the prominent greater trochanter, is the seat of problems that can be quite significant.

**Contusions.** Contusions directly impact thereover, creating a local situation that is in no way different from that described for the olecranon bursa: local bleeding in an area that can of itself produce even more swelling. Collections of up to 100 cc. of serosanguineous fluid can be aspirated from the area, not entirely from the bursa but also from the contiguous dead spaces, after the growing accumulation disrupts the true anatomical limits of the bursal sac. Be that as it may, these accumulations center around the bursa, and, if the underlying trochanter is intact (which can be easily checked by direct palpation for bony tenderness and crepitus as well as by x-ray), one aspiration, pressure thereafter, and controlled activity for at least 1 week to avoid reaccumulation should suffice. Even if a second aspiration proves necessary, so be it; under no circumstances should the area be opened for drainage, unless one is prepared to deal with a chronic serosanguineous, occasionally purulent drainage that may go on for months.

**Chronic Bursitis.** One must recognize the chronic bursitis that sometimes develops, usually in association with an unusually mobile tensor fascia lata tendon that continually snaps over the bursa and trochanter, hence the *"snapping hip."* This combination is seen as an entity on occasion, usually in sthenic long-striding distance runners, whose easy lope is characterized by a certain fluidity of hip motion. This peculiar gait, together with the incessant and unending repetitive nature of the activity, cannot help but aggravate the bursa, and it is surprising that the problem is so infrequently seen. Again, as with other bursitis problems, the complaint is usually based on the most minimal findings, simply because excessive athletic demands render it more noticeable. As with other bursitis problems, the complaint should be judged for what it is worth, not as one secondary to a grossly thickened bursa that is both acutely and chronically painful but as one secondary to the most minimal early reaction within the bursa, hence responsive to the most minimal treatment. Thus, a careful reprograming of the daily track workout-schedule, retaining the overdistance work at half speed, while increasing the short interval speed work for a week, may be all that is necessary without resorting to injections or surgical excision of the bursa. Injection with a long acting steroid may become necessary if this reprograming fails; however, in all the cases so far encountered injection has never been required.

## PRIMARY DISLOCATION OF THE HIP

Case 7, G. C.: A first team fullback of outstanding ability was involved in a pass-defense drill toward the end of a long afternoon practice session, a drill that was strictly non-contact and was designed to familiarize the defensive backs with their regional responsibilities in multiple defensive alignments. Moving with his usual aptitude to the correct positon, at half speed and under control, he collided with the play-acting end, who was running his own exact offensive pattern. The collision was inadvertent and was of little force. Because it was unexpected, however, G. C. fell backward heavily, his left leg and thigh twisted beneath his body weight. Pain and disability were immediate, and examination within 60 seconds revealed the hip to be held in adduction and internal rotation with a palpable fullness in the left buttock. Immediate diagnosis of a posterior dislocation of the hip was made, but in view of the degree of pain already present in a boy known for his physical "toughness" no attempt was made to reduce the dislocation. Instead, immediate transportation to the hospital under the care of our chief orthopedist was arranged. Reduction under general anesthesia was easily accomplished and post reduction course was completely uneventful. Since this occurred during the pre-season practice sessions, there was hope in some over enthusiastic quarters that a return to action could be anticipated for that season, but sober appraisal of the facts, particularly the small but significant incidence of femoral-head necrosis or deformity following these dislocations, led to a decision to limit weight bearing for at least 3 months and to follow the hip, clinically and by x-ray, for at least a year before allowing full-scale football competition. The following season all athletic expectations were fulfilled, and G. C. became an integral part of a winning season. Now, as a practicing geologist, he is active in the most strenuous field work without problems.

The above case illustrates a number of worthwhile points with which to close this chapter. First, this was strictly a non-contact drill, hence any physician who wishes to protect his patient from "contact work" had better be sure to appreciate what non-contact means in football. Second, this was at the end of a long and rigorous day of practice, thus illustrating the increased tendency toward injury when athletes are tired. Third, this was a totally unexpected impact and shows why the slogan, "Be Ready," is dinned at our athletes over and over by our head trainer. Fourth, this was a practice, routine and midweek, not a game or even a scrimmage, yet for the remainder of that entire season no injury of comparable magnitude occurred, thus underlining the fallacy of providing medical coverage for games only. Fifth, diagnosis was the simplest part of the problem, as it usually is in problems involving major orthopedic disability. Sixth, reduction under anesthesia was quite simply accomplished with a minimum amount of trauma, as against the possibilities of serious complication should such reduction have been attempted in a writhing, screaming, fighting athlete of impressive muscularity. Finally, despite criticisms from others not directly involved the decision was made limiting a return to athletics, in order to assure the most secure future, not for the sake of football. We are convinced that this was and is the only kind of decision that should ever be made.

# 16

# *Injuries to the Upper Leg*

Included here will be a discussion of injuries and disabilities encountered in the area between the hip and knee, excluding only those that have been covered in Chapter 15. Little reference will be made to fracture, because any fracture of the femur is unlikely to present much of a challenge in diagnosis and because treatment of such a major injury requires hospitalization and specialist care according to strict clinical indications and standards, with no consideration whatever for athletic needs.

Discussion of upper leg injuries can be divided according to the three major anatomical areas that are the three major functional units: the quadriceps group anteriorly (extension), the adductor group medially (adduction of thigh), and the hamstring group posteriorly (flexion of the knee). By virtue of its specific functional and anatomical identity each group is subject to injuries and disabilities that are unique to it.

## QUADRICEPS INJURIES AND DISABILITIES

Anatomical review of the quadriceps area reveals the most powerful muscle group in the entire body, occupying the entire anterior surface of the thigh and responsible for its normal contour. The four functional units within this group are the rectus femoris, the vastus medialis, the vastus lateralis, and the vastus intermedius. All are distinguished by their total length, their bulk, and their common power, power exerted through the quadriceps tendon (patellar tendon) to the tibial tuberosity. Because these muscles are so bulky and long and possess so common a function, direct injury of any kind results in a functional disability that is strikingly dramatic both to inspection and palpation as well as to simple testing.

**Clinical Evaluation.** Inspection, palpation, and functional testing should form the basis of any evaluation of quadriceps injury or disability. *Simple inspection* on occasion reveals a swelling and loss of

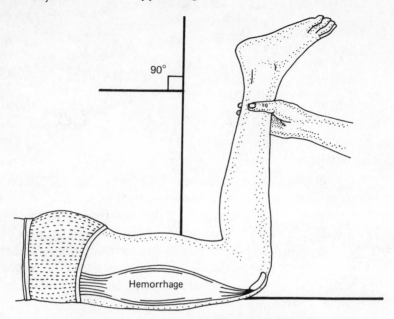

THE FLEXION TEST & QUADRICEPS CONTUSION

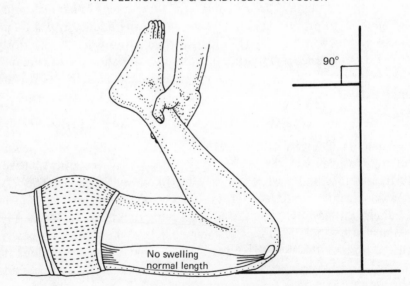

THE FLEXION TEST & FULL FUNCTION

Fig. 16-1. Functional quadriceps tests.

muscle definition, that in the trained athlete can be most striking, and at the same time is effective in localizing the site of injury. *Simple palpation* in the supine position, with the leg fully extended and relaxed, often reveals a palpable mass within one or another of the muscles in the group, a mass that ofttimes can be outlined, accurately measured, and baseline degrees of hemorrhage and overall consistency established. Most important, because of the common function of the entire muscle group *a single simple functional test* can provide a strikingly accurate guideline not only to disability as of the moment but also to clinical progress, functional recovery, and prognosis.

In the test shown in Figure 16-1, advantage is taken of the fact that any alteration of quadriceps function either acutely or chronically will by hemorrhage or scar, respectively, limit the total working length of the entire muscle group, without the examiner depending on such variable factors as pain, pain threshold, or size of mass and degree of induration.

The athlete is placed in the prone position, thereby locking his pelvic girdle and lumbosacral spine, and the precise degree to which his heel can be brought to his buttock is measured. This is done first on the normal side, since some athletes are quite tight bilaterally, then on the injured side. As soon as any scar or hemorrhage in the quadriceps is stretched beyond the point of tolerance, the lumbosacral spine arches and the buttock rises to prevent further excursion, an end point that can be seen from a distance, an end point that will thence forward accurately reflect the slightest change for the better or for the worse in injuries and disabilities that may be too small and too deep to be seen or palpated, and an end point that can be used unhesitatingly to guide every phase of treatment and rehabilitation.

### Acute Strains

Of the specific athletic problems that are commonly encountered within this large muscle group, the most frequent and the least challenging are *acute strains,* varying in severity from the "sore quads," that are so much a part of any return to athletic activity after a sedentary interval (as any occasional athlete will readily attest), to the acutely painful and disabled thighs of the competitive athlete who has attempted too much too soon. Such athletes do not suffer symptoms during overexertion, but within 2 to 4 hours none have any doubt whatever that they have overdone it. Local swelling is usually not remarkable but overall spasm is to a varying but ever-present degree.

Most typically—these unfortunates experience their greatest difficulty in going down stairs, usually managing this important maneuver by inching down sideways.

Examination reveals little by direct inspection and palpation, but the *flexion test* demonstrates a constant degree of limitation, which accurately reflects the true degree of disability. The next consideration is the extent of activity permissible, not of any great importance to the middle-aged enthusiast but of key interest to the competitive athlete. It is here that the flexion test is of the greatest value. If flexion is limited to less than 90 degrees, no running or jogging can be permitted until such time as this limitation subsides; whereas, if flexion can be carried up and beyond 90 degrees, a light jogging program effectively shortens disability, so long as it remains under control and is never allowed to give rise to any subjective "tightening" in the affected thigh. This means that, for example, the baseball catcher, sore from too many squats and half crouches at the beginning of the season, cannot be allowed to return to this type of activity until he has not only "run the soreness out" in a series of supervised, controlled workouts but has also demonstrated an increasing flexion that very nearly brings his heel to his buttock. A total of 2 to 4 days may be necessary to accomplish these objectives, but it must be devoted nevertheless. Otherwise, the swollen and friable muscle may be torn by premature overexertion—a rare outcome but one that need not be risked with proper management.

## Quadriceps Muscle Tears

Regardless of its rarity the *quadriceps muscle tear* proves much more troublesome to manage, with a correspondingly longer period of disability. It develops typically after a history of strain, seldom if ever de novo. Disruption of muscle continuity is accompanied by bleeding, which in muscles of this great length and bulk can become a serious problem of itself (see "Quadriceps Contusions" below). Ice, compression, and elevation are mandatory and must be continued for just as long as bleeding persists, as evidenced by progressive changes in the flexion test. The subsequent course of treatment requires as close management as any bleeding within the quadriceps, avoiding local heat as much as possible and restoring activity by supervised exercise precisely as is outlined below. The degree of initial tearing is never great, because functional disability is so rapidly limiting and the groups involved are so inherent bulky, but local scarring must inevitably result. Even in minimal amounts scar tissue within the quadriceps always proves chronically troublesome. Hence, any effort to avoid scarring, in spite of a few extra days lost after a minor strain, is eminently worthwhile.

## Quadriceps Contusions

Beyond the more minor and less troublesome problems that arise in the quadriceps muscle group, attention must be directed to the biggest bugbear of them all, *quadriceps contusion,* the *"charlie-horse."* This is a contusion through, around, or in the absence of, a pad, a contusion that can impact at any point along the entire anatomical length of the muscle group, can occur medially, anteriorly, or laterally, and can prove the most permanently crippling of all contusions. It occurs in the most innocuous of non-contact sports through an unfortunate combination of circumstances, and it occurs with uniform frequency in all the contact sports, padding or no. Its occurrence does not imply that the usual protective padding is inadequate; nothing less than a full suit of medieval armor would completely eliminate these incidents. It does, however, emphasize the absolute indispensability of padding, padding that must be worn to be effective, padding that must be worn properly. Again we emphasize the necessity of proper fitting of the shell pant and the proper wearing of the hip pad, to keep the properly fitted pant from sagging and thereby allowing the thigh pad to slip around uselessly. One needs to see just one instance of massive bleeding, with hemorrhage from groin to knee and total loss of extensor function, to appreciate the hazards of each and every quad contusion, no matter how minor it may appear at the outset.

The contusion itself, a result of routine blunt impact, is no more than just that, a contusion, formed by the bleeding of crushed and disrupted muscle fibers. But, because of the bulk and length of the muscle contused, bleeding here proceeds at its own pace, governed by local factors of vascularity and compressibility that cannot be anticipated except in the crudest terms. As anyone who has performed surgery within this area can attest, the large venous channels that abound throughout may, on the one hand, be disrupted by a minimal impact that is barely noticeable, yet bleed unimpeded until the entire muscle compartment from groin to knee is filled with a tense mass that so tautens the overlying fascia lata that occasional distal vascular insufficiency may develop with some minimal blanching of the toes—fortuntely, such arterial impairment has never progressed beyond this point, and pressure relieving fasciotomy has never been necessary either in our own experience or elsewhere within the framework of competitive athletics. On the other hand, a massive impact may give rise to an immediate disability and a palpable, grapefruit-sized mass within the muscle, which does not then progress further but recedes steadily in the next 72 hours to complete resolution. And somewhere between are the myriad bumps that occur daily throughout a contact sport season, giving rise to temporary local soreness and subjective "tightness" without much more symptomatic or functional significance.

It is a matter of considerable import to differentiate between these contrasting pictures, keeping in mind that the least may become the worst with little warning. *The functional flexion test* plays an invaluable role here, because, if a contusion of the quadriceps is symptomatically minor and local palpation fails to reveal a definite mass, this same flexion test, by demonstrating 90 degrees or more of flexion, will clear the boy to return to full work immediately after a preliminary running trial of 5 minutes for any further "tightening."

If, however, a mass can be felt and there is definite limitation to less than 90 degrees, ice, compression and elevation are immediately instituted; if within two hours swelling has not increased, limitation has not increased, and the subjective complaint has subsided, elastic compression, continued ice, and elevation are continued for another 48 hours. But if any of these signs has worsened, bedrest, elevation of the leg, ice, and crutches for limited ambulation become mandatory. Then, using daily palpation of mass and the flexion test, the degree of hemorrhage can be serially evaluated, and ice and compression either terminated or prolonged beyond the minimum 48 hours.

Once bleeding has stopped (i.e., the situation has remained stable enough for hemostasis to be reasonably certain), a graduated program of activity can be initiated, avoiding any local heat and/or counter irritants for at least 10 days. Walking, then jogging—always under supervision, always with a check on any possible rebleeding—can then be initiated until alternate jogging for 50 yards and walking for 50 yards can be tolerated for a period of 2 hours. Then and only then should active running begin. Running, in turn, is preceded daily by the flexion test, now used as a *stretching exercise* by the injured athlete himself. On his first running day he should jog until he feels "loose," then by himself try to bring his heel to his buttock by gently pulling on his ankle. This may take 5 minutes to achieve the first time, but never longer thereafter. After such preparation, he can then be sent off to sprint and run without concern for further aggravation. When this last stage has been satisfactorily completed, the athlete can redon his pads, hit the bucker and sled a few times, then finally rejoin his fellows, wearing a special pad over the contusion and under his regular padding.

This is the program we have used with uniform success, in essence allowing the athlete and his injury to determine the course, be it rapid or slow. It is cautious but safe. Sometimes with this method an apparently minor contusion may limit competition for 2 weeks, much to our puzzlement, but in retrospect this may be the precise injury that if pushed could balloon up into the massive "charlie." For this we should be thankful.

**Massive "Charlie-Horse."** Despite increasing pain, the alarming loss of quadriceps function, and the worrisome pressure effects, the *massive "charlie-horse,"* shows no real correlation with degree of initial impact or with extent of initial findings. Most frequently they balloon up during the first 24 hours as a complete surprise to the athlete, who thought the initial injury was unworthy of mention. It has been our impression that these massive cases are more likely to develop in contusions on the anterior or medial aspect of the quadriceps. Certainly, contusions of the lateral aspect do clear up more rapidly and are accompanied by the least disability at any one time, but this observation is of limited worth, since we have also seen massive hemorrhages originate in the most minor lateral contusions. Treatment must be intensive in all cases, if not for the injury per se then in anticipation of what might happen in any one of them!

Once such massive hemorrhage has finally ceased, the rebleeding tendency remains for up to 5 or 6 days. Loss of quadriceps function is the most alarming to the athlete, but fortunately it always returns, if not in 2 weeks, then in 4. Resorption of the mass is a long, slow process, spanning weeks to months, while the mass becomes harder and harder, commonly exhibiting a *"stippling" of calcium* by x-ray within 6 weeks or so. Throughout this entire interval limited weight bearing and close observation must be continued, even after the first appearance of calcification. Not infrequently this type of calcification disappears as silently as it appeared, without any palpable change in the mass. But even then, particularly if the mass is within the vastus intermedius along the femoral shaft, a truer type of *myositis ossificans* can appear as a dense, steadily maturing bony spur. Local heat and judicious passive and active motion must be *gently* initiated, as soon as the danger of rebleeding has subsided on the 7th to 10th day, but no thought whatever should be given to a return to athletics then, or for 6 months to a year to come.

Persistent functional disability remains the most worrisome problem. Flexion may remain limited up to a year after injury and quadriceps strength may remain similarly impaired, whether or not calcification has developed. To avoid such disability, some have advocated multiple aspirations in the acute stage, a totally useless procedure; others have administered parenteral enzyme preparations, which either has accomplished nothing whatever in our experience, or has been suspiciously associated with rebleeding in the 2nd week on minimal stimulation. Some have even advocated surgery to provide both a decompressing fasciotomy, never a necessity in even the worst of our cases, as well as an opportunity to control the bleeding directly, a patently hopeless measure of desperation. Others have advocated late surgical excision of the resultant calcification, when in our experience these calcifications have never been a source of functional disability and have required only a special pad and careful pre-practice "stretching" exercises to render them completely innocuous.

**"Low Charlie."** Another specific variation on the quadriceps contusion deserves some mention, not because treatment is different from that outlined above, even to the key functional test and its implications, but because its site gives rise to symptoms that may be mistaken for significant knee injury—the *"low charlie,"* the contusion of the vastus medialis just above the knee joint. The muscular component of this particular bruise conforms to the usual signs of swelling, spasm, and limitation. However, because of its contiguity with a true extension of the knee joint, the suprapatellar bursa, it can bleed thereinto, hence into the knee joint, thus giving rise to false signs of actual knee joint injury. We have found that patient treatment of the quadriceps bruise on its own indications, ignoring the bursal collection, has never led to anything but the prompt return of a fully recovered athlete in precisely the time anticipated. In contrast, we have seen an instance in which, because of intercession by family-selected specialists at home, recovery was interrupted midway, the knee aspirated, the tocsin sounded, x-rays scrutinized, felt splints and crutches ordered, even arthrograms obtained, all while the contusion became progressively scarred and fibrotic; fibrotic scarring, then, produced a limitation of flexion that stimulated another two week spate of diagnostic maneuvers, and finally culminated in a three month ban on all competitive athletics. All this because of a quadriceps contusion that happened to be low enough to bleed the wrong way!

## HAMSTRING INJURIES

Passing to the second of the three anatomical and functional compartments of the upper leg, we must consider the equally massive and powerful muscles of the posterior thigh, the semi-membranosus and the semi-tendinosus medially, and the biceps femoris laterally, which frame the popliteal fossa by their distalward divergence, but all of which originate proximally from the ischial tuberosity. Because of their function as the primary flexors of the knee joint, as well as secondary extensors of the hip, any disability in these muscles has a disastrous effect on any competitive effort in the weight-bearing sports. It should come as no surprise, then, that problems referable to the hamstring area are not only among the most frequent but remain the most persistent and the most difficult of all muscle injuries to treat satisfactorily.

The athlete, demanding the utmost propulsive power and efficiency from these muscles more than from any other, has nurtured and developed his hamstrings to a degree that can be almost incredible—this is particularly true of the trackman, whose entire competitive being centers around these three muscles. Nor should it be unexpected that the average sprinter should know more about his hamstrings than any doctor or trainer. This merely emphasizes the demand and the dependence the competitive athlete places upon these three muscles and ought to prepare the physician in athletics for the innumerable complaints and symptoms referable to them. Sometimes it seems that track men talk about their hamstring just to have something to talk to the doctor about, while getting around to what is really bothering them. At other times it seems that the "sore hamstring" was created by and for trackmen, just to plague doctors and trainers with a condition that in its myriad variations and its infinite degrees of functional disability can render them as confused and groping as the well-known "blind dog in a meat house."

**Clinical Evaluation.** A doctor must devise a series of objective examinations that he can apply in all instances of hamstring complaint or symptoms, if only as a means of creating some sort of order out of this confusion. As always he must obtain an accurate history to determine acuteness or chronicity and, in the case of the latter, some information as to what the original incident was like and what treatment was then applied. He should carefully inspect and palpate the entire posterior thigh, with the patient prone and his lower leg supported on something, even the examiner's own thigh in the absence of anything else—without this support the hamstrings will be holding up the entire lower leg and foot, negating any findings of spasm or mass. The examiner should then turn the athlete on his back and, holding the knee at full extension, test passive flexion at the hip to the normal maximum of 90 to 95 degrees. Having completed his sequential examination, the examiner can then accurately evaluate the problem, be it chronic or acute. Acute and chronic strains and acute tears are discouragingly frequent, over and above those complaints that seem to have no basis in fact whatever, and it is this sequential examination that separates one from the other and provides information that allows the examiner to formulate a logical program of rehabilitation and treatment.

## Contusions

Significant *contusion* in the hamstring area is rare. The reason why this should be so is a little puzzling. Be that as it may, contusions are rarely seen on the posterior aspect of the thigh and respond to local ice and compression with gratifying rapidity and minimal disability.

### Hamstring Strain

*Hamstring strain* characteristically deevlops gradually, beginning as a soreness or "tightness" in the area that progressively hampers activity until the athlete is forced to discontinue his efforts. As with all muscle strains there is no gross disruption of continuity and no gross bleeding. Instead, there is overall spasm and soreness most marked at an anchor point on the skeleton, here the proximal ischial tuberosity area and/or a musculotendinous junction here easily palpable in all three muscles.

The degree of abnormality in these findings varies from case to case, but, if there is no real spasm, all muscles are loose, there is no soreness in the ischial tuberosity area or any musculotendinous junction, and, particularly if the straight leg raising test is in the 90 degree range, something else is definitely going on. In fact, the examiner had better talk to the coach and trainer to discover how the practice workouts are going, whether the upcoming meet is expected to provide too much competition for the athlete's taste, and also check a hundred other possibilities.

**Hamstring Tear**

If the onset of hamstring pain is acute, for example in the middle of a sprint, or the victim volunteers that he thought someone kicked him in the thigh (so sudden and explosive is the pain), one is dealing with a *hamstring tear or "pull."* There is spasm and an acutely tender mass in that part of the muscle where hemorrhage is already under way, and subjective pain most often localizes to that spot. If the tear is extensive, the mass is equally extensive, and disability is such that weight bearing is impossible. In lesser cases, there is a mass no bigger than a walnut with very little spasm or pain.

**Treatment of Hamstring Injuries**

In all cases having palpable evidence of bleeding and a painful spasm commensurate therewith no further competition can be allowed, and compression and ice must be imediately instituted. Subsequent thereto careful daily evaluation of the mass and its resolution as well as of the progress of muscle spasm provides an accurate guideline to recovery. As soon as bleeding has definitely stopped, walking should be started, at first normally then with an exaggerated high "knee action." This is followed by a jogging-running program that is gauged to local findings and subjective tolerance. During this recovery period it is not unusual to note a classical ecchymosis that first appears at the apex of the popliteal fossa and extends distalward, secondary to the distalward flow of extravasated blood hitherto obscured within the heavy muscles. This should not be viewed as alarming but as further confirmation of the initial severity of injury.

Nowhere in this program is there any room for a deliberate forcing of activity. A hamstring "pull" simply cannot be "run out" despite the beliefs of some in the athletic world. Any attempt to push such an injury inevitably leads to a complete tear of the muscle and a subsequent scarring that permanently hampers all future activity. Instead, patient, controlled exercise to tolerance uniformly promotes rapid resolution of the acute process and formation of the most supple and functional scar. Of even greater interest, it takes a much shorter time than might be otherwise possible. The athlete with a true hamstring "pull," with bleeding that later appears at the popliteal fossa, can be returned to full competition in 2 weeks without once risking additional, possibly permanent damage. In contrast, forcing, then tearing a hamstring may result in a whole season—possibly a whole career—lost, should the tear prove extensive enough.

During this period of rehabilitation the athlete should be instructed in the *"hurdler's stretch" exercise,* a track modification of the classical "split" of acrobatic dancing. Just as the victim of quadriceps injury adopts his flexion-test-stretch as part of his normal everyday warm-up, so should the "hurdler's stretch" become an integral part of the runner's everyday warmup.

## The Tight Hamstring

The *chronic, tight, scarred hamstring* is one of the most distressing aftermaths of improperly treated hamstring injuries. Once scar is established in any or in all of the hamstrings by such ill advised extremes as prolonged bedrest for all acute pulls and strains, or the tearing of a hamstring clear across its belly because of an enforced running program, the scar itself becomes a source of chronic tightness as well as recurrent strains that usually center either just proximal or just distal to the mass. A day of ice and prompt active rehabilitation will usually suffice, but so frequent are these episodes that some boys simply cannot run full-speed again, while others become so conscious that they are about to "pull" again, that they cannot be depended upon. Patient reassurance, local heat, massage, counter-irritant wraps, and cautious psychotherapy are all part of what must be resorted to in these instances. Regardless of method, one must strive to keep these boys running without interruption; any significant layoff inevitably tightens scarred hamstrings even further.

There is no simple answer to the problem of chronic hamstring injury. The doctor and trainer must work carefully with each case, probing every possible avenue. One must not give up and accuse the athlete of being "psycho." Apprehensive he may be for one of many obscure reasons, but he is still trying to run.

Case 8, S. J.: A highly rated All-State fullback on routine freshman football screening was found to have a fibrotic, scarred mass, 10 x 15 x 5 cm., occupying the entire mid-belly of his left biceps femoris. On close questioning, he described a classical "hamstring pull" toward the end of his junior season in high school, for which he received heat treatments for 2 days, then an enforced return to full duty. Despite pain and disability he limped through the rest of the season, but found it impossible to run full speed thereafter, despite which, as a high school senior, he was voted to All-State honors. However, still unable to run full-speed, he was never able to compete successfully on the college level despite a positional shift into the line, and graduated with his permanent scar and permanent disability unchanged.

## ADDUCTOR INJURIES

This muscle group, forming the normal contour of the medial thigh, has already been discussed in relation to the pelvic girdle and so-called "groin-strains." Strains from forceful abduction of the thigh on the hip can occur further distalward and, certainly, contusions can and do occur, but neither is of any great significance in athletics, responding quite satisfactorily to routine local measures. There is, however, a specific *contusion-strain* seen in the the area of the adductor tubercle on the medial femoral epicondyle, and it is of particular importance because of its frequent confusion with intrinsic knee injury, usually a medial collateral strain. The causative mechanism most often encountered is a forceful adduction plus an impact on the ground, hence there will be a bone bruise of the medial femoral condyle, which may remain tender for months, as well as a strain of the adductor tendon insertion. This last may also include a periosteal avulsion leading to subsequent calcification, the *Pellegrini-Stieda disease*. However, if the history of injury is obtained in sufficient detail, as it must always be, confusion with true knee injuries is avoided, and local treatment—ice, compression, and active rehabilitation—returns the athlete, suitably padded, to full activity in 3 to 5 days. Any subsequent calcification, though arresting by x-ray, has proved of little significance other than as an item of interest, for disability has never been a factor therefrom and surgery has never been indicated.

# 17

# The Knee in Athletics

Any attempt to limit discussion of knee injuries might be viewed as heresy in this era of mass information, in which the "football knee" is so widely recognized and the knee injury to the star athlete is so widely reported by the news media. It would seem that one can no longer handle any athletic injury competently without first gaining recognition as an expert in the surgical treatment of knee injuries, nor rank as an expert in the surgical reconstruction of permanently damaged knees without presuming to be an equally qualified expert in every phase of athletic medicine. We shall, however, limit our discussion to knee injuries as they occur in a controlled athletic program. We shall do so without reproducing x-rays, without quoting detailed operative reports, without describing ligament sutures or tendon transplant techniques. These details pertain to orthopedic surgery and must be kept in proper perspective by any doctor primarily responsible for the health of athletes in a controlled program. Certain results can be reasonably expected, but there is no miracle to knee surgery. If one were to compare it objectively to simple, routine cholecystectomy, its delicacy would not seem so technically outstanding or so strangely curative.

If the actual knee surgery is not technically difficult, what is the value of an orthopedic consultant in the treatment of these admittedly difficult and unfortunately common problems? The answer concerns judgment, that rare blend of diagnostic and surgical acumen that is in many ways comparable to that necessary in evaluating an acute appendicitis. In the latter, for example, a classical case can demand operation with a certainty that a second-year medical student can recognize immediately, and the procedure itself is within the surgical range of the average intern. Yet the decision whether and when exploration is indicated can still be one of the most challenging and difficult that the experienced general surgeon can encounter. The simplistic approach, by which the difficult diagnostic problem (hence the acutely injured knee) calls for operation immediately, is as logical as removing the appendix of every child with a non-specific stomach ache. Nevertheless, it is heard all over the country.

What are the indications for arthrotomy? Is it to provide an opportunity to look around the joint, because impatience would not allow a proper work up and an accurate diagnosis? Does it mean the elimination of arthrography as a helpful diagnostic tool, because such a study might delay surgery? Or is it a final logical step, indicated by an appraisal of all the facts and findings, with a judicious weighing of the advantages and disadvantages of surgery?

The results of major knee surgery, no matter how anatomically satisfactory or functionally sound, may fall far short of ideal on the athletic field. Many boys never recover from the psychological effect of knee surgery, some never recover from the physiological effect. Many orthopedists will say that this is all mental and the fault of the boy, not the surgery. But should not this have been taken into consideration beforehand? Certainly if arthrotomy is clearly indicated as the one means of recovering 100 per cent function, so be it, but can one accurately evaluate and predict this, while operating indiscriminately on all cases within 12 hours of injury? It has even been said that a negative arthrotomy does no harm whatever and that after such a "limited" procedure the athlete can return to full activity in so short a time that he will have lost no time at all. Even if this were true, which seems doubtful, is this any justification for unnecessary major surgery?

This is not to deny that certain instances of major knee injury do require immediate surgery, to repair gross ligament damage that is apparent from the moment of injury. When a knee is "hanging by a string," so to speak, with obvious total disruption of a collateral and/or cruciate ligament, there can be no question nor hesitation about prompt reparative surgery, and close scrutiny of the criteria for immediate surgery according to O'Donoghue will confirm that such cases were never questioned. But in 18 years there have been only four cases in the Yale intercollegiate athletic program that fit into this category—two in hockey—with but two instances in football on the freshman, junior-varsity, or varsity level. Does this mean that we play a special brand of football in the Ivy League, or does it mean that too many knees are being operated upon far too early by enthusiasts using O'Donoghue's criteria without the experience and judgment to apply them?

To add further to the controversy, let us point out an article, little noted by the "experts" in the field, but nevertheless a cogent plea for sanity. Written by the dean of college team physicians, Dr. Harry R. McPhee, a man of unparalleled experience in the field of athletic injuries, it reviews a total of 211 separate knee injuries in 194 athletes, personally seen and followed over a span of years from 1933 to 1956 among 768 varsity and junior-varsity Princeton football candidates. Of this total there were but 23 knee operations. Of the 153 cases responding to direct communication, 79 per cent reported no knee problems of any kind after graduation and only one eventually required knee surgery 11 years after college. (Student Medicine, *10:* 422–430, 1962.)

What then of the physician primarily responsible for the well being of all the athletes? How can he choose among the radical and conservative factions? To this there is no easy answer, except that he must be guided by his own principles. If he is fortunate enough to find an orthopedist with the rare combination of technical skill and sober, painstaking judgment, he can work closely with him from the beginning, together examining each knee injury and together following each operative case through the long rehabilitation process. If, however, he is surrounded by a more sanguine breed, to whom immediate surgery is the only answer, then he must exercise the greatest restraint in his referrals.

## EXAMINATION OF THE INJURED KNEE

Before he can make any decision, however, the physician must know how to evaluate the true extent of any knee injury. Complete and painstaking examination must be undertaken at the time of injury and thereafter with every advantage taken of x-ray and other diagnostic measures.

Complete examination includes: first, *an exacting history* of the precise mechanism of injury, something that must be obtained before the athlete can forget it; second, *a thorough inspection of the entire knee joint* for swelling or deformity; third, *a sequential series of tests* that must include *a complete test of range of motion from hyperextension to full flexion, abduction and adduction in full extension as well as 15 degrees of flexion, the "drawer" sign, and rotation of the lower leg on the femur with the knee flexed to twenty degrees.* No knee can be examined without each of these maneuvers, nor can any injury be correctly evaluated by any single one without the others. Each maneuver has a specific meaning and the presence or absence of findings in each one of them is of lasting significance. *All areas must be thoroughly palpated,* checking for tenderness along the medial and lateral joint lines, the medial and lateral collateral ligaments, the medial femoral condyle (to check on adductor tendon pathology). *True joint effusion* must be differentiated from prepatellar effusion and, finally, *the fat pad area* checked for suggestive thickening or tenderness. Only after this complete examination can a working diagnosis be formulated, and a program of future rehabilitation or consultant referral decided upon. (See Fig. 17-1.)

## Contusions

We shall consider the types of knee injuries encountered in the light of the history and examination given above. First of all, the various types of contusions must be recognized. For this there must be a *specific incident of impact,* which is nearly always possible to determine within the first minutes of evaluation. If the blow was neither sufficiently forceful nor remarkable to cause any counterjoint motion, the athlete will be the first to state this with a positive knowledge that can be depended upon. The site must then be carefully located and inspected, keeping in mind possible confusion with contusions on the femoral condyle and associated neighborhood symptoms that might falsely suggest collateral ligament strain. The "low charlie" with its penchant for suprapatellar bursal bleeding must also be kept in mind. In the area of the prepatellar bursa any impact must be suspect as a source of a ballooning *prepatellar-bursal hemorrhage* that can be quite alarming in volume for the unwary. This is particularly true if there is a history of past bursal injuries, for then the total bursal accumulation can approach 100 to 200 cc. of sanguineous fluid in a taut serosal sac that may extend 5 to 6 cm. above the upper limits of a patella. Similarly, *bruises of the bony surfaces of the condyles or of the patella itself* can occur with local characteristics typical of the bone bruise yet distinctly separable from true ligamentous or internal knee damage, firstly, by the absence of any true instability, effusion, or joint line or ligament tenderness, and, secondly, by the presence of a full range of motion.

## Minor Ligament Strains

In contrast, *minor ligament strains* are evidenced, first, by a history of counterjoint force, and second, by distinctly localizeable tenderness along the length of the medial or lateral collateral ligaments. Occasionally this tenderness is limited to a narrow area, precisely along the more vulnerable anterior distal limb of the medial collateral, without demonstrable tenderness elsewhere. Such specific tenderness is diagnostic even in the absence of demonstrable instability either in full extension or at 15 degrees flexion.

More commonly, there is *some degree of demonstrable laxity yet a distinct elasticity* on abduction or adduction at 15 degrees flexion; there is *no lateral motion on full extension.* This is the most commonly encountered type of ligament strain, and in a few days is as tight and stable as ever, flexed or fully extended. Moreover, in the *medial collateral strain,* because of the close application of medial joint capsule around the ligament, a subsequent minor effusion may be anticipated without indicting internal structures; this effusion promptly disappears on active rehabilitation. The *lateral collateral strain* is very rarely accompanied by an effusion. In either case, as long as the joint lines remain clear of tenderness, as long as the "drawer" sign remains negative on daily testing, as long as there is full range of motion, and as long as there is full hyperextension in the standing position, internal derangement need not be seriously considered.

## Ligament Tear

In the complete or near-complete *collateral ligament tear* all the above signs are present to a correspondingly greater degree. Adduction or abduction is grossly remarkable without any sense of elasticity at all, and full quadriceps stabilization in extension does not alter the degree of lateral instability, which may amount to 15 to 20 degrees, depending on the courage of the examiner. In cases of complete collateral tear any remaining stability is provided by the medial joint capsule itself. If this is partially torn, there may be so little support that the true limits of lateral angulation of tibia on femur can be too frightening to demonstrate. Nor is such a demonstration necessary, for the diagnosis cannot be more certain; nor is there the least doubt as to immediate disposition, namely, *emergency surgical repair.*

Case 9, R. P.: A 20-year-old junior fullback with bruising size and speed was hit by a legal and effective tackle, which impacted his bent right knee from the antero-lateral direction, snapping it forcibly into hyperextension and hyperabduction. Disability was immediate, and examination on the field revealed a joint which could be "opened" with alarming ease along its medial aspect, even in full hyperextension and with full quadriceps contraction. The diagnosis was unquestionable, and emergency orthopedic surgical repair requested. Within 4 hours, under general anesthesia, surgical repair of a completely disrupted medial collateral ligament was carried out, which procedure required reimplantation of the superior limb into the femoral condyle.

Postoperative recovery was totally without complication and rehabilitation progress thereafter was such that stability was completely re-established, quadriceps strength surpassed that of the contralateral side, and all running and cutting maneuver were totally without visible impairment. However, the next football season proved disappointing; despite complete recovery by every objective measure, the unique combination of speed and power never returned.

## Cartilage Injury

If there is *joint line tenderness and limitation of extension or hyperextension by five or more degrees,* a cartilage injury must be suspected. Unfortunately, x-rays are of no value, revealing only bony pathology, which is not in question, or calcified loose bodies, not primary considerations. Very rarely an avulsion of tibial spine may confirm clinical cruciate damage, but even this will not clarify the question of meniscus injury. One is forced to suspect without definite knowledge, but is this such an unusual situation in medicine? Certainly, every opportunity should be afforded the knee to spontaneously resolve under these specific circumstances, since in our experience and in that of McPhee (cf. above) a large proportion of these subside spontaneously, full range of motion returns, joint-line tenderness disappears, and the boy can then return to full athletic participation with no problems whatsoever in later life. This does not mean that one can forget about these knees; an even closer watch must be kept over these cases for the least sign of recurrent difficulty. Nonetheless, a little extra care and observation is ofttimes all that is necessary to avoid a needless arthrotomy.

## Anterior Cruciate Integrity

Finally one comes to *the "drawer" sign* and its true meaning, the presence or absence of anterior cruciate integrity. Immediate on-the-spot examination may often be the most revealing, before any reflex spasm of the hamstrings can develop to completely obscure a possibly positive sign. A definite positive sign with an accompanying effusion can mean but one thing, and surgical repair should be seriously considered within the first 24 hours. However, we have yet to see such an isolated, straightforward finding.

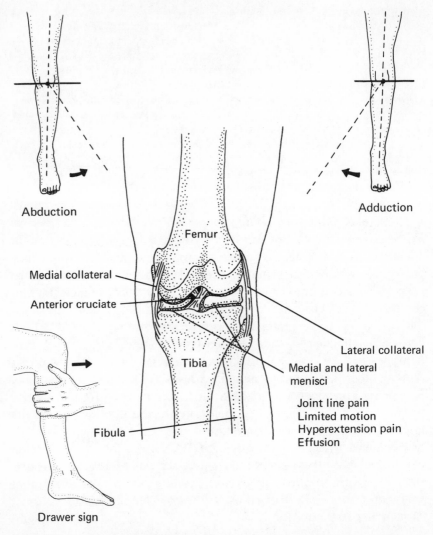

Abduction

Adduction

Femur

Medial collateral

Anterior cruciate

Lateral collateral

Tibia

Medial and lateral
menisci

Joint line pain
Limited motion
Hyperextension pain
Effusion

Fibula

Drawer sign

Fig. 17-1. The left knee (anterior view) and check points in examination.

## THE INITIAL TREATMENT OF ACUTE KNEE INJURIES

The usual acute knee presents a mixture of the various signs described above with, for example, a moderate effusion, some medial collateral instability on partial flexion but none on full extension, some medial joint-line tenderness, but no loss in range of motion. To recommend surgery upon a knee such as this would seem unreasonable even to the most enthusiastic orthopedist, but should operation eventually become clearly indicated, as evidenced by subsequent episodes of unmistakable medial cartilage impaction after varying periods of symptom-free activity, someone is sure to accuse the physician of ignorance and procrastination. As stated earlier, however, the classical cases of cartilage injury are as child's play, while those requiring immediate ligament surgery are as clearly indicated. It is in this vast majority of subacute problems that judicious observation, not precipitate surgery, must be the answer.

Treatment in all cases of acute knee injury is basically the same, and is designed to stop bleeding and to support damaged soft tissues until resolution can begin. Some advocate the plaster knee cylinder; we favor a supporting elastic adhesive strapping, felt splints, ice, compression, and elevation, with crutches for ambulation. Our reasons are based mainly on the ease with which the local area thereafter can be palpated and inspected daily or even twice daily. In the key 24 to 48 hours after injury localizing signs may develop that will be extremely significant in determining the true extent of internal damage. Also, the rapidity of resolution of certain initial signs may provide a very early guide toward an active rehabilitation program. Thus, an effusion in the first 24 hours that subsides by 50 per cent in the second 24 hours is most encouraging, while any effusion that continues to mount despite treatment can mean just the opposite. Any effusion in the first 24 hours may obscure true joint-line, hence cartilage tenderness which may then emerge in the second 24 hours as the effusion subsides.

Any variation and combination of symptoms and signs can develop and can be accurately followed and interpreted by these changes. For this reason, *no attempt is made to aspirate any early effusion.* It is better to utilize the presence and volume thereof as a direct reflection of resolution progress within the knee joint. Should it subside under observation only to return on ambulation, an internal derangement is more definite. If it disappears and does not return, as is more usual, one has another indication of a lesser extent of internal damage. In either case, the objective is to keep any knee suspected of *cartilage damage* under a *strict regimen of controlled exercise,* increasing activity only as effusion or local pain may tolerate, while at the same time increasing activity in lesser injuries all the more rapidly as these same local signs progressively subside.

As soon as local swelling or hemorrhage has stabilized under close 48-hour observation, *ligament strains without significant instability* can be started on weight bearing of a graduated nature on up to full weight bearing, followed by light jogging and then full-speed running, as ligament soreness and/or effusion permit, supporting the knee at all times with a carefully applied strapping.

With dependence so-placed on these local symptoms to guide the rehabilitation, *local anesthesia is distinctly contraindicated*. It has never been missed, because once motion starts, proper control leads to an accelerated subsidence of local discomfort rather than an aggravation thereof, and the sum total is a strong knee fully rehabilitated at about the same time that a similarly injured knee under alternative treatment might be coming out of the plaster cylinder for another two weeks of rehabilitation. The supporting adhesive strapping, applied daily for every workout, is continued in all cases of ligament strain for the remainder of the season. Although this may seem laborious and cumbersome, we feel a good deal more secure with it, and so does the athlete —in fact all chronic knees with demonstrable instability are similarly supported for every workout, because the external appliances of varying design and cost do not do the job as well.

**Post-Traumatic Quadriceps Atrophy**

Of additional importance, particularly in cases of ligament strain but also in all cases of acute knee injury, is the remarkable rapidity of quadriceps atrophy immediately thereafter, sometimes visibly evident within three to four days and characteristically apparent in the lowermost portion of the vastus medialis, just above the patella. This atrophy is all the more remarkable because of the extraordinary development of this muscle mass in the competitive athlete—ironically, this is the last segment of quadriceps to develop even after the most strenuous competition over many years, yet it is the first to go after injury. Functional restoration must be rapidly accomplished, in order to stabilize the injured knee. Hence, it is our policy to start quadriceps weight work within seven days of injury if local symptoms permit, as is more often the case than not. Once begun, it should be continued as part of the athlete's daily routine for at least 4 to 6 weeks or until no signs of atrophy can be measured or palpated. By this means it is not unusual at the end of the season to find an athlete with a functionally and anatomically stronger knee on his injured side than on his normal side, a result worth striving for.

## THE RETROPATELLAR FAT PAD

The fat pad situated behind the patella is normally impalpable and is invisible by x-ray; so it is usually ignored as a source of significant knee symptomatology. Nevertheless, a specific picture referable thereto, the *"pinched fat pad,"* is quite common in athletics. In fact, it is more frequently seen in sports than is true internal derangement.

The history is completely non-specific and atraumatic, the symptoms variously developing after running, jumping, punting, and a host of other normal athletic activities. The uniform complaint is of vague deep discomfort in the retropatellar area on hyperextension. Thorough examination always fails to reveal any ligamentous instability, joint-line tenderness, or evidence of internal derangement, yet there will be a slight, almost undetectable effusion, and a loss of the last 5 degrees of hyperextension, accompanied by an increasing discomfort directly behind the patella. Careful palpation in this area will reveal an ill-defined soft-tissue thickening and induration on both sides of patella and patellar tendon and deep thereto, and this vague mass is consistently tender. In the absence of any other sign or symptoms, these findings are diagnostic of a bruising, as it were, of that portion of the fat-pad that protrudes into the joint space, but is normally clear of impaction on full extension of the joint. Under normal circumstances it remains unnoticeable, but under the stress of competitive athletics, the incessant demand on reptitive knee action is certain to pinch that pad sooner or later. Once caught, hemorrhage gives rise to minimal effusion, while swelling of the pinched tag renders it all the more protuberant and thus more prone to further impaction.

It is important to recognize these cases at the outset, because despite the minimal symptomatology and the virtual absence of true functional disability further strenuous weight bearing assures increasing symptoms. Accordingly, athletic prohibition and local ice must be resorted to for just as long as the palpable thickening and hyperextension discomfort persist. Since resolution may take between 3 to 6 days, during which no workouts can be permitted, complaints will be loud and long, but with steadfast medical forbearance no further recurrent problems need arise. If the athlete is a punter in football and the complaint is on his kicking side, this prohibition must be extended even further, until at least 2 to 3 days of hard running have adequately tested resolution of the acute process.

It must be stressed that this is a *diagnosis of exclusion.* Every other possibility must be seriously considered before it can be entertained. There must be a palpable induration and tenderness in the fat-pad area alone, otherwise significant internal derangement will be mistakenly diagnosed as a "pinched fat-pad," a dangerous error. But given the diagnostic signs and symptoms as enumerated, proper treatment will clear up these episodes with gratifying rapidity and without recurrent tendencies.

## ACUTE AND CHRONIC PREPATELLAR BURSITIS

The usual history and findings in a *prepatellar bursitis* have already been touched upon in the section on the examination of the acutely injured knee. The comments about the olecranon bursa and its problems (see Chap. 13) are equally applicable here. It must be re-emphasized that a history of impact directly over the bursa is all-important. Blunt impact to this particular area, followed by acute swelling, is truly diagnostic, the only other remote possibility being a fracture of the underlying patella, which is not only exceedingly rare within a controlled athletic program, but is far more painful initially and thereafter.

X-rays are occasionally helpful but rarely necessary. One need but palpate the swollen bursa, always external to the patella, to make the diagnosis, mindful of the greatly increased limits of this anatomical structure in cases with a history of one or more previous episodes of acute swelling. Treatment should be undertaken immediately, discontinuing all athletic activity for the moment. *Compression and ice,* applied in the usual manner as soon as swelling is brought to medical attention, will normally suffice. *Needle aspiration* may be necessary occasionally, but spontaneous resorption is sufficiently frequent to warrant at least 24 hours of close observation before doing so. *A long-acting steriod* can be instilled at the completion of initial aspiration, should such eventually prove necessary. This, in our experience, has virtually eliminated the necessity for further aspirations. Regardless, firm compression and limited activity must be continued in all cases for at least 24 hours to assure maximum resolution of the acute process.

The usual prepatellar hemorrhage requires close observation and treatment for at least 2 to 3 days. Recovery varies according to local signs and symptoms, seldom requiring more than another day or two of rehabilitation but always requiring continuing elastic support and added protective equipment for at least a month.

Of even less concern is the *chronic prepatellar bursitis,* a condition frequently well established for years before the athlete arrives at school. Aspiration may be necessary to relieve local pressure in massively swollen and taut bursae, but local elastic-bandage pressure will suffice in most cases without more being necessary. There is no cure for the chronicity and in the contact sports constant reaggravation must be an assumed risk. With proper additional padding and elastic-bandage support (to be worn without fail) no instance has proven significantly troublesome. Cortical steroid instillation is helpful in persistently recurrent cases and has effectively "dried up" several of these chronic bursae, but it is not always necessary and should therefore be kept as a reserve weapon rather than as a primary therapeutic tool. Much more important is the proper padding of the area for all games and workouts thereafter, something that is no less essential in these chronic cases than in the acute cases. Particularly in football, the standard knee padding is inadequate in the face of the hypersensitive nature of these irritated bursae, and special means must be employed to dissipate inevitable impacts.

## THE OPERATIVE KNEE

The acutely injured knee that requires operation is most difficult to define, since definition depends so much on the particular orthopedist concerned, his diagnostic and surgical abilities, and a host of other factors. There can be no question that certain conditions do require surgery, no matter who the orthopedist may be. These are: first, the *torn meniscus* with impaction or persistent effusion and disability; second, the *torn cruciate,* anterior or posterior; third, the *completely torn collateral ligament,* medial or lateral; and fourth, the *intraarticular loose-body* secondary to osteochondritis dissecans or chondromalicia patellae. Any case that on initial examination raises the suspicion of any of these four conditions should be seen promptly by the orthopedist, and treatment decided upon. On the other hand, any case that fails to exhibit definite evidence of any of these possibilities, in particular those without evidence of collateral or cruciate ligament damage (hence not necessarily operative cases), should be watched carefully, if possible with the orthopedist. Immediate surgery is clearly indicated only in cases of major ligament damage, not in any of the other possible operative indications. Too often we have seen instances of precipitate surgery performed elsewhere in the face of non-ligamentous knee problems, where the wrong compartment has been explored and the wrong cartilage removed, while the knee has remained as symptomatic as ever.

Barring severe ligamentous injuries, diagnosis of which is relatively simple, all cases of questionable cartilage damage or possible lesser injury deserve a painstaking attempt at proper evaluation, sometimes over a 2 or 3-week period. During this interval signs and symptoms may develop, that may lateralize completely counter to intial impressions or may disappear altogether never to return. Even cartilage impaction can disappear spontaneously. To deny an injured athlete this grace period does not make sense, when there is nothing to lose and everything to gain.

## THE POSTOPERATIVE KNEE

Any physician in a position of medical responsibility for a football squad, much less for an overall year-long athletic program, encounters many athletes with knees that are postoperative. He is sure to carry 5 to 10 such postoperative knees at all times on an average sized football squad. He must be prepared to evaluate these chronic problems as part of his responsibility, regardless of parental or home physician clearances or recommendations. To do so, he must examine each knee thoroughly, establishing a base line range of motion, stability, and quadriceps strength and bulk. Before making up his mind, he must determine with exactitude the operative procedure performed, the reasons for it, and the opinion of the operative surgeon on the candidate's present athletic capabilities. It is the physician's responsibility, not that of any one else, to determine whether any postoperative result is truly capable of withstanding the rigors of competitive football or any other contact sport. Any untoward outcome will be his and the school's fault, not the parents', the athlete's, or the home physician's or surgeon's. This is particularly true when an athlete reports for football with medical clearance from home, carrying a knee cage that is either illegal according to the rules or is completely inadequate to support a knee that is grossly unstable. (We have seen several instances, wherein candidates reported within 2 to 3 months of operation, with advanced quadriceps atrophy, constant effusion, yet written clearances to play football!)

No matter who the surgeon, certain immutable standards must be met to allow any athlete to compete successfully in a vigorous contact sport. The first is time, something that cannot be shortened, no matter how uneventful the postoperative recovery. It has been our experience that in football any major arthrotomy (with the single exception of the tiny exploratory incisions customary for the removal of loose bodies) requires at least 6 months of active rehabilitation before pre-season practices begins. Otherwise, sooner or later during those gruelling 2-a-day sessions, effusion and pain develop that limit further effective competition.

**Repaired Ligaments.** If in addition to this irreducible time factor the surgery included repair of significant ligament damage, that repair must also be carefully tested. Postoperative instability of the collaterals, apparent on full extension and maximum quadriceps support, cannot be externally supported for such a sport as football, regardless of what knee cage or what rigid or semi-rigid support may suffice for normal activities. In sports the sweating alone assures enough "slippage" to largely negate their effect. Nor can the most expert tape job accomplish adequate support in these permanently disabled knees, effective though it may be in the minor laxity, demonstrable only in partial flexion. There can be little argument that cases such as these should be categorically barred from football, despite the fact that hockey, a different type of contact sport, is not similarly barred.

What should be done with postoperative ligament repairs that are stable to all testing? In these instances there is no cause for concern, and nothing further need be done, other than to confirm in writing the surgeon's specific clearance for all contact sports. Unfortunately, we have yet to encounter a postoperative ligament repair that has not proved permanently unstable to examination, regardless of where or when it was done. Such cases doubtless exist, judging from the enthusiasm with which these primary repairs are being done, but we have not seen any. Two hockey injuries, repaired by immediate surgery, recovered good knee function, but not to football standards, nor have any of several from the secondary school level demonstrated adequate stability for football. This is not intended to prove or disprove the treatment concept, which makes good surgical sense, but to point out a fact that we hope will change as more of these procedures are done. In the meantime, it is important to remember that any knee injury that disrupts major ligament continuity is of itself a permanently crippling injury, to a degree dependent upon many factors, only one of which is prompt and skilled attention. Consequently, the ultimate aim of any treatment, immediate or delayed, should be to restore a badly damaged knee to a status that will assure a normal everyday life. If this primary aim is successfully accomplished and, by good fortune, football also becomes a reasonable risk, all well and good. Failing this last, however, has the treatment really failed? Football, after all, demands the utmost stability in the knee joint for an athlete's very survival, so the standards must be arbitrarily rigorous and uncompromisingly applied. But football is not the only sport in the world. Those postoperative knees should be judged accordingly, not by football standards alone.

**Meniscectomy.** As to the more frequent postoperative meniscectomy, the same time factor remains immutable. Again and again we have seen earnest candidates report with knees more recently postoperative than the necessary 6-months recovery period. Every one without exception has been forced to discontinue his efforts in the face of an increasingly painful synovitis and effusion. On the other hand, with a good vigorous rehabilitation program, no visible or measurable quadriceps atrophy, and a 6 months or longer post-operative recovery period, athlete after athlete has successfully competed in football and other sports without the least difficulty. We do not regard a fully rehabilitated meniscectomy as functionally different from any other normal athlete. We take no precautionary measures, we recommend no particular local support, we anticipate no difficulties, nor do we encounter any.

**Osteochondritis Dissecans.** The athlete with an established *osteochondritis dissecans* and a history of loose-body removal presents another type of problem. He can return to full activity quite rapidly, since his is a small exploratory incision, but the concern here is for recurrent and unpredictable locking, negating much of the athlete's team efforts. In one such instance, an otherwise remarkably equipped and able young man underwent repeated surgery for recurrent loose bodies, each time developing further disabling symptoms just as he was beginning to make his mark with the team. Finally, in sheer disgust, he transferred his considerable abilities elsewhere, only to "lock" his knee again when jumping out of bed! Such a situation can be discouraging, yet it must be recognized that at any one time such an athlete is not functionally disabled and cannot, therefore, be barred from athletic participation. What, however, is he doing to his joint surfaces? Or, as is occasionally seen, there is the highly publicized football player who has undergone medial and lateral meniscectomy on one or even both knees, during one or another of which procedures *articular chondromalacia* has been noted and curetted, yet has continued to progress thereafter. He may exhibit little if any functional disability at any one time. What, however, is he doing to his joint surfaces? Should athletes such as these be symptomatically treated from episode to episode, or should they be taken in hand and advised of the problems they may be actively creating for themselves in later life?

## ACUTE AND CHRONIC PATELLAR DISLOCATIONS

A rare but easily recognized acute injury is the patellar dislocation, usually lateralward and usually accompanied by a striking degree of acute pain and disability. Examination is diagnostic. The gross deformity, presented by a knee whose patella has displaced lateralward out of the condylar notch and is locked lateral thereto, is impossible to miss. Immediate reduction can be simply accomplished on the spot before spasm and swelling develop. Any delay makes reduction more difficult and more painful. The knee is hyperextended to provide maximum relaxation of the structures involved, following which the patella is grasped and levered over the lateral femoral condyle with a steady medialward pressure. Reduction is rewarded by an immediate relief of acute pain. Attention can then be turned to further treatment measures. X-rays should be taken to obtain some baseline evaluation of possible chip fractures, posterior patellar avulsions, and the like, but these do not require immediate attention. Felt splints, compression, and ice should be applied to minimize the inevitable swelling, and the knee then immobilized in slight flexion (15 to 20 degrees) to safeguard reduction, with crutches to eliminate any weight bearing. Orthopedic consultation should be immediately sought, for some orthopedists feel that the only definitive treatment is surgical while others do not, and the physician had best not be caught in the middle.

With or without surgery the principal concern in these cases should be the likelihood of chronic recurrence. So common is this that in a 4-year active intercollegiate athletic program there will always be two or three athletes with this specific problem. On the whole, however, the main difficulty has not been with the recurrent dislocation itself, for each recurrence is more easily handled than the primary episode, in terms of both reduction and rehabilitation. Instead, the obstacle has been one of accurate information. More often than not we have discovered these cases only through a recurrent episode which has either spontaneously slipped back or already been reduced by the victim himself. We are thus left with the problem of future disposition rather than immediate treatment. Surgery is never a serious consideration here, because the athlete will have gained sufficient experience to know that despite the temporary discomfort with each episode, his disability will last no more than 3 or 4 days, if that. He is usually quite willing to go along as he is, without any further interference, and this may account for the fact that these recurrent cases are so rarely brought to our attention for definitive disposition. On the other hand, the same athlete is usually quite willing to accept certain local measures if they will reduce the probability of future dislocation. It has been our policy, therefore, to recommend that these cases be either strapped, which locks the patella in place, or wrapped snugly with elastic bandage over sponge rubber to pressure the patella in the notch and prevent its distressing lateralward excursion. Whether by purely statistical probability or not, these alternative methods have succeeded in eliminating the problem of recurrence in all cases that have come to our attention.

## THE CHRONIC POST-TRAUMATIC KNEE

Even more than the postoperative problem, the chronic post-traumatic knee secondary to injuries dating back through secondary school to childhood is encountered with distressing frequency. Certain standards must be adopted to properly determine athletic disability in these cases (alluded to in a previous chapter). To repeat the essentials, *there must be full mobility, fully-developed quadriceps musculature, and functional stability.* Of these three criteria, the first two need no discussion; the third is rife with potential pitfalls for the unwary.

One must define stability as it applies to athletics. To do so one must return to basic medical principles for a knee that is subjectively unstable in normal everyday activities is certainly not one that should be subjected to the rigors and risks of any competitive contact sport (certain professional athletes notwithstanding). Fortunately, there is an anatomical corollary to such functional instability, in that these same subjective symptoms are uniformly associated with either cruciate or collateral instability of gross degree, hence the "drawer" sign is markedly positive or lateral instability is obvious, even with full extension and maximum stabilization by the quadriceps.

What of *external support* in these instances? The most elaborate devices of steel, canvas, and fitted leather have failed to stand up under the constant daily pounding of competitive weight bearing sports. Daily adhesive strapping, applied by skilled trainers, has been found to be the most efficacious. However, if permanent disability is such that gross ligamentous instability is demonstrable, even this will prove inadequate. The maximum ligamentous instability that can be tolerated in the contact sports is that which can only be demonstrated in partial flexion, not in full extension. This is our principal guide. Any compromise therefore requires more than a little rationalization, no matter what the temporary pressures, because a knee that does not meet this standard is permanently disabled and will persistently plague its owner. To subject it to even greater permanent damage is unreasonable—youthful overexuberance, parental pressure, or overenthusiastic medical advice notwithstanding.

In the non-contact weight-bearing sports much the same overall standard should apply. Whatever the activity, it must be under control, must allow for external support to the damaged knee, and must be well tolerated under all competitive conditions.

In knees that meet these last criteria of functional stability external support by strapping is mandatory for all contact-sport activity and strongly recommended for the others. It is of interest to note that, once an athlete with a knee problem starts a program of daily strapping, he will almost always continue voluntarily with it into other sports, a significant measure of his own concern. By using these support methods, the incidence of recurrent problems has been minimized to a significant degree. This has highlighted another important facet in a controlled overall program: in the treatment of athletes from all sports many will be seen who participate in several throughout the year, always with the same chronic knee problem, which then becomes so familiar to examination that a very accurate objective baseline can be established, that immeasurably enhances evaluation of any further acute or chronic difficulties.

## OTHER CHRONIC KNEE PROBLEMS

**Osgood-Schlatter's Disease.** Osgood-Schlatter's disease of the tibial tubercle is occasionally encountered, presenting a picture that ranges from an acute inflammatory reaction with apparent sequestration to a quiescent non-tender protuberance. In the former instance, all athletic activity that places excess demand on the patellar tendon, hence the tibial tubercle must be barred. In the latter local padding alone should suffice. As to the vast middle ground, the guiding principle should be the least treatment to fit the symptoms rather than the most, since the process is self-limited. Radical surgical treatment for the sole purpose of assuring athletic competition is somewhat out of proportion and perspective.

**Chondromalacia Patellae.** Another chronic problem, chondromalacia patellae, may be encountered, particularly in runners on the track team. The complaint is one of discomfort with every step, worse on sprinting, but still noticeable on going down stairs, squatting, and on every other motion that forces the patella into its groove. Examination often demonstrates a palpable, almost audible grating, when the patella is forced into its bed while the knee is flexed and extended. X-rays are diagnostic in the advanced cases, but are frequently negative in the early ones.

The treatment should be expectant, then surgical, in that order. The reason for delay in surgery is to evaluate its true need. Some cases suggest the diagnosis but do not exhibit changes sufficiently advanced to show on x-ray; these may very well clear up spontaneously after a 2-week layoff. If changes are demonstrable by x-ray and symptoms are truly disabling, surgery may be necessary, and any further athletic participation will depend upon the orthopedist's local findings and whether he feels that he has resolved the problem.

**Osteochondritis dissecans** must be considered not only from the postoperative standpoint (as discussed above) but also from its long-term implications. It is a process—or disease if you will—that is characterized by chronicity. Rarely can an orthopedist "cure" such a case. The unfortunate athlete must resign himself to a chronic situation that will intermittently become acute because of disabling loose body impactions within the joint. It is easy enough to remove these as they develop and hope the situation is ended, but is continued vigorous competition really the best thing thereafter? The greatest temptation is to assure such an athlete that all is well and to urge him to go back to that which he so desperately wants. Certainly one cannot flatly advise him to terminate his athletic career with any real factual data on hand to support such an arbitrary stand. But it has been most enlightening in our experience to discover how great is any athlete's concern about the future of his knee, no matter what his apparent enthusiasm, and to realize how eager he is to find someone who will advise him honestly. More often than not his athletic enthusiasm is but one side of him, that which he turns to his parents, to his coach, to his friends, and to the surgical specialist, while his other side is accessible only to those who have known him throughout the pain of his acute disability and have worked closely with him through the daily rigors of active rehabilitation, sharing his discomfort and discouragement—the trainer and the team-physician. If that physician will talk over the future with him, presenting him with the true facts and the probable odds on his future permanent disability, he will find that the athlete will have been waiting hopefully for just such a statement from one he feels he can trust. The athlete will then be in a position to make the wisest decision about future sports participation. After all it is his knee; he is going to have to live with it, and no one else is going to share his future discomforts. It should be a choice that he alone makes.

## THE ROLE OF FOOTBALL CLEATS IN KNEE INJURIES

In the past few years there has been increased concern over the role of ancillary equipment in the production of knee injuries in football; in particular, the role of the customary conical football cleat. Originating with Hanley at Bowdoin, who demonstrated a convincing correlation between the conical cleats, firmly fixed in the ground, and subsequent knee injury, there has been a flurry of activity directed toward modification of the cleat.

It is Hanley's contention that knee injuries occur even in the open field and without impact, because the entire foot, particularly the heel, is firmly locked on the ground, thereby transmitting disruptive torsional forces to the knee. If impact to the knee area is added to this, the result is certain to be doubly disastrous. The logic of this theory is not significantly altered by the fact that in our very small series of cases impact, not counterjoint torsion alone, has always been necessary to produce significant injury, because the fixed foot has still been an essential part of the mechanism. Furthermore, it has always been remarkable to note the low incidence of knee injuries in hockey, in which the foot is anything but fixed. This is in spite of the two major operative cases mentioned previously, because both of these instances were due to a rare combination of circumstances that could just as easily have snapped other major bones or joints at another time.

In more recent years Torg has pressed for a simple shortening of cleat length on the basis of well documented studies in the Philadelphia High Schools, and 1971 marked the first year of an overall NCAA ruling that shortened all cleats by edict to ⅜ of an inch. Again, the effect of such a change on the overall incidence of significant knee injuries remains to be demonstrated on the college level, particularly in view of the added variable, as mentioned previously, of artificial surfaces and their special shoe requirements, but we stand ready to be convinced by what seems a logical concept.

# 18

# *Injuries to the Lower Leg*

The lower leg is an anatomical and functional unit that transmits muscular power to the foot and ankle either from the upper leg and knee, as a rigid, hinged extension thereof, or from within itself, as prime mover of ankle, foot, and toes. It is exceptionally well adapted for its multiple tasks; at the same time it is subject to local problems that, because of its essential role in athletics, can be disastrous to the serious competitor. Examination of the entire part is relatively straight-forward, for review of the anatomy demonstrates a key fact: The two supporting bones, the tibia and fibula, are grossly palpable from one end to the other, particularly the weight bearing tibia.

Examination includes accurate appraisal of bony integrity, which can be diagnostic even in the not uncommon instances of fibular stress fractures. Furthermore, the muscular compartments are so distinctly separable by anatomical site and by separate function that accurate appraisal of each compartment is simply accomplished.

The anterior tibial group dorsiflexes the foot and extends the toes, the peroneal group everts and fixes the foot on the ankle, and the gastronemius-soleus flexor group plantar flexes the foot and toes, each a separate function that can be tested passively and against active resistance. These muscles are extraordinarily developed in the competitive athlete and can be accurately defined as separate groups, thus further localizing specific problems. The same deliberate, sequential examination that has been applied to other areas is even more satis-factory in the lower leg; namely, a careful detailed history, a thorough, painstaking palpation, and a simple series of functional tests. At the conclusion of examination, diagnosis should be quite clear cut and definite.

## Injuries to the Fibula

If one excludes fractures in the malleolar area as part of the ankle (to be discussed in Chapter 19), there are several specific problems involving the fibula proximal thereto, that should be recognized. Most are due to direct impact, because the fibula is not strictly speaking a weight-bearing bone, subject to weight-bearing stresses and torsions. Impacts are painfully common in the contact sports and strike more often from the lateral, external aspect of the lower leg, directly over the length of the bone. All such impacts must be evaluated first for *direct fracture,* sometimes with angulation from sheer force. The subcutaneous nature of the fibular shaft usually allows the diagnosis to be made or strongly suggested enough to warrant a diagnostic x-ray.

Short of clinically obvious fracture, which must be treated without concern for future athletics until solid healing has taken place over at least a 6-week period, there is the *fibular stress fracture and the directly related fibular periostitis.* These most commonly appear at the junction of middle and lower third and are characterized by a vague history of persistent soreness, aggravated by running and usually developing in track men after a change in running surface. Examination sometimes reveals a tender and thickened area on the shaft of the fibula, which may or may not be crepitant and often appears normal on x-ray. At other times examination reveals a specific and consistent "sore spot" on the smooth bony shaft, again with a normal x-ray. Regardless, all running must be terminated while the area is checked repeatedly, always with another film in 10 days. If this is again negative, but local findings remain as before, a third x-ray may be necessary in another 10 days, which then will show fracture-line absorption, callus formation, and periostitis, all of which were absent in the previous films. Ironically, making the diagnosis does not necessarily alter treatment, for often the belated appearance of x-ray changes coincides with a steady resolution of local symptoms and signs during the enforced rest. The athlete may, therefore, return to his labors at roughly the same time that the x-ray diagnosis is finally made. The layoff is symptomatically necessary in any event, while the final x-ray diagnosis justifies the time lost if nothing else.

As a result of direct injury, one occasionally encounters a fibular head that has been loosened from the tibiofibular ligaments, exhibiting bizzare but limited range of false motion, without any particular discomfort to the athlete. Local swelling and tenderness in the acute stage may be such as to obscure the basic problem, but routine ice, compression, and elevation prove uniformly effective in controlling these symptoms, leaving the athlete with a painless but *abnormally mobile fibular head.* Such abnormal mobility can prove chronically annoying in the running sports, because it moves about and clicks with every step (at times almost audibly). Surgical repair of the ligaments for permanent fixation of the fibular head would seem the most reasonable choice, but has been unanimously turned down by all our athletes as being more than the condition demands. They soon discovered that a simple sponge-rubber and snug elastic bandage over the area not only holds the errant bone quite adequately without adverse peroneal nerve pressure symptoms but also eliminates the annoying clicking.

If this false motion or any other pathology on or about the fibular head is associated with *peroneal nerve symptoms* as it winds around the fibular neck, surgery should be considered. The only significant peroneal nerve injury seen over the years, however, has been in a coxswain who habitually leaned his lower leg lateralward against the gunwale of the racing shell, thereby developing a mysterious peroneal weakness that disappeared only when the area was padded and the habit overcome.

### Contusions of the Lower Leg

As can be appreciated by anyone who has "barked his shin," contusions of the lower leg, despite shin guards and other protective devices, are common and painful. There is never any doubt as to the history of impact. Once the possibility of direct bony injury has been eliminated by direct palpation, there remains only the routine treatment with ice, compression, and elevation. Some concern has been shown by some over the *anterior tibial compartment contusion,* since this is a closed space and inordinate swelling therein can certainly lead to muscular ischemia and necrosis that requires fasciotomy for relief. However, as was stated in reference to the massive quadriceps contusion, bleeding and swelling to this degree has not been seen in 30 years of intercollegiate and intramural athletics, and with prompt ice and elevation should not be seriously anticipated.

On the other hand, contusions of the lower leg can present other problems of unique significance. *Contusion* over the anatomical length *of the greater saphenous vein* frequently ruptures this large vascular channel, resulting in swelling and ecchymosis that can be initially alarming. Local pressure, elevation, and ice will suffice but, because of the definite tendency for such an area to thrombose, a *local phlebitic reaction* may develop. This secondary phlebitic reaction is identical to localized saphenous phlebitis. It is palpably tender and warm, and may ascend up the vein for a variable distance. There is no need for anticoagulants or other intensive measures, since this is a local reaction to local trauma. If treated by bedrest, elevation, and local heat, it subsides satisfactorily in 5 to 7 days. If it can be avoided by anticipation, however, the time saved rewards the effort. Any contusion over the saphenous area, therefore, should be immediately started on ice, compression, and elevation, studiously maintained for at least 24 to 48 hours if only to avoid secondary phlebitis. Ambulation should then be started progressively, just as in a postoperative vein stripping, but strenuous running should be completely barred for at least another day or two, to assure that resolution and absorption are well underway. After a total of 4 days, running can be initiated under direct supervision, with immediate cessation should swelling recur. If no swelling develops, full contact may be allowed, with a protective pad which must be worn for at least two to three weeks. Thanks to this precautionary program, no particular difficulties have been encountered, the only instances of significant post-traumatic phlebitis appearing in those athletes who failed to report initially and continued to play until swelling, redness, and palpable thrombosis developed. These required up to a week of strict bedrest and local heat to clear up, hardly a worthwhile price to pay for something that can be avoided with a little foresight.

**Fascial Tears**

Disruption of the deep fascia overlying active muscle groups can develop anywhere, but because of the high incidence of blunt impact to the lower leg these tears are most common along the posteromedial and antero-lateral crests of the tibia, where impact is particularly prone to tear the fascia overlying either soleus and long flexors medially, or anterior tibial laterally. These tears are not palpable initially. Their presence is suggested by a more persistent bleeding and a greater local reaction than might otherwise be expected. Within a week, when local induration subsides, there is a palpable defect in the fascia, through which muscle can be felt to bulge. Fascial tears in other areas exhibit much the same history and present much the same basic problem; namely, the rationale for surgical repair. Though direct repair would seem most logical, these rents are not clearly defined, the surrounding fascia is often attenuated, and simple closure of the defect must be under such tension that some type of fascial graft is usually necessary. Alternatively, without reparative surgery what is the functional problem presented by the defect? Symptoms develop only during exercise, when the underlying muscle normally swells within its fascial sheath yet slides freely beneath it. With a rent this same swollen muscle protrudes through, thus impinges on the defect margins with every motion, creating more swelling, more impingement. Therefore, any external pressure should suffice that holds the muscle down below the level of the fascial rent, where it can thus slide freely and not impinge thereon. A local sponge rubber pad, held in place with an elastic bandage, has proven uniformly effective in completely terminating symptoms from these fascial defects. The moment the pad is inadvertently omitted before strenuous activity, local symptoms promptly recur. This method is crude, but it is effective. Contrasted to a technically difficult surgical procedure that requires a large working incision as well as a separate donor-site incision, it offers an alternative that for the athlete makes a great deal of sense.

### Strains of the Gastrocnemius and Soleus Muscles

**Calf Strains.** As the principle plantar flexors of the foot and ankle, the powerful gastrocnemius and soleus muscles are subject to frequent and crippling strains, usually in the area of the musculotendinous junction of the gastroc with accompanying deep spasm of the underlying soleus. These calf strains are almost always seen at the beginning of an athletic season, in those who have left their conditioning work to last and are desperately trying to catch up. The immediate result is a painful cramping of the entire muscle group that effectively terminates all such misdirected effort. Examination uniformly reveals a "tight calf" maximally tender at the exact point of strain. Occasionally a palpable tender mass indicating some actual bleeding can be made out; more often the entire muscle group is tight and sore, particularly along the visible and palpable musculotendinous junction.

Treatment is mostly vocal, since nothing really helps such sore calves to any extent. Local heat frequently causes swelling and more pain; ice usually cause more painful cramping, and hot whirlpools provide only temporary relief. All running should be terminated and the athlete checked daily until the spasm subsides, usually a matter of 2 to 3 days. Then he can be started out on a more logical and controlled running program, walking first, then jogging, then running easily for distance. Though such a program would seem to assure recurrent cramping and strain, such is never the case as long as the resumption of exercise is withheld until the calf is palpably as loose as its opposite counterpart.

**Soleus Strain.** Of more unique interest is the soleus strain that occurs as an entity, independent òf the gastrocnemius. Though rare, it is seen with recognizable frequency and is characterized by a cramping in the calf that is persistently recurrent and not associated with poor overall leg conditioning, as is gastroc-soleus strain. It usually appears in the middle of a season, is uniformly disabling, and is distressingly difficult to treat. On examination the gastrocnemius is loose and non-tender, whereas the underlying soleus is tight and acutely sore—in fact, its entire anatomical structure will be easily palpable, proximally in the popliteal fossa as it peeks over the divergent heads of the gastrocnemius, laterally and medially where its margins protrude beneath the massive belly of the gastrocnemius, and distally along the deeper aspect of the common Achilles tendon! Treatment is not too satisfactory. Every physical therapy modality— whirlpool, heat, hot packs, or massage—tends to make the area subjectively worse, and even the most cautious exercise results in immediate cramping. Instead a complete layoff should be instituted, checking the muscle at frequent intervals until all tenderness has subsided. A series of dorsiflexion stretching exercises should then be started up to tolerance. After all of 10 days to 2 weeks or more a graduated program of controlled running can be resumed.

**Strain of Gastrocnemius Head.** Most important of calf injuries in a differential sense is the high strain of the gastrocnemius heads, a result of a sudden hyperextension of the knee. Because counterjoint motion of the knee is involved, there should be immediate concern for the knee joint. Before all else the knee must be thoroughly checked for possible damage. However, with a particular and specific history of a snapping hyperextension it is not unusual to find nothing whatever in the knee, but, instead, a *specific tenderness and swelling in one or both heads of the gastrocnemius,* high up in the popliteal fossa and palpable only when the knee is passively flexed. Palpation of the tender swelling elicits an immediate reaction from the injured athlete that is remarkable in its consistency. With this the diagnosis is defined. Treatment is as for any strained muscle: ice and rest for 2 days, then a gradual active rehabilitation. Most important, the badly frightened athlete and others can be reassured that there is no true knee damage and that full activity can be anticipated after 5 to 7 days of active rehabilitation.

## "Shin Splints"

The term "shin splints" has been used as a catch-all for all conditions occurring around the anterior tibial crest as well as for vague problems in the posterior flexor compartment. Its use has led to confusion in any intelligent discussion of the subject. Many consider that the term applies to strains in the anterior tibial compartment, a specific picture that can, because of the closed-space nature of the compartment, give rise to the "anterior tibial syndrome," described in contusions of the area but here related to simple strain. Some associate the symptoms with posterior tibial irritation, deep behind the posteromedial crest of the tibia, and others with a periostitis in the same area.

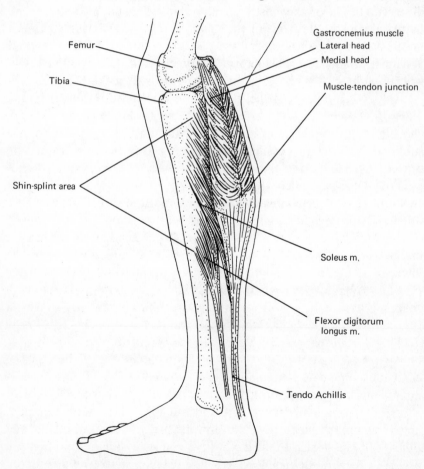

Fig. 18-1. The medial leg and "shin splints."

In general, the *symptoms of "shin splints"* are related to a change in running surface or an alteration in running drills, and these are factors necessary for the diagnosis. The pain is typically deep seated and throbbing, is much worse at night, and is not relieved by any specific physical therapy modality—in fact it is increased by all of them. Continued running usually makes the disability worse, at best alters it not at all, and never relieves it, no matter how closely the workouts are supervised. Prolonged layoffs are sometimes beneficial if sufficiently prolonged, but not consistently enough to make the 2- to 3-week time loss a practical measure. In all, this is the characteristic clinical picture of "shin splints," the picture that trainers, athletes, and coaches associate with the term, yet one that is still too diffuse to define or discuss accurately.

One must, therefore, try to redefine and reduce this symptom complex to a common denominator, that will fit all the above characteristics of history and complaint and at the same time eliminate distinct and separate conditions such as anterior tibial strains. On doing so, one is left with but one condition that fits all the symptomatic characteristics, a complaint that invariably localizes along the *postero-medial crest of the tibia in the middle to lower third,* a specific tenderness that is palpable as a distinct swelling and, at times, a local bony roughening, with a soreness and spasm that extends for a variable distance into the immediately contiguous muscles. Review of the local anatomy then demonstrates a constant muscular origin from this exact region on the tibia, that of the *soleus muscle proximally and the flexor digitorum longus* distally.

Analysis of each case reveals that every one is directly related to running "duck-footed," that is, with feet everted and externally rotated, thus transferring a significant portion of the forceful plantar flexion of both foot and ankle from the powerful gastrocnemiussoleus groups through the Achilles tendon to a less efficient mechanism off the medial forefoot and medial aspect of the hallux. In consequence, classical strain symptoms must be anticipated at certain predictable bony anchor points, and anatomical review again pinpoints *medial soleus and flexor digitorum longus attachments* as the logical focus of this strain. This then, is the classic "shin-splint." (See Fig. 18-1.)

All this is theoretical. Proof must be based on the efficacy of specific measures directed toward "duck foot" eversion. Encouragingly enough, strapping the ankle with the foot pulled toward inversion and instructing the runner to work out lightly with a conscious effort to run "pigeon-toed," have never failed to work. Repeated daily sessions of closely supervised running must be an integral part of this specific rehabilitation program for a further 7 to 10 days. Once the "duck footing" is consciously overcome by the athlete, the entire problem tends to solve itself progressively with each workout. The special tape support should be continued throughout this key period, though it is of less and less importance with each day of improvement. It had best be applied daily for at least a month, if only as a constant reminder to the athlete to keep his feet pointed forward in the normal manner.

Our theory on the pathophysiology of "shin splints" and their treatment is not original. It was worked out over many years by the head trainer at Yale, Mr. O. W. Dayton, but it does make anatomical, mechanical, and physiological sense. "Duck footing" is always directly related either to changes in running surface or to an ill advised attempt to compensate for a primary calf soreness that stems from poor conditioning. Signs of strain then appear with predictable regularity along the medial middle to lower third of the tibia. The diagnosis is easily made, and with treatment as outlined the complaint disappears.

## Achilles Tendinitis

The tender, swollen tendo Achilles, crepitant to palpation and acutely disabling, was a familiar sight to military surgeons, when the Army combat boot first came into wide use during World War II. At that time it was attributed to pressure on the area from the heavy boot counter. The same classical swollen tendon, painful on every motion of the foot and ankle and equally disabling, has no such easy explanation in athletics, in which it is a common problem. Sometimes an ankle taping with too great pressure over the tendon (just as the combat boot counter) can give rise to symptoms. More often than not the condition appears suddenly with no explanation. It must be recognized as a totally disabling condition, that must be allowed to subside completely before athletic activity can be safely resumed. A lift in the heel to relieve the constant aggravation with each step can be prescribed as initial treatment; otherwise, little can be done. Response to strict athletic prohibition usually is encouragingly prompt, with the acute process disappearing within 5 to 7 days. Any attempt to shorten the period by restoring activity in the presence of minimal local findings immediately brings back all symptoms and signs. Local steroid injection can be symptomatically effective, but does not immediately alter the actual inflammatory process, thus has been suspiciously associated with cases of spontaneous rupture of the entire tendon from too vigorous reactivity following this dramatic local relief. As with so many similar conditions, we have preferred to let the athlete live with his disability, providing both ourselves and him with a visible and palpable index of progress, without at any time risking ill advised overexertion and subsequent tendon rupture.

## Plantaris Tendon Rupture

The thin, cord like plantaris muscle, deep in the posterior aspect of the calf, is subject to but one ailment that is symptomatically noticeable in the midst of the overwhelming functional predominance of the overlying gastrocnemius and soleus muscles: spontaneous rupture. Uniformly a sudden development, it is usually described as an explosive pain deep in the calf—"Like I was shot"—stemming from a sudden uncoordinated effort at movement from a complete standstill, and it has been reported at times as actually audible. Audible or not, the acute pain is deep in the calf and is further aggravated by forceful dorsiflexion of the foot. Thereafter, because of secondary bleeding (particularly if the tear is high up toward the fleshier portion of the muscle) deep irritation and soreness of the calf can develop, that may raise the question of a positive Homan's sign, hence a deep thrombophlebitis. The onset, however, is classical, the disability is classical, and in a few days a minor ecchymosis is seen on either side of the Achilles tendon to further confirm the diagnosis. Treatment is purely supportive, avoiding heat for the first 48 hours to minimize any deep bleeding. A felt lift under the heel to minimize pain on walking is often helpful. Crutches are seldom necessary but walking must be aided by a cane, since symptoms continue for several weeks despite the total unimportance of the structure itself. We have yet to see this condition in an athlete and have, therefore, not yet had to contend with the prolonged subsequent disability. There is never permanent functional loss, but the time lost from all strenuous activity can be discouraging. In competitive athletics, the usual 3 to 4 weeks disability can mean nearly half of a competitive season, a disastrous loss for so small and useless a structure.

## Calcaneal Bursitis

As the final item in our survey of lower leg injuries, the calcaneal bursa might better be discussed in relation to the foot and ankle, yet its position, just superficial to the calcaneal spur and the attachment of the tendo Achilles, renders any inflammatory reaction as disabling as any problem in the lower leg. A typical superficial bursa, it is subject to all the problems of any such bursae; so direct puncture and laceration must be anticipated. Because of its position it is even more prone to impact from errant kicks and hockey pucks. Acute collections of blood are seen, which demand treatment identical to that for any other blood filled bursa: early aspiration and compression. Similarly, blisters have an unfortunate tendency to develop over this protruding area because of pressure from the shoe counter; as blisters often will, some get secondarily infected and a *purulent bursitis,* requiring intensive local and systematic treatment, may then develop.

Most annoying of all is the *thickened chronic bursa with recurrent swelling,* that can develop following acute injury but more often results from constant shoe counter pressure over an unusually prominent calcaneal spur. So persistent can this problem become that surgical excision of the spur and bursa may become necessary. At other times repeated injections of cortical steroid may be resorted to. If caught early, these latter problems will improve with some judicious padding and little else, and this is much to be preferred to any radical surgery.

# 19

# *Ankle Injuries and Disabilities*

Any attempt to review such an oft-injured area as the ankle joint must include discussion of fractures and fracture-dislocation. It is our intention to limit such discussion to the particular problems of accurate diagnosis before x-ray, leaving the myriad classifications of fracture deformity to the orthopedist, who is primarily responsible for definitive treatment. This is not to say that the complex definitions of eversion, inversion, supination with adduction, and supination with rotation are not important in the understanding of how these various bony injuries occur and why, but, if there is x-ray demonstration of bony disruption, it is the orthopedist's task to restore continuity to as close to anatomical as possible. If closed manipulation will suffice, all well and good. If open operation is necessary, so be it. Regardless, the ankle joint must be restored to maximum function, whether it be in a banker, lawyer, housewife, or athlete.

## Clinical Evaluation of Ankle Injuries

It behooves the physician on the spot to examine every ankle injury from the viewpoint of "fracture–no fracture" before he considers anything else. He will find that this all-important differentiation is never more easily made than under these circumstances, for at no other time does he have the opportunity to examine an ankle literally within seconds of injury. He will inspect and palpate a joint that has yet to swell, hence retains all bony and soft tissue landmarks. To add to his good fortune, the ankle is normally a subcutaneous joint accessible to thorough inspection and palpation from all but its posterior aspect. In particular, the lateral and medial malleoli are ideally situated and conformed for a firm, probing examination that can very accurately delineate fracture-line tenderness, crepitus, and even the tender localized irregularity of an incomplete fracture. The important peroneal, posterior tibial, anterior tibial, and Achilles tendons are easily palpable in their normal anatomical course, so they can be thoroughly checked by exacting palpation as well as by active and passive motion tests.

**Delayed Evaluation.** Should examination of the ankle be delayed beyond two or three hours, these particular advantages are completely lost. Faced with such a swollen joint, the physician must obtain x-rays before all else. But before this post-traumatic swelling has occurred he will often be able to so positively eliminate bony injury that further treatment measures can proceed without x-ray. This last statement will be met with disapproval by many doctors, who staunchly believe that failure to x-ray every ankle injury is negligence. As with everything else in medicine, however, ankle injuries vary in severity, from the minimal swelling and soreness, that can return to full activity after but 1 day of intensive treatment, to gross tears of major supporting ligaments. These differences can be very accurately delineated within this limited period of time. Certainly, *after swelling has become established accurate evaluation is no longer possible, and every ankle should then be x-rayed,* but careful clinical judgment can and should be employed before that time.

**Severity of Injury.** The first thing that must be established is the initial severity of injury and the precise interval preceding examination. The mild sprain, which the athlete has "walked off" on his own, resuming his activity until increasing soreness forces him to seek medical advice, is one degree of severity; the acute tearing sensation with immediate crippling pain and disability is another. A minor initial episode, that precludes further activity, but permits measured and deliberate weight bearing, yet within 5 minutes exhibits marked swelling, is another recognizable variation.

The first instance is the least severe and with intensive local treatment should result in full athletic activity within 2 or 3 days. The second is a severe ankle injury that requires the most careful examination to rule our fracture and even with the most vigorous efforts sets its own pace in recovery. The third, despite an initial swelling that equals if it does not outstrip the worst variety of sprain or fracture, with proper treatment recovers full strength and function in almost as short a time as the first.

**Clinical History.** Examination, therefore, cannot be of full value unless an accurate history is obtained simultaneously. A precise review of the exact circumstances of injury, an exact description of the forces involved, a clear subjective review of the type of counterjoint stress—whether inversion, eversion, or hyperextension—must be extracted from the injured athlete before he forgets them. Particular local circumstances must be identified; for example, was the ankle strapped, was the ankle wrapped? Any history of injury, recent or long past, must be painstakingly extracted, for pre-existing ankle injury can have a profound effect on initial findings, definitive treatment, and subsequent course. The particular advantages of a prior acquaintance with the athlete's history as well as a baseline familiarity with his ankle mobility and strength are here clearly demonstrated.

**Steps in Injury Evaluation.** As to the actual on the spot evaluation, a *sequence of logical steps* should be followed. The first is *thorough palpation of all bony points* over their entire accessible surfaces, palpation with increasing pressure until one can be satisfied that no true crepitus or fracture line tenderness exists. This means not only thorough palpation of the entire surface of both malleoli but also an equally thorough *palpation of the entire distal third of both tibia and fibula.* If this proves negative, then the *malleoli should be forcefully levered in the anterio-posterior plane* by firm external pressure, to further rule out fracture. Finally, if all else fails to arouse suspicion of bony injury, *the ankle should be gently everted and inverted to the limit,* not to test pain in the ligament areas but to provide a last and positive check on ankle-mortise integrity.

Having thus surveyed the injured ankle for bony injury and found none, the physician can turn to the damaged soft tissues. *Any amount of swelling should be carefully noted, in particular the relation of swelling to the time of injury.* This provides an index of the extravasation that might be anticipated. In the ankle more than in any other area bleeding of itself can cause lasting symptoms that must be avoided whenever possible. Bleeding is not, however, dependably correlated with the actual degree of soft tissue injury. A rapidly ballooning ankle may be a simple reflection of a minimal ligament stretch that has at the same time involved a larger blood vessel. Initial examination within minutes will correctly assess these facts. Thereafter, acute tenderness and disability are more directly related to the extent of extravasation and the subsequent inflammatory reaction than to the actual soft tissue damage. *Consequently, significant areas of maximal tenderness must be carefully outlined and identified at the very outset:* even 3 or 4 hours later such will be totally useless. The talofibular, posterior and anterior, and the calcaneofibular ligaments should be palpated carefully on the lateral side, the deltoid and posterior talotibial ligaments on the medial side. The posterior tibial tendon area should be palpated firmly along its course behind the medial malleolus, if the sprain is of the eversion type. The long and short peroneals should be palpated in like manner along their respective course behind the lateral malleolus, if the sprain is of the inversion type. (See Fig. 19-1.)

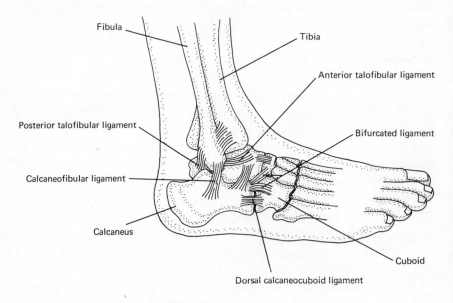

LATERAL RIGHT ANKLE & FOOT

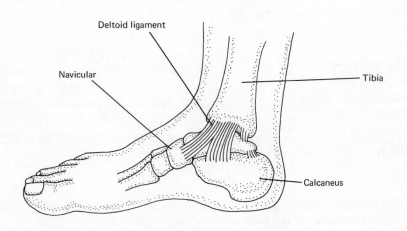

MEDIAL RIGHT ANKLE & FOOT

Fig. 19-1. Ligaments of the ankle and foot.

## Contusions of the Ankle

If we turn now to the more specific injuries encountered in and around the ankle, we find that contusion is seen in all its forms, particularly in hockey in which the puck and the sticks are a menace to feet and ankles. Because of the anatomical characteristics of the area *these contusions are uniformly "bone bruises,"* with all the persistence and annoying chronicity associated therewith. *Local ice, compression with elastic bandage, and elevation constitute the routine treatment,* to be continued for 24 to 48 hours and normally followed by a prompt return to full activity. Because of the juxta-articular site of these bruises, bleeding frequently dissects into neighboring ligaments and capsular elements, giving rise to symptoms of sprain without any history to suggest sprain. It is occasionally of value, therefore, to supplement routine treatment with a *supporting ankle strapping,* as a symptomatic adjunct. *Some type of external padding,* usually a sponge rubber affixed outside of the skate or shoe, should be insisted upon thereafter, to minimize the disproportionate pain of further recurrent impact over the persistently tender area.

## Acute Sprains of the Ankle

*The inversion sprain* is the most common of ankle sprains, the one with which trainers and athletic physicians are woefully familiar. The result of a common mechanism, this sprain exhibits evidence of tissue damage predominantly on the lateral side, to a degree proportionate to the initial severity of the injury. Excluding bony tenderness then, the physician finds the most constant area of tenderness *directly over the anterior talofibular ligament, less frequently over the calcaneofibular ligament* (Fig. 19-1). An area of lesser tenderness is not infrequently found on the opposite side of the ankle in the anterior talotibial area, where the abnormal inversion has effectively pinched and impacted these structures. If examination is early enough to precede obscuring hemorrhage, localization is amply demonstrated.

*In the eversion sprain tenderness is maximal over the deltoid ligaments,* initially in the anterior limb thereof but with increasing damage extending further posteriorward (Fig. 19-1). Localization is no problem, as long as the area is examined early enough.

The *hyperextension sprain,* much the most resistant to treatment, exhibits signs of *tenderness and swelling on both sides of the ankle, in the anterior talofibular ligaments and the anterior limb of the del-*

*toid ligament*. There are even signs of tenderness and swelling deep in the soft tissues posteriorly, indicating a probable impaction of capsular and posterior ligament elements by the abnormal motion.

**Treatment.** Treatment of all these varieties of ankle sprain is basically the same. The first objective must be the *control of bleeding,* hence swelling. The usual routine of ice, elastic bandage compression, and elevation must be applied from the moment the injury is reported. Further inadvertent eversion or inversion of the injured ankle is minimized by a *Gibney adhesive strapping,* an open-face strapping that allows swelling to take place without interference or constriction, while at the same time providing secure support to those structures in the greatest need. In the less severe types of ankle sprains, in which the first hour of ice and elevation has controlled virtually all swelling and local tenderness indicates the most minor degree of soft tissue damage, the ice bag is strapped over the outside of the compression bandage and Gibney strapping and the athlete allowed to return to his room without crutches: he is, however, given firm instructions on constant elevation and a minimum of ambulation. All others are placed on crutches, and those with the more severe sprains are admitted to the Infirmary for intensive and constant ice and elevation.

As soon as swelling has "peaked" under treatment (usually within 36 to 48 hours) and has begun to subside, as evidenced by a daily reevaluation, *graduated weight bearing* is begun with the added support of *modified figure-of-eight encircling adhesive strapping.* Great care is exercised at the beginning of this initial stage of activity to instruct the injured athlete on what constitutes useful weight bearing (i.e., toes pointed straight ahead and the foot "rocking through" on the ankle, rather than twisting or dragging). Continued daily examination reveals a surprising diminution of symptoms and swelling with this regimen, and tenderness, which on the 3rd day usually coincides with the total area of extravasation, will by the 5th day have relocalized in the precise area of original damage, where a palpable thickening and fibrosis will be evident. As soon as unsupported walking can be accomplished without any visible trace of a limp, the athlete is ready to begin a program of active rehabilitation. Until that time, however, he is barred from any activity. It is a rule of thumb that a boy can begin reconditioning only when he can walk normally and not a moment before.

## Active Rehabilitation of the Injured Ankle

2 or 3 days after injury in the case of minor sprains and five to seven in the case of more severe sprains, *a very careful program of controlled exercise* is begun, first with alternate light jogging and walking, then with the former increased to tolerance until 300 to 400 yards can be covered without visible or subjective distress. As long as pain does not increase between daily sessions and as long as daily re-examination of the ankle reveals no recurrent swelling, the jogging can be alternated with straight ahead running, then with sprinting, until sprints of up to 100 yards can be comfortably tolerated. Serpentines are then added to the program, running the athlete along what is essentially a sine wave course at increasing speeds and thereby placing a graduated stress on the injured ankle, which can then be further challenged by "sharpening" the curves until a complete 100-yard zig-zag course can be run at full speed. Then and only then is the athlete allowed to return to full activity.

Throughout the entire program he will not have been forced to do anything to which his ankle would not have been given ample opportunity to adjust at its own pace. Any evidence of increased swelling or pain results in an immediate readjustment of the work program; any recurrent limp is immediately corrected or its basis thoroughly investigated.

Such a program is time consuming and laborious, particularly to the trainer, who must remove and reapply strapping daily, then twice daily, supervise the projected exercise program, and yet keep in mind overall team progress and what special work the injured athlete can and cannot afford to miss. The physician must be constantly alert to the slightest evidence of reaggravation and adjust requirements accordingly. He must not under any circumstances allow external pressures and circumstances to accelerate the graduated program to the athlete's physical detriment. The reward will be a fully conditioned athlete, who can return to his duties in a remarkably short time as compared to the average clinical outpatient with an identical injury. Unfortunately, the reward is not without its disillusionments, since both the doctor and trainer can be sure that the injured athlete, who returns after 5 days of intensive effort on their part and his, will be considered by most critics to have been scarcely injured at all. And there is always one boy, who, after smoothly and painlessly completing every step of the above program without incident, will run onto the playing field before thousands, exhibiting a brand-new and monstrous "gimp" never before seen— immediately convincing everyone in the stands that a broken ankle has not only been neglected but is being further abused for the sake of athletics!

In this treatment program we have not mentioned local heat, whirlpool, or other physical therapy modalities. Aside from a rarely necessary modicum of local heat to "loosen" up the injury site just prior to a programmed workout, none of the various modalities have proved either necessary or desirable. If a program of constant supervision and controlled rehabilitation, adjusted daily to tolerance, cannot be adequately administered, the only practical alternative must be daily physical therapy treatments, including all applicable techniques. For the average clinical problem it is indispensable. But with a controlled program we have found little use for it.

Similarly, the injection of local anesthetic, "spreading agents," or cortical steroids is of no particular value in a controlled program. The keystone to the entire exercise plan is the athlete's physical tolerance, hence his local symptoms in relation to the resolving injury. Any artificial alteration of these key local symptoms will totally destroy guidelines and possibly engender a permanently damaging acceleration of the entire rehabilitation program, a consideration of far greater significance than the temporary presence of some minor local discomfort, which in our experience ceases to be of any import after the 2nd day.

**The Chronic Ankle Injury**

On the college level the physician must be prepared to deal with a large number of athletes who give a similar history of significant and recurrent ankle injuries. Some are the final result of severe initial injury and the most thorough treatment, even including plaster casts for 3 to 4 weeks; others are the result of no treatment at all. Most exhibit a common laxity of their lateral ligaments, to a point that some will be able to invert their feet to a remarkable degree. Though this range of motion may be striking to those inexperienced in this field, it is actually of little concern. Athletes with ankles such as these are extremely unlikely to suffer significant ankle sprains thereafter, because there is little left to sprain. Instead, with *daily ankle strapping* by skilled trainers, a service which is constantly available throughout all athletic areas, these athletes can take part in all sports without notable problems. *External support is absolutely essential* no matter what the sport, not because there is any real functional disability without it, but because these "weak ankles" without support, inevitably "turn under." Despite the fact that these recurrent episodes are quite innocuous under routine treatment, lasting no more than 2 or 3 days, they can be annoying.

What of the truly unstable ankle, as exhibited and proven by stress x-ray films? Again, we must try to redefine related athletic disability and the meaning of an unstable ankle by x-ray. Demonstration of anatomical hypermobility of the talus within the ankle mortise is one thing, and the stress x-ray demonstrates this graphically, but it is equally clear that many athletes of the type described in the previous paragraph would exhibit the same hypermobility. Why then have we not ordered such films on each of these young men? We have not because they are neither disturbed nor hampered by their ankle problems and, taped or not taped, are capable of far more skilled and violent activity than most normal human beings. Therefore, their problem, admittedly demonstrable by x-ray and physical examination, is whatever doctors want to make of it and of no real interest to them.

If an athlete with this degree of hypermobility in the ankle joint were to complain of demonstrable swelling and recurrent pain on every effort within his sport despite daily and adequate tape support or, worse, if he were to complain of similar symptoms in his normal activities, then we have a truly unstable ankle. Surgical stabilization by whatever tendon transfer or tunneling may be preferred must then be considered. But we have seen instances in which skilled athletes have been urged into these operative procedures simply to eliminate the necessity for daily ankle strapping or some such minimal indication. As a result, they have indeed acquired an ankle rigidity that is occasionally visible on normal gait and always starkly apparent on full speed running and cutting. The effect of such stabilization procedures on subsequent athletic performance has therefore been uniformly disastrous. If there is significant permanent ankle disability, as evidenced by persistent swelling and pain on minimal exertion, ankle stabilization should be seriously weighed. Judging, however, from the many athletes in all sports who despite demonstrable instability have successfully engaged in their chosen activity with no more than a daily adhesive strapping, such extensive surgery is rarely necessary.

## The Value of Ankle Wraps

The rigid policy of ankle wraps or ankle strapping on every ankle for every workout and game has been firmly entrenched in athletics since the early 1930's, tracing back to Thorndike's original statement, "once a sprain, always a sprain," and his recommendations in favor of this overall policy. So prevalent did it become, that many football veterans of the 1930's can remember on-the-spot checks by coaching staffs at odd moments during a routine practice, with all delinquents deprived of supper. ("Hit 'em where it hurts!") Over the years many have given up the practice for one or another reason, while others have remained steadfast, notably the professional football clubs, who uniformly assess automatic fines to enforce their ruling. (Again, "Hit 'em where it hurts!") However, many, including ourselves, have wondered just what such a blanket policy does secondarily to the knee joint. If the foot is fixed with the ankle effectively locked by a good sturdy wrap or strapping, while impacting torsional forces applied, something has to give, and it might be the knee first. There are no conclusive figures to back up this feeling, but it does make enough sense to warrant serious consideration. Furthermore, it is far more preferable to treat a sprained ankle than a knee injury. And what, in fact, happens when ankle strapping is limited to those athletes with demonstrably "loose ankles"? Instead of encountering a spate of crippling ankle injuries, we have noted no significant change, either in total time lost or in severity of injury, since abandoning this arbitrary policy. Many will disagree with us on this policy change (in effect for 18 years now), but we are happy with it, and knee injuries have not been a frequent problem perhaps for this reason.

## Peroneal and Posterior Tibial Tendinitis

An ankle complaint is encountered on occasion that does not necessarily stem from direct injury, though it may develop a few days thereafter. The complaint is of pain and discomfort, worse on certain ankle motions, and tenderness is uniformly localized over the course of either the posterior tibial tendon, running behind the medial malleolus, or the peroneal tendons, running behind the lateral malleolus. *Palpation of the involved area* reveals a distinct fusiform swelling of tendon sheath, an acute tenderness, and *a peculiar "squeaking" crepitus on motion of the involved tendon.* Ankle sprains or contusions, both of which give rise to bleeding that can dissect into and involve these tendon areas, can frequently precede the development of these problems, but this is not uniformly the case. Some instances arise de novo with no explanation whatever.

**Treatment.** Treatment is tempered by certain athletic considerations, in that immediate relief by injection means an immediate resumption of activity unless the doctor is willing to follow and supervise that athlete every minute of the day. We prefer to *treat these cases expectantly,* applying ice to the local area for lack of anything better, while completely limiting the athlete's activities until symptoms and signs subside. Fortunately, since these are athletes and the problem is almost always associated in some way with athletics, such a prohibition usually results in a very rapid subsidence of symptoms and local findings in a matter of three or four days, after which a graduated program of rehabilitation to tolerance returns the young man to full activity in another 2 or 3 days. Adhesive strapping to limit ankle excursion is of considerable value, but it must be most skillfully applied; otherwise, direct pressure over the involved tendons aggravates matters. Although this overall approach has met with uniform success up to the present, there will doubtless be *recalcitrant cases. Locally administered cortical steroid* with a rigid subsequent control over activity will have to be employed with these.

## The Ankle After Fracture

An occasional athlete is seen who has suffered a recent fracture or fracture-dislocation of the ankle that is sufficiently long past to assure adequate bony union. He has, or should have, written permission from his orthopedist to engage in vigorous athletics and preferably his last x-ray if not all of them. The key is the ankle itself. More often than not, the necessary immobilization to assure bony healing has led to marked atrophy and weakness of all the muscles, only some of which may have been remedied by the time he appears as an athletic candidate. Worse yet, if massive soft tissue damage was also a part of the original injury as, for example, in a fracture-dislocation, there will be a brawny, leathery mass of solid scar tissue binding all ankle motion in dorsiflexion, plantar flexion, eversion, inversion, and rotation—walking and running can then be accomplished only with a limping gait.

In essence, the problem is little different, though much greater in degree, from the scarred ankle that always develops from prolonged boot immobilization for acute sprain, followed by intensive whirlpool and heat lamp treatments, all without the benefit of active rehabilitation. It must be overcome the same way. With the situation as outlined, we simply encourage the athlete to wade into the thick of it, limp and all. Occasional soreness and minimal swelling may develop as a result of overstretching the tight tissues, but this will be a steadily diminishing problem as time passes.

Despite the most vigorous contact athletics and equally strenuous conditioning between, a year may be necessary before ankle motion, strength, and normal running will return. If the athlete in the meantime can protect himself and operate effectively, all well and good, limp or no limp. Naturally, close supervision will be necessary at all times, checking the ankle at frequent intervals. But, sooner or later, time and violent exercise will do the job!

Case 10, C. S.: A flanker back, with great speed and quick hands, was hit at the goal line by the single safety man with a clean, legal tackle on the last play of the last scrimmage of the pre-season double sessions. He heard and felt his ankle "go" and, consequently, moved not one muscle thereafter; examination revealed an obvious bimalleolar fracture-dislocation of the ankle with lateral displacement. Because of an arbitrary ruling by our training staff he was wearing high-top shoes, as were all squad members during practice, and the dislocation was held quite stably by the high shoe. No further splinting was considered necessary, and the athlete was immediately transferred to the hospital and staff orthopedic care. Reduction was easily accomplished by closed manipulation, and post-reduction films showed good position and a satisfactory ankle mortise. After 12 weeks in plaster, gentle physical therapy was begun and a rehabilitation program initiated. 20 weeks after injury, C. S. was running, but his ankle was a mass of dense tight scar tissue that prevented motion in all directions except within a limited range. Nevertheless, 24 weeks after injury he won a position on the varsity baseball squad and competed thereafter in all phases of the sport satisfactorily. He had a visible limp, however, on all running or jogging. 50 weeks later, he returned to football, still with a limp, now visible only intermittently but reflected in a persistently limited range of motion in the ankle, and an improved but still considerable fibrosis. Performance was satisfactory, though not outstanding; complete rehabilitation and football success were attained only in his senior year, 2 years after injury.

Here illustrated are a number of important points. First of all, the injury was a result of perfectly normal circumstances and could have happened to anyone. It represents the type of major injury that will not be changed by rules makers, equipment designers, or medical experts. Secondly, the reaction to major injury was typical, in that the athlete knew that something was definitely wrong, hence remained utterly motionless until help arrived, a pattern that is common to all significant injuries—by and large, the athlete who is writhing about and screaming is probably not hurt seriously (though he may be hurting), while the boy who lies stock still, afraid to move a muscle, had best be looked after quickly! Thirdly, the now discontinued high top shoe here demonstrated its value, and the oft-heard argument concerning the weight saving and added speed offered by the "low-cuts" loses all importance against one such instance as this. Lastly, the prolonged convalescence is typical of major skeletal injury in the athlete. 20 weeks of recovery after an injury such as this is perfectly reasonable and the functional result—varsity baseball—might under average, non-athletic circumstances be labelled "good." For athletic demands, however, 2 full years were necessary to restore full effectiveness despite the most vigorous activity. Even then, speed and "niftiness," prime requisites in virtually all athletics, never did return completely.

# 20

# Foot Injuries and Disabilities

As the ultimate weight bearing surface of the upright hominoid, the foot bears the brunt of all physical abuse heaped upon it from above and thrust into it from below. In the weight bearing sports problems in the feet become so magnified by their crippling effect on total performance that the slightest sprain or contusion can eliminate an athlete from competition as effectively as a major long bone fracture.

Anatomically, the tarsals and metatarsals are virtually subcutaneous on the dorsal surface, a factor of great advantage in the clinical appraisal of injuries. On the plantar surface, however, considerable pressure is necessary to outline the metatarsals until one reaches the distal heads, which are more easily palpated. The tarsals remain almost inaccessible to direct examination from their plantar aspect, while, in contrast, the os calcis is easily palpable from its lateral and medial aspects though equally inaccessible from below or above. In all, inspection and palpation of the foot can be quite accurate when combined with an accurate history and complaint.

More important from the athletic point of view are the normal weight bearing arches. Our discussion of these, the longitudinal and the transverse, will be short, since whole monographs have been published on the subject. Suffice it to say that these arches are normally present and are considered essential for the normal weight bearing mechanics of the human foot. However, in athletes, who are in a younger age group, hence have not had sufficient time to develop symptomatic static problems, these arches may or may not be present, with little correlation to size, build, or ability. The longitudinal arch may be completely absent in some of our fastest track sprinters, while a ponderous football tackle, who can barely get out of his own way, may have longitudinal arches that are classical. Similarly, a marked flattening of the transverse arch, with dropped metatarsal heads and early hammering of the toes, may be found in some athletes who run 10 miles daily without symptom, while another competitor, with an apparently normal transverse arch, will require a metatarsal lift in his street shoes and all his athletic shoes in order to avoid a crippling and recurrent metatarsalgia. In years to come these static deformities may gradually become more classically symptomatic, but for our purposes findings of arch deformity are significant only if accompanied by symptoms.

**Metatarsalgia.** *Metatarsalgia* is indeed a problem, particularly in trackmen despite the many who should have symptoms but do not. The complaint is typically one of pain under the metatarsals and along the shafts of the bones, and soreness is most marked under the heads, on the plantar surface. Examination must be painstakingly thorough, grasping each metatarsal shaft individually and checking its entire length for the slightest roughening or tenderness, as well as forcefully levering each to elicit the least bone pain. If in spite of such vigor no specific bony tenderness can be elicited but, instead, soreness and sensitivity seem to be centered between the bones, a mechanical strain and stretching of the soft tissues can be safely postulated. *A felt pad should be applied, just proximal to the plantar aspect of the metatarsal heads,* pushing them gently upward. This usually relieves all symptoms. The initial complaint can range from severe and crippling pain to an annoying soreness that increases during activity. In any case symptoms will clear up on felt pad elevation in two to three days if not immediately.

**March Fractures.** If bony tenderness is elicited or there is palpable and tender roughening of any of the metatarsal shafts, x-rays should be obtained. If these show nothing, they should be repeated in a week; if still negative, in another week. *The stress fracture, better known as the "march fracture,"* can reveal its presence by the late appearance of a healing fracture despite numerous negative studies theretofore. In the meantime *the same routine treatment, a metatarsal lift, will suffice,* since, should symptoms subside entirely, no further x-rays need be scrutinized. Even if the opposite is true, nothing more is necessary, for with persistent soreness the athlete neither wants nor can return to full activity. In fact, by the time that a definite area of bony thickening and reaction is detectible, the symptoms have usually subsided to a tolerable level and athletics can be resumed to tolerance. In one such instance, not in an athlete but illustrative nonetheless, a student decided to use one of the more popular physical conditioning home programs, which included running in place for a certain length of time. The eager novice undertook this part of the program in bare feet on a concrete floor and for three weeks hobbled about to classes on a pair of exceptionally sore feet, which were, however, beginning to recover quite satisfactorily by the time he was first seen. X-rays then revealed two healed march fractures in one foot and three in the other!

**Spasm of Plantar Fascia.** As to specific longitudinal arch problems, *deep spasm of the plantar fascia* is occasionally seen, appearing suddenly in the arch and standing out cord-like to inspection, let alone palpation. The pain associated therewith can be quite acute and crippling. There may be an accompanying ecchymosis at the exact point of maximum tenderness, usually at the calcaneal end of the aponeurosis. Problems of this sort seem to be directly related to extraordinary demand, as in trying to drive the heavy football blocking sled by the usual short chopping steps, with cleats firmly planted and the foot dorsiflexed to its extreme to maintain traction. *Local ice and crutches may be necessary* for the most severe of these strains and tears. Fortunately, most are mild and respond readily to a cessation of strenuous activity for a few days and a *longitudinal arch support*. Interesting to note, these acute plantar arch symptoms have rarely been encountered in athletes with long-standing flat feet, but rather in those with normal or high arches. The explanation may be in the symptomatic early breakdown of the arch, either precipitated or accentuated by abnormally stressful demand, hence possible only with normal or high arches.

**Contusions and Abrasions.** Aside from the above problems, which are directly related to forces as they are transmitted through the foot to the ground, there are the innumerable contusions and abrasions that result (for example, in football) from being stepped on by the rigid, steel-tipped cleats of friend and foe. Rarely do these injuries penetrate the skin; when they do, they should be handled as any dirty puncture or laceration. More often, *a simple contusion of the dorsum* results, which, because of the subcutaneous nature of the bones on the dorsum, is as initially painful and as annoyingly persistent as any other "bone bruise."

*Treatment* is in no way different, once the possibility of direct fracture has been ruled out either by thorough examination or by x-ray, and consists of the usual *ice, local compression wrap, and elevation, with protective padding strapped outside the shoe* for at least 2 to 3 weeks. Fortunately, a single day of ice and elevation will almost always suffice and with adequate padding thereafter no disability need be anticipated. In contrast, contusions of the plantar aspect, namely *the "stone bruise"* under the metatarsal heads and the *"heel bruise"* under the calcaneus, have already been specifically alluded to as particularly bothersome. *The heel cup* is specifically designed to transfer weight around the bruised area in the heel. But the "stone bruise" requires the greatest ingenuity—the *usual felt metatarsal lift,* carefully adjusted and applied anew daily, usually proves to be the most effective. Continued athletic activity must be guided by local symptoms, but aspiration and/or injection of steroids has never been necessary.

**Forefoot Sprain.** The most common sprain in the foot is the so-called "forefoot sprain" of the calcaneocuboid portion of the ligamentum bifurcatum by forceful inversion and internal rotation of the foot on the talonavicular joint. (See Fig. 19-1.) Swelling is usually immediate and considerable, pain is acute and disabling, and weight bearing often proves impossible, necessitating crutches. Despite this alarming onset examination reveals swelling to be localized over the calcaneocuboid area, and tenderness well localized to the same area. *Ice, compression, and elevation must be applied from the first.* Despite the victim's skeptical disbelief he will be able to walk normally within 2 days and, if need be, run in 3. *Supported by daily restrapping* with the routine encircling figure-of-eight adhesive ankle strap, recovery in this particular sprain is as dramatic and gratifying as any in athletics. What's more, it is uniformly predictable. The supportive strapping should, of course, be continued for at least 2 weeks to lend necessary reinforcement, but in no instance has there been any evidence of permanent calcaneocuboid laxity.

**Sprain of the Great Toe.** Other than the forefoot sprain, the only joint injury worthy of special mention here is the sprain of the great toe or, specifically, *sprain of the first metatarsal-phalangeal joint,* not because it is different from any other sprain but because it has a specific and serious effect on athletic function. A result of excessive plantar flexion of the metatarso-phalangeal joint, or extreme dorsiflexion thereof—seldom from lateral or medial deviation—it presents a typically swollen joint, without crepitus or bony tenderness, hence seemingly routine and easily dismissed with not more than the usual strapping for immobilization and local ice to reduce local swelling.

Although such treatment is indeed ideal and local symptoms and signs do subside quite rapidly, every attempt to resume running thereafter will be met with an immediate recurrence of pain, swelling, and disability, simply because the hallux is the weight-bearing toe and its proximal joint must bear the brunt of every running step. Walking can be quite simply accomplished by keeping the great toe off the ground, but running in this manner is utterly impossible. Consequently, the athlete must be prepared to miss up to 10 days to 2 weeks of practice and games while his injury slowly resolves to completion, before any running, even with strapping support, can be tolerated.

In direct contrast, *sprains of the other toes* can be quickly appraised for possible fracture, then strapped to one or more healthy neighbors, and the boy sent back to full duty without the slightest problem. With such treatment, recovery is neither prolonged nor accelerated, and complete resolution of local reaction may be anticipated in 10 to 12 days. In the meantime the athlete will have lost no time, will have suffered little or no discomfort, hence is likely to have forgotten about his injury completely. But, not so, with the sprained great toe!

**Ingrown Toenail.** Finally, a word about the ingrown toenail seems in order, not a definitive statement on recommended treatment but a discussion of some of the factors that must be taken into consideration. Unguis incarnatus is notably a chronic problem, characterized by acute and chronic granulation tissue and paronychial inflammation, the direct results of a corner of toenail that has penetrated the epidermis and is deeply imbedded in the soft tissues as an infected foreign body. A vicious circle is set up thereby, for the more the nail grows and digs in, the more inflammatory response is produced; the greater the inflammatory response, the more the local swelling and the progressively deeper the penetration. Treatment should be directed toward: first, removal of the foreign body, namely the toenail corner; second, adequate drainage of the acute and chronic infection; third, prevention of recurrence in the face of a constantly growing toenail. In view of these factors certain arbitrary surgical techniques have been developed over the years directed toward the accomplishment of all three aims at once. As a result, radical removal of nail and matrix is the accepted routine surgical treatment for this condition. Lastingly effective it is, while at the same time temporary removal of the imbedded nail, to accomplish but two of the objectives, namely removal of the foreign body and establishment of adequate drainage, has been universally condemned as falling woefully short of the third aim, the prevention of recurrence.

However, within athletics, certain other considerations must be taken into account. Firstly, the problem is unlikely to come to medical attention until a competitive schedule is well underway, hence time lost unnecessarily may result in failure as a competitor. Also, these are always young men, far too young to have the permanently deformed feet and toes that often constitute the true basis for chronic toenail problems. Finally, their necessary daily showering keeps their feet much cleaner than most. Consequently, a compromise was made early in our experience, simply removing the imbedded toenail corner and loosened nail adjacent, to provide immediate, though temporary drainage, with the plan in mind to perform more definitive surgery after the season. As expected, infection subsided rapidly, the area healed up nicely, and local discomfort disappeared. Subsequently, however, the growing nail not only failed to imbed itself again, but moved on out over the healed and normal bed to a completely free and normal end point. Since that occasion, repeated experiences have ended precisely the same way, indicating that, perhaps, with early control of local swelling and inflammation and the subsequent healing and resolution in the area, recurrent unguis incarnatus is not the necessary outcome in these younger men but may actually be an exception.

# 21

# *Major Fractures and Dislocations*

Significant fractures and dislocations in sports do not differ from similar injuries, no matter what the precipitating factor, nor should any special consideration be given to the athlete in the proper treatment of them. *The ideal treatment for any fracture or fracture-dislocation is the only treatment, athletics notwithstanding.* A text on clinical orthopedics is the only proper place for the discussion of these injuries, not a book on the particular unique aspects of primary medical care as it applies to athletes and competitive sports.

Some attention, however, must be given to those problems of initial emergency treatment that must be handled by the physician on the spot before the orthopedic surgeon can assume responsibility, over and above the problems of initial diagnosis discussed elsewhere. If the physician happens to be an orthopedist as well, there may be no problem, but even in such instances he cannot leave the rest of the squad to render complete, definitive treatment as well as emergency treatment.

### Initial Management of Major Skeletal Injury

Once it is determined that a fracture does exist and that immediate transportation to the hospital is necessary for appropriate x-rays and ideal specialist care, preparations must be made toward the accomplishment of this objective. The first thought must be toward an *adequate immobilization of the part,* to stabilize fracture fragments and prevent further soft tissue damage or an even more disastrous compounding. An adequate splinting must be applied with whatever means are at hand; basswood splints, cage splints, inflatable splints, molded plaster splints, even folded newspapers will do, but the principal concern must be to secure immobilization of the joints above and below the fracture, immobilization that will withstand any problems in transport to the nearest hospital. The injured part should not be encircled with constricting wrappings that might impair circulation for even the briefest time.

**Gross Angulation and Overriding.** If there is *gross angulation* without serious overriding of fragments, hence little or no danger of compounding, this gross angulation *can be gently straightened* as the splint is applied without fear of increasing local damage. If the fragments are subcutaneous, however, the greatest of care must be exercised. In an unstable fracture of both bones of forearm or lower leg the danger of compounding is quite high, even more so *if there is significant overriding;* therefore, *gentle traction may be necessary* during application of the splint, to reduce and hold the overriding for the hospital trip. The Thomas ring splint for upper and lower extremities comes to mind in this situation. If it can be applied easily and firm traction rapidly established with the usual windlass method, all well and good, but any type of firm and bulky splinting will do as well, as long as traction is maintained during application.

**Compound Fracture.** The next question that arises is that of the obvious compound fracture with gross contamination. If at the moment of examination there is nothing more than a puncture wound externally, the bone end having already returned thoroughly contaminated into the depths of the injured part, there is unfortunately little to be done; applying a sterile dressing over the wound and a thorough splinting is all that remains, because deep contamination is already well-established. However, what of the compound fracture with the compounding fragment protruding through its puncture wound, thoroughly contaminated? Here there is every reason to cover the bone end with a sterile dressing and leave everything as is, making no attempt whatever to pull the contaminated bone end back into the wound. The only possible exception to this would be in the rare instance of distal vascular insufficiency secondary to the angulation or overriding accompanying the compound fracture—in such an instance, and only in such an instance, immediate reduction must be accomplished by traction, despite the serious deep contamination, simply to save the extremity.

**Major Dislocations.** These same considerations apply to *major dislocations.* In general, a single attempt at reduction is always worthwhile in primary dislocations, for the sake of pain relief if nothing else. *In the more routine dislocations,* reduction is desirable early, but, if there is any problem at all, less soft tissue damage is done by a *gentle manipulation under general anesthesia* than by weights or tugging, twisting, and wrestling with a young man who is likely to be much stronger than the doctor and his assistant together. However, in dislocations of the elbow and, most particularly, the tibio-femoral dislocation, vascular damage may become rapidly irreversible before anatomical reduction can be accomplished in the usual deliberate manner. In these specific instances—*in the elbow if there is any sign of distal insufficiency, in the posterior tibio-femoral dislocation even if there is none at all—an immediate reduction must be aggressively sought,* pain or no pain. Parenteral narcosis may be all that is available; regardless, reduction must be accomplished at the earliest possible moment.

**Meniscus Impaction.** Meniscus impaction, as an acute traumatic entity, without other evidence of significant knee pathology, presents a similar problem. *Manipulation* to reduce the impaction and restore full motion is certainly reasonable, if it can be easily accomplished *by gentle means and not by force.* A single attempt without anesthesia, flexing the knee over counterleverage in the popliteal fossa and rocking it gently in this position to disengage the meniscus, then extending the leg with the joint abducted or adducted (whichever the case may be) to hold open the joint space, may result in complete relief of all symptoms and signs. *Under no circumstances should this maneuver be forcibly done.* If there is the slightest sign of impaction as the knee is extended, the effort should be immediately terminated; otherwise, the impaction will be further crushed, torn, or converted into a "bucket-handle." Even irreversible joint-surface damage can occur. For the same reasons *no more than one unsuccessful attempt* should be made. Instead, ice, compression, felt splints, and crutches should be adopted as the initial treatment of choice, with bedrest and constant elevation in the Infirmary or hospital as a further alternative under orthopedic supervision.

**Spine Injury.** The most frightening injury of all is that to *the cervical spine.* The boy should be moved supported as is, if there is no evidence of cord or medullary damage already. The slightest alteration, even toward what might seem a more reasonable and comfortable position, may be the final one that converts the case into quadriplegia. If definite cord signs are already present and the neck is not fixed in any one position, the neutral position should be supported either by sandbags or by hand until the hospital is reached, thus assuring an adequate airway at least. A boy with *fractures of the dorsal and lumbar spine,* below D-5 or D-6, would best be transported face downward, to preserve the normal lordotic curve. Those with fractures above this level would best be moved in the supine position.

In summary, certain positive steps must be taken by the physician, no matter what his particular specialty background, to assure that cases with major fractures or dislocations arrive in the orthopedist's hands in the best condition possible. Even if he knows nothing else of surgery or orthopedics, of this he must be sure and certain.

## Return to Competition After Major Skeletal Injury

As pointed out in the section on ankle injuries, the return to full athletic competition following major ankle fracture can be difficult indeed, simply because the demands are so much greater than in average workaday living. It was emphasized that definitive treatment should not differ from that afforded everyone so injured. The sole difference is in the total length of time required for rehabilitation, and it is here that the physician responsible for the care of athletes must be primarily concerned. It is not at all unusual to have unfamiliar candidates or known athletes report after major fractures or dislocations with medical assurances from home that all is now well and that full activity is now not only permissible but desirable. Yet, in truth, the athlete is an athlete no longer, so long have his activities been limited. Such a boy certainly cannot be allowed to return to full activity until he has done the necessary conditioning work. If it takes him 2 months or even the whole season to manage the simplest conditioning exercises, so be it! Much criticism will be heard and there will be parental rumblings about waivers and medical certificates to allow their boy to play immediately, but the only possible course is clear. It matters not how severe the injury was initially, nor how miraculous the treatment and recovery; if the boy falls short of functional requirements, he falls short. Moreover, it is absolutely essential that some definite statement be received in writing, to the effect that the injured boy is officially released to athletic activity; otherwise, should trouble arise, the physician will be all alone again!

Any athlete returning to competitive athletics either as a postoperative or post-trauma case must be thoroughly evaluated from the responsible physician's own viewpoint and standards, not those of the family doctor or specialist. Only then can rehabilitation begin, at a pace to be determined by the physician responsible and to a point that must satisfy him and not any one else. In general, after major injuries it takes an athlete 2 days for every day in plaster to recover athletic proficiency even under the best of circumstances. If the injury involves a major joint surface, it is closer to 3 days for every 1 in plaster. This time requirement cannot be altered, no matter how optimistic or enthusiastic everyone may be, and it is one that the physician and trainer must honor even when no one else recognizes it. It is the physician in control who must carry the responsibility, no one else.

# 22

# *Athletic Taping*

The use of adhesive tape is widespread throughout the sporting world, but the multiple techniques applied to varying needs remains a mystery to most doctors. Indeed, it is always a revelation for any physician to witness for the first time the application by a skilled trainer of a routine ankle strapping. The ability to place multiple strips of ordinary surgical adhesive tape over various contoured parts, without constriction, without wrinkles, without areas of disproportionate pressure, is an art that takes years of experience.

The physician cannot hope to duplicate such highly skilled efforts, but he should know what techniques are available. If he must carry on without adequate help, he must tape as best he can. He must turn to the various manuals, expressly published to provide the detailed techniques in graphic form. However, certain basic taping procedures should be understood by every doctor in the field, so that he will know what can be done for certain injuries.

Thus the routine shoulder cap strapping (see Fig. 22-1), which duplicates the upward pull of the deltoid and relieves the strain on structures supporting the glenohumeral joint, is useful in rotator cuff strains, deltoid strains and contusions, distal trapezius strains, and the "shoulder pointer," as well as the generally sore shoulder following subluxation of the glenohumeral joint.

On the other hand, the Watson-Jones strapping (see Fig. 22-1) is expressly designed for the acromioclavicular strain and separation, exerting pressure over a felt pad downward on the distal clavicle against counter pressure through the long axis of the humerus to the scapula by way of the glenohumeral joint, hence looping around the flexed elbow over another felt pad, directly in line with the humeral axis.

Also worthy of note is the elbow cinch strap (see Fig. 22-2), which utilizes the great strength of twisted adhesive to limit elbow extension in cases where such limitation is desirable; e.g., in recent hyperextension episodes. In like manner, the hyperextended thumb can be "cinched" to the index figure to prevent hyperextension, as long as thumb mobility is not a necessity (see Figure. 22-2). Obviously, a quarterback or center cannot operate effectively so taped, but linemen

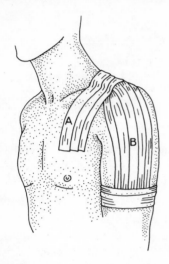

A:  ANCHOR STRIPS

B:  WORKING STRIPS

ROUTINE SHOULDER-CAP STRAP

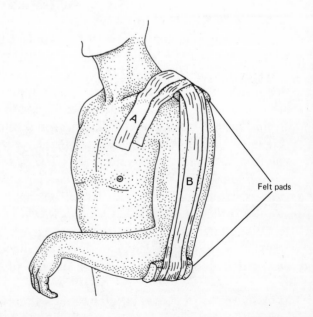

Felt pads

WATSON-JONES STRAP

Fig. 22-1.  Shoulder strapping.

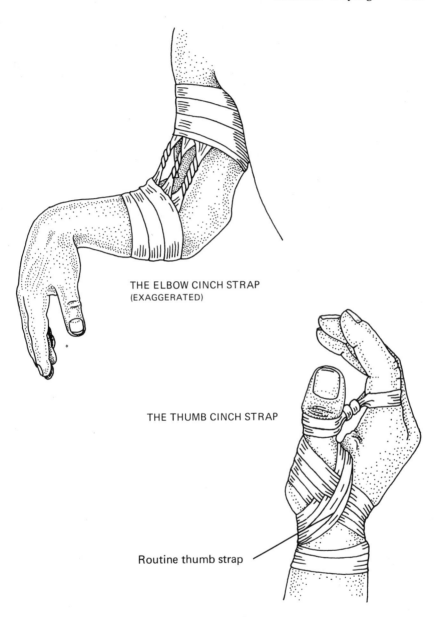

THE ELBOW CINCH STRAP
(EXAGGERATED)

THE THUMB CINCH STRAP

Routine thumb strap

Fig. 22-2. Cinch strapping for athletics.

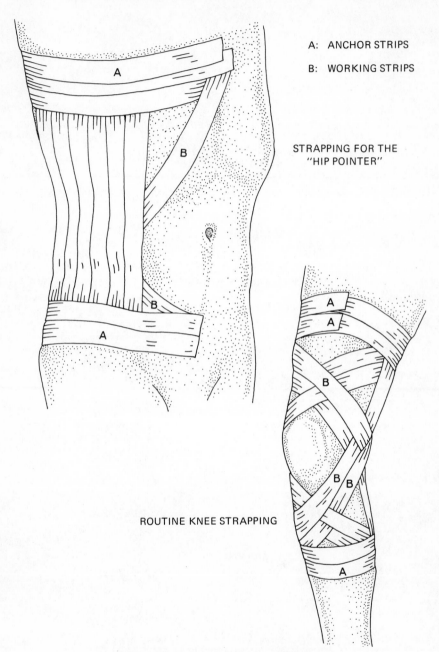

A: ANCHOR STRIPS

B: WORKING STRIPS

STRAPPING FOR THE
"HIP POINTER"

ROUTINE KNEE STRAPPING

Fig. 22-3. Special strapping for specific injury.

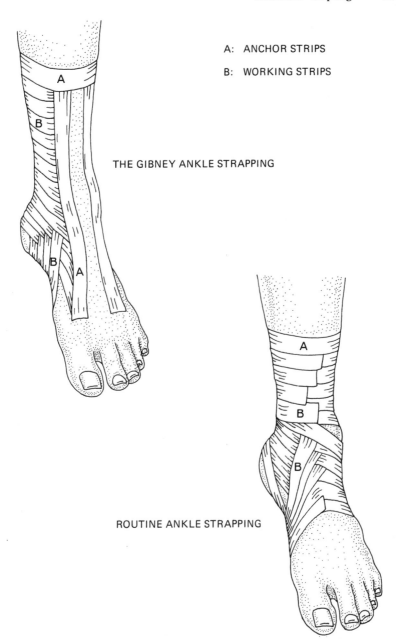

A: ANCHOR STRIPS

B: WORKING STRIPS

THE GIBNEY ANKLE STRAPPING

ROUTINE ANKLE STRAPPING

Fig. 22-4. Strapping for the injured ankle.

and defensive personnel can manage quite well. To further reinforce the metacarpophalangeal joint, a figure-of-eight taping can be applied, using the wrist as a base. One would think that taping of this sort would result in swollen and cyanotic thumb and forefinger. An unskilled application will lead to this, but this is extremely rare.

The "hip pointer" can be helped by strapping that pulls the athlete over to the injured side and limits motion, and this can be accomplished by a specific strapping (see Fig. 22-3). One must guard against tape sensitivity in such broad area of application, especially in the fair-skinned athlete, since this particular taping should be left in place for at least 3 days.

As to strapping for the injured knee, there are many methods, only one of which we have illustrated. It must be very skillfully applied to avoid constriction in the face of swelling, hence is much more useful as a supportive strapping during rehabilitation exercises and post-injury competition. Also, because of the fixation of the patella with this particular technique it is exceptionally effective in preventing recurrent dislocation.

The ankle is another area in which skill and experience can result amazing virtuosity in strapping. Application of either type as illustrated (see Fig. 22-4) takes the average skilled trainer no more than 30 seconds per ankle, without a wrinkle and without disproportionate pressure points. The Gibney boot strapping, open-faced over the dorsum, is used only as a stabilizer for acute injury, providing room for subsequent swelling yet preventing inversion and eversion, the two motions that must be avoided. The routine figure-of-eight ankle strap, with or without heel-lock, is, on the other hand, expressly designed to provide maximum support for all purposes, hence is the ideal strapping for rehabilitation as well as for long term support.

Other strapping methods abound, and for these as well as the detailed techniques of actual application the reader is urged to consult the manual on taping procedure by O. W. Dayton, the head trainer at Yale University.

*Appendix*

# Intercollegiate Tackle Football Injuries: A Five-Year Statistical Study

In the past 15 years, perhaps as a result of the nationwide saturation coverage of football by television, there has been an increasing pressure toward better medical control of injuries incurred by the participants in this violent sport. At the same time it has become increasingly clear that many expert medical opinions and recommendations have all too often been based on subjective personal recollections or on isolated observations of over-dramatized traumata involving headlined stars, rather than on a sober appraisal of carefully collected, accurate squad data. To remedy this shortcoming, a number of studies have emerged that have attempted to provide some factual information, upon which valid recommendations might then be based; such studies have included California high schools,[2, 8] Oregon high schools,[7] Georgia high schools,[3] a large Air Force program,[1] a touch-football program,[6] and more recently the NCAA, ACHA, and NATA sponsored National Tackle-Football Survey, a study which is still in progress. Equally significant has been the ongoing work of Robey Blyth, and Mueller on North Carolina high-school football players, a preliminary report of which has been recently published.[11]

In all these studies an honest attempt has been made to establish a statistically significant total of participants, to assure some validity in the collected data. Accordingly, all studies have been based on either a detailed third-party review of insurance forms,[2, 8, 7] medical records, [3, 1] and/or a painstaking epidemiological survey by direct interview.[6, 11] However, in no instance on a major-college level, has an entire study, from the moment of injury and examination through diagnosis, treatment, rehabilitation, and subsequent return to full participation, been reported as a unified entity, personally controlled and recorded by the solely responsible team-physician. A thorough report from Harvard University [13] comes closest to this particular ideal, but is diluted by the inclusion of all intramural tackle-football participants, whose motivation and skill are so variable that serious distortion of injury frequency, time loss, and treatment response is inevitable; our own experience with a counterpart intramural tackle-football program indicates injury frequency and time loss to be tripled, indeed often quadrupled.

It is therefore the purpose of this report to present a series of injury statistics, accumulated over a 5-year period of varsity and junior-varsity football at Yale University in a program, personally supervised and controlled by the author to assure uniformity of diagnosis and treatment from the moment of injury to the moment of return to full participation. All data has been extracted from material personally recorded, collected, and collated, and every attempt has been made to include all information that might be considered of value for immediate as well as future application, epidemiological and otherwise.

## MATERIAL AND METHODS

**Total Sample:** This figure encompasses all candidates for both junior-varsity and varsity football at Yale University from the years 1966–1970 inclusive. Injury data exists of comparable accuracy and detail back to 1958, but, in reviewing same, it has become apparent that the changing rules in intercollegiate football, particularly modifications in the early 1960's toward total platooning of offensive and defensive squads, have so altered the overall injury picture as to render this earlier group of figures valueless for the present day. In fact, the contrast is so striking that we have included, where noteable, analogous figures from a single year of two-way football (1960), to underline this particular difference, which difference nullifies our originally projected 10-year study (1960–1970).

Significant difficulty is also encountered in determining an accurate figure even for the 5-year total sample for a number of disparate reasons. Firstly, the entire squad roster for any 1 year begins with the sum total of all candidates invited back to pre-season practice on September 1st, yet may also include a few enthusiasts who arrive unexpectedly from distant homes (hence are never turned away), and is further distorted by the inevitable few who report back, then turn right around for home, sometimes before the first practice! Secondly, there is a steady attrition, from the 1st day onward, that may account for 10 to 20 candidates before the mid-September end of two-a-day practice sessions, very little of which is related to injuries incurred but is more a result of motivation-loss. Thirdly, this anticipated attrition is further distorted by the arrival in mid-September of a number of bona-fide junior-varsity candidates, who return to classes and to football at the same time without any real hope of "making the varsity" but are full-fledged members of the squad nonetheless.

In all, the total squad-roster depends entirely on the particular pre-season day and, as the season progresses, how the team is doing or, even more significant, the offensive or defensive depth chart. Thus, a normal starting figure over the past 5 years has varied from 95 to 105, falling thereafter to around 75 to 85 by mid-season. However, since this final level does reflect to some degree overall injury losses, *a fair total sample must reflect this pre-season high, that is, one hundred (100) a year or five hundred (500) in 5 years,* with no numerical attempt to be more exactly accurate.

**Injuries:** Included in this study are all conditions of a surgical nature that resulted in 1 or more days loss of practice time or game opportunity, no matter the surrounding circumstances.

**Diagnosis:** All diagnoses listed are as anatomically and physiologically accurate as possible, conforming in the main to the *STANDARD NOMENCLATURE OF ATHLETIC INJURIES* [12] but further detailed wherever possible. Each and every diagnosis was personally made by the author, and the appropriate individual treatment plan worked out and followed in detail with our head trainer, Mr. O. W. Dayton. Treatment response and rehabilitation progress have provided a constant, unerring check on the original accuracy of diagnoses, and all diagnoses in this study, therefore, have been confirmed either by subsequent course or, where indicated, by surgery.

**Days Lost:** By definition and by Athletic Department Regulation, previously agreed to by the Athletic Director and *all* coaches, all injuries and illnesses in our intercollegiate athletic program were immediately categorized into:

1. *Full disability:* not allowed to practice or participate in any way other than passive observation.
2. *Competitive disability:* not allowed to participate in scrimmages or games, but otherwise may participate in a graduated, supervised rehabilitation and practice schedule.

A complete disability list was kept accordingly, modified daily to maintain constant, accurate control over the activities of *all* intercollegiate athletes (not only football), and it is from these lists that most of the data for this study has been extracted.

**Treatment Methods:** Without exception all listed injuries were handled according to principles outlined and treatment detailed in the first edition of this book.[5]

## RESULTS

**Table I: Overall Summary**

A cumulative total of 273 injuries was incurred by the JV and varsity football squad between 1966 to 1970 inclusive. Using an overall total of participants of 500 for the same period, as discussed above, *the index of injury incidence was 0.546 for the period,* a somewhat higher figure than in other studies; this difference, however, may be more apparent than real in the light of the overwhelming preponderance of minor injuries included in the overall total (Table II and II A).

Table I
Overall Summary
*Varsity and JV Football, Yale University, 1966–1970*

| | | Practice | | | | Games | | | | |
| | | Pre-sea | Season | | | | | 1st/2nd | | |
| Year | Total | Con | Non | Con | Non | Reg | Sub | Half | Surgery | Comments |
| 1960 | 24 | 6 | 4 | 4 | 6 | 2 | 1 | 2/1 | 4 | See Table XI |
| . . . . . . . . . . . . . . . . . . . . . . . . . . . . . . . . . . . . . . . . . . . . . . . . . . . . . | | | | | | | | | | |
| 1966 | 30 | 8 | 12 | 4 | 2 | 4 | 0 | 2/2 | 1 | See Tables II–XII |
| 1967 | 59 | 14 | 11 | 3 | 12 | 18 | 1 | 6/13 | 1 | See Tables II–XII |
| 1968 | 60 | 11 | 7 | 7 | 3 | 21 | 11 | 10/22 | 2 | See Tables II–XII |
| 1969 | 48 | 17 | 21 | 0 | 2 | 8 | 0 | 6/2 | 0 | See Tables II–XII |
| 1970 | 76 | 15 | 16 | 9 | 6 | 23 | 7 | 11/19 | 0 | See Tables II–XII |
| | *273* | 65 | 67 | 23 | 25 | 74 | 19 | 35/58 | 4 | |

100% of total injuries
0.546 incidence rate

| | | |
|---|---|---|
| Practice Injuries 1966–1970: | | *180* |
| | Contact . . . . . . . . | 88 |
| | Non-contact . . . . . . | 92 |
| Game Injuries—1966–1970: | | *93* |
| | 1st half . . . . . . . . | 35 |
| | 2nd half . . . . . . . . | 58 |

Of interest are the yearly figures and their variation and, for contrast, their comparison to the figures of 1960; there is no explanation for these seasonal variations, there having been no significant rules changes, equipment changes, or technique changes between 1966 and 1970. Yet, despite this the low of 24 in 1960 contrasts strikingly with the high of 76 for 1970; clearly the difference lies in the two-way football of 1960, although the element of overall skill might be questioned, since the undefeated 1960 squad was undeniably one of our most skilled senior aggregates. However, if skill were a principal factor or secondary thereto, overconcentration of total exposure to a select group of the most skilled, 1968 should have been an equally low-injury year, yet the figure for that comparably successful season was 60, the second highest yearly total.

The overall figures for injuries in practice, 180, as against 93 in games is not surprising in view of the ratio between 60 practices and nine games, but even more arresting is the practice-injury ratio of contact (88) to non-contact (92). In short, there are more or as many injuries suffered in non-contact activities, such as pass-offense and pass-defense drills, agility drills, hitting the bucker, offensive and defensive timing drills, than (or as) in half-line, goal-line, two-on-one, or full-scale squad scrimmages: the utter futility of providing medical coverage for scheduled scrimmages and games only is herewith demonstrated and underlined. Furthermore, as the 1960 figures indicate, frequent intra-squad scrimmages, a coaching method largely dispensed with by our present staff between weekly games—welcomed medically (132 pre-season practice injuries vs. 48 season practice-injuries)—yet an integral part of the previous staff-planning (up to 3 to 4 intrasquad scrimmages per week, throughout the season), were without an untoward effect on overall injury figures; in fact, the high number of game injuries in recent years could be a result of insufficient violent contact through the preceding week, an argument repeatedly used by the "hard-nosed" school of coaches.

The total number of game injuries has been further broken down into halves, demonstrating a definite increase in incidence in the 2nd half, a correlation even more striking in Table III; the obvious relation of increased frequency with increased fatigue is a tempting one here, but, as will be seen in the subsequent detailed analyses, this may again be more apparent than real, inasmuch as length of play as a regular clearly increases exposure throughout the game, to reach its highest point in the 2nd half, fatigued or not! In the same vein the overwhelming preponderance of injury in regulars vs. subs (74 to 19) simply underlines the fact that, by definition, a substitute plays very little, hence is exposed that much less in terms of overall risk, with specific exceptions (see Table VII, Hamstring Injuries).

The most striking figure in Table I is in the final column; in 1960 four surgical procedures were carried out, one shoulder and three knees, while in the 5 years under study, 1966–1970, there have been but four altogether, this in contrast to reports of many more surgical knees in a single college-football season! [9, 10] A more detailed analysis of these cases will be found in Table XI, but, suffice it to say, no candidate has subsequently undergone surgery elsewhere without our knowledge, hence the recognized possibility that our program is missing disabled athletes in real need of corrective surgery appears insubstantial.

**Table II: Diagnostic Breakdown and Analysis**

Contained within this imposing categorization are all diagnoses for time-loss injuries as well as other related problems leading to time loss, omitting only purely medical conditions, such as mononucleosis, acute respiratory disease, and the like. All high-frequency diagnoses are further analyzed in detail in subsequent Tables (III–XII) and are marked by asterisks (*). Of the remaining, the low incidence of 2nd and 3rd degree A-C separation in our series, 1 in 5 years, is consistent with experience prior thereto, as is the low incidence of 1st degree A-C separation, a scant 2 in 5 years. The high incidence of pulls and/ or contusions of the 11th and/or 12th ribs in most recent season is remarkable and mysterious, involving different positions, offensive and defensive, interior line and perimeter, to a total of 6; all were uniformly disabling for 2 to 5 days, with full recovery thereafter. And related thereto regionally, low-back contusions and strains, not paid much heed as a source of football disability, nonetheless accounted for 14 time-loss injuries, including one lumbosacral strain that forced discontinuation of football!

**Table II A: Analysis "Other" Category, Table II**

Table II A details further comment on each case in the "other" category, but additional amplification seems indicated in certain instances. Thus, a single furuncle of the anterior thigh occurred in 1966, of little significance except that the candidate failed to report it until it had been subjected to the rigors of a JV football game; by

Table II
Diagnostic Breakdown and Analysis
*Varsity and JV Football, Yale University, 1966–1970*

| Diagnosis | (1960) | 1966 | 1967 | 1968 | 1969 | 1970 | Total | Incidence |
|---|---|---|---|---|---|---|---|---|
| Drngmnt, Knee, surg | (3) | 1 | 1 | 2 | 0 | 0 | 4 | 0.008 * |
| tr, med coll, Knee | (2) | 1 | 10 | 8 | 7 | 8 | 34 | 0.068 * |
| tr, lat coll, Knee | (1) | 0 | 1 | 0 | 0 | 0 | 1 | 0.002 |
| Contusion, Knee | (0) | 1 | 3 | 1 | 3 | 6 | 14 | 0.028 |
| Sprain, Ankle | (1) | 3 | 8 | 10 | 5 | 7 | 33 | 0.066 * |
| Peroneal Tendonitis | (0) | 0 | 1 | 1 | 0 | 0 | 2 | 0.004 |
| Achilles Tendonitis | (0) | 0 | 0 | 0 | 0 | 2 | 2 | 0.004 |
| Contusion, Quad | (0) | 5 | 5 | 5 | 3 | 5 | 23 | 0.046 * |
| train, Quad | (0) | 2 | 0 | 0 | 0 | 1 | 3 | 0.003 |
| Strain Hamstring | (0) | 3 | 0 | 1 | 3 | 4 | 11 | 0.022 * |
| Contusion A-C | (1) | 2 | 1 | 2 | 3 | 4 | 12 | 0.024 * |
| Seprtn, 1st deg | (0) | 0 | 1 | 1 | 0 | 0 | 2 | 0.004 |
| Seprtn, 2nd & 3rd dg | (0) | 0 | 0 | 0 | 1 | 0 | 1 | 0.002 |
| Contusion, lwr leg | (0) | 1 | 3 | 3 | 0 | 3 | 10 | 0.020 |
| Concussion, cerebri | (0) | 1 | 2 | 4 | 0 | 2 | 9 | 0.018 * |
| Groin Strain | (1) | 0 | 4 | 0 | 5 | 2 | 11 | 0.022 * |
| Strain Gastroc | (0) | 2 | 0 | 0 | 1 | 2 | 5 | 0.010 |
| Contusn iliac crst | (0) | 0 | 2 | 3 | 2 | 2 | 9 | 0.018 * |
| Contusn ribs | (1) | 0 | 1 | 1 | 0 | 3 | 5 | 0.010 |
| nj ribs XI a/o XII | (0) | 0 | 1 | 0 | 0 | 6 | 7 | 0.014 |
| Rib sep a/o fract costochndrl | (1) | 0 | 1 | 1 | 0 | 0 | 2 | 0.004 |
| Shin Splints | (0) | 0 | 0 | 0 | 2 | 0 | 2 | 0.004 |
| Strain neck | (2) | 1 | 1 | 2 | 0 | 2 | 6 | 0.012 |
| Strain lumbosacrl | (0) | 0 | 4 | 0 | 1 | 4 | 9 | 0.018 |
| Contusn lumbosacrl | (0) | 0 | 1 | 0 | 1 | 3 | 5 | 0.010 |
| Metatarsalgia | (0) | 0 | 0 | 0 | 0 | 2 | 2 | 0.004 |
| Fractures | (3) | 1 | 2 | 1 | 1 | 3 | 8 | 0.016 * |
| Dislocations | (1) | 1 | 0 | 1 | 2 | 0 | 4 | 0.008 * |
|  |  |  |  | (sblx fg) | (sblx thmb) | (2 sublux) |  |  |
| OTHER, (SEE TABLE II A) | (3) | 6 | 5 | 11 | 7 | 10 | 39 | 0.078 * |

TOTAL (Two double injuries)      275

TOTAL (CORRECTED)      273   0.546

then there was clinical evidence of deep disruption of the inflammatory barrier from repeated direct trauma, and the resulting deep cellulitis necessitated intensive antibiotic and local therapy and an 8-day loss. The single nasal laceration, also in 1966, was typical of the type inflicted by the Riddell helmet despite the rubber snubber and, once established, continually recurred throughout the season with a thickened, scarred nasal bridge as a final result. The 3 headaches leading to time loss in 1967 were typical pre-season headaches, with which all team-physicians and trainers are familiar, differing only in intensity and in the fact that these particular 3 required more than the usual half-day to clear; the combination of dehydration, violent contact, and newly fitted helmets with extra-snug suspension-sweatbands, all combined to produce this familiar pre-season phenomenon, in this instance affecting all three candidates at once in an unusual vignette of discouragement and futility.

### Table II A
### Analysis "Other" Category

#### 1960
1 laceration, knee, deep, involving prepatellar bursa, (7 days lost)
1 sterno clavicular strain, mild, (3 days lost)
1 acute psychosis, (hospitalized, no trauma, left school for 2 years)

#### 1966
1 lateral meniscus, chronic since high school, returned 30 days w/o operation
1 infected blister, (2 days lost)
1 furuncle thigh with cellulitis, (8 days lost)
1 sprained wrist, mild, (3 days lost)
1 laceration nose, bridge, extensive, helmet, (5 days lost)
1 plantar strain, (5 days lost), (combined with strained hamstring)

#### 1967
1 strained thumb, mild, (1 day lost)
1 abrasion sclerae, (2 days lost)
3 headaches, (no concussion, early pre-season, 1 day rest sufficient)

#### 1968
1 laceration brow, deep, (combined with ankle sprain)
1 pulmonary contusion (single frothy hemoptysis, neg. serial films, 2 days lost)
2 Contusions, ankle
1 contusion hand
1 cellulitis hand
1 laceration hand
1 contusion abdomen, (observation 36 hrs.)
1 contusion deltoid

1 contusion toe
1 laceration tongue, through and through, layer repair, (3 days lost)

### 1969

1 acute appendicitis, (classical signs pre-season, uneventful append. return 21 days)
1 "pinched fat pad" knee, (no other signs, symptoms, 1 day lost)
1 contusion hand
1 contusion deltoid
1 contusion biceps
1 laceration chin
1 sun-lamp burn, (self-administered, 1st-degree of face & eyes, 2 days lost)

### 1970

2 forefoot strains, classical, (1 to 2 day lost)
2 contusions elbow
1 infected blisters, multiple
2 subdeltoid bursitis, (one intensively treated w/o result @ home, hence quit, the other in previous traumatic-dislocation, glenohumeral, 1 year before, also gave up football)
1 contusion deltoid
1 strain thumb, mild, (3 days lost)
1 abrasion sclerae, minimal, (1 day lost)

In 1968 a severe abdominal contusion in a running back, suffered during a pre-season scrimmage, gave rise to considerable concern, but careful and repeated observation over a 36-hour period was rewarded by a complete clearing of all symptoms; the initial impact was tremendous, and after the victim recovered his "wind" he complained of persistent pain in both upper quadrants, without rigidity or rebound, without shoulder pain, and with normal peristalsis—examinations at half-hour intervals thereafter for 2 hours of normal findings and vital signs, followed by repeated abdominal evaluation for the next day and a half, sufficed to eliminate the real possibility of hepatic or splenic damage.

Even more remarkable was the tongue laceration listed for 1968 in a running back with the pernicious habit of running with his tongue protruding despite numerous warnings; inevitably, violent contact was eventually made with the victim's jaw. His teeth penetrated the inferior aspect of the tongue two-thirds through to the superior surface and divided several large veins and a branch of the lingual artery. There was an accompanying deep laceration of the superior surface, similarly penetrating one-third of the tongue-substance. After ligation of the bleeders with plain catgut, layer-repair was carried out under local anesthesia. Healing was rapid despite one episode of recurrent bleeding, requiring re-ligature at 48 hours.

The sun-lamp burn in 1969 is worthy of comment as a typical example of a perennial problem among our undergraduates, athlete and non-athlete. Loss of laboriously acquired "summer tans" reaches distressing proportions about mid-November, with the growing determination to "do something about it" culminating in sun-lamp burns all over campus, hence, not surprisingly, in this personable yet introspective squad member. Lastly, some amplification of the two cases of season-terminating subdeltoid bursitis seems in order. Both occurred in 1970, one in a defensive end, the other in a running back with a history, as listed in Table XII, of a subcoracoid glenohumeral dislocation in the same shoulder during the 1969 season. In both cases, recurrent past episodes and repeated outside evaluation by their personal orthopedists made objective assessment difficult. Specific treatment by cortical steroid injection was requested by both cases, and both personal decisions to give up the sport were made on the advice of their respective orthopedists without consultation with us and without objective disability by our standards.

### Table III: Ankle Sprains

All ankle sprains incurred in our football program are thoroughly evaluated within moments of the injury; ice, compression, and elevation immediately instituted; and a close personal supervision by doctor and trainer begun. As soon as swelling has peaked and bleeding has stopped, weight bearing is started in a graduated program of increasing stress as tolerated, supported only by adhesive strapping and without local injections, fomentations, whirlpool, or the like. As soon as the athlete can sprint full speed and cut full speed, he is restored to full activity, with continued adhesive-tape support for an additional 3 to 4 weeks. Hence, as in all discussions henceforward, full-disability days are simply those before active rehabilitation begins, while competitive-disability days are those required to complete the active rehabilitation program to our satisfaction.

As to the widespread use of prophylactic ankle strapping or ankle wraps, it has aways been our feeling that such support can only transfer untoward torsional forces upward to the next joint, the knee, and we would much rather deal with a sprained ankle than an injured knee. The low time-loss figures (2.1 days full disability, 2.2 days competitive disability) would bear this out. In fact, the sprained ankle rarely keeps an athlete out of action for more than 5 days total, while the acute medial collateral strain of the knee (Table IV) averages nearly a week at best. And it remains questionable whether even without prophylactic ankle support our total incidence of ankle sprain (33 in 5 years) is significantly higher than in those programs that demand such support.

A further examination of the positions played by those suffering ankle sprains confirms the accepted fact that mobility is a prime requisite; 30 of the 33 occurred in positions requiring great lateral mobility. Nor is contact a significant factor, since 15 of the total occurred during non-contact drills. Even more remarkable, 15 of the total occurred during pre-season practice; the relation of this last figure with violent activity in as yet unadjusted pre-season candidates is clear.

The 12 ankle sprains incurred during games remains lower than the 21 practice sprains and should be even lower, were it not for three suffered in one game, the only game our squad has ever played on Astroturf; unfamiliarity with this highly publicized artificial surface, the total lack of "give," the unexpected traction even with soccer-type cleats, all combined to amass the greatest number of single-game time-loss totals in our experience, what with the further unfortunate fact that the sprains so incurred clearly differed from the usual eversion, inversion, or rotatory types, but, instead, were a result of "jamming" the joint, with persistent pain, synovitis, and prolonged disability.

The preponderance of 2nd-half sprains (9 to 3) again raises the question of fatigue as a factor as against the equally significant increased exposure in playing both halves as a regular; such a differentiation had best be left to the epidemiologists!

## LEGEND FOR TABLES III–XII

      MG: middle guard

        O: Offense,  D: defense

e.g.OE: offensive end

      DT: defensive tackle

also RB: running back

      QB: quarterback

      LB: line-backer

Table III

Ankle Sprains

*Varsity and JV Football, Yale University, 1966–1970*

| Year | Tot | Pos | Practice Pre-sea Con | Pre-sea Non | Season Con | Season Non | Games Reg | Sub | 1st/2nd Half | Days Lost Full | Comp | Comments |
|---|---|---|---|---|---|---|---|---|---|---|---|---|
| 1960 | 1 | HB | | | | | | | | 2 | 1 | A lucky year |
| 1966 | | DE | | x | | | | | | 0 | 2 | |
| | | OC | | x | | | | | | 1 | 2 | |
| | | RB | | | | x | | – | | 1 | 2 | |
| | 3 | | 0 | 2 | 0 | 1 | 0 | – | 0/0 | 2 | 6 | Average: 0.6 days full / 2.0 days comp |
| 1967 | | OC | | x | | | | | | 1 | 1 | |
| | | OG | x | | | | | | | 1 | 3 | |
| | | RB | x | | | | | | | 2 | 3 | |
| | | RB | | | | x | | | | 6 | 2 | |
| | | DE | | | | x | | | | 20 | 8 | |
| | | DE | | | | | x | | 2nd | 2 | 0 | Tibiofib diastasis, mild |
| | | LB | | | | | x | | 1st | 1 | 0 | |
| | | RB | | | | | x | | 2nd | 2 | 0 | |
| | 8 | | 2 | 1 | 0 | 2 | 3 | 0 | 1/2 | 35 | 17 | Average: 4.3 days full / 2.1 days comp / (corr) 2.0 full / 1.1 comp |

| Year | Pos | | | | | | Depth | Days full | Days comp | Surface |
|---|---|---|---|---|---|---|---|---|---|---|
| 1968 | LB | | x | | | | | 2 | 1 | |
| | OT | | x | | | | | 0 | 2 | |
| | OE | x | | | | | | 0 | 1 | |
| | RB | | | | x | | 2nd | 2 | 7 | |
| | LB | | | | x | | 2nd | 3 | 2 | |
| | QB | | | | x | | 1st | 0 | 2 | |
| | RB | | | | x | | 2nd | 0 | 1 | |
| | MG | | | | | x | 2nd | 0 | 2 | |
| | DE | | | | | | | 3 | 7 | |
| | OT | | | | | | | 3 | 2 | |
| **10** | | $\overline{1}$ | $\overline{2}$ | $\overline{0}$ | $\overline{4}$ | $\overline{1}$ | $\overline{1/4}$ | $\overline{13}$ | $\overline{27}$ | Average: 1.3 days full / 2.7 days comp |
| 1969 | RB | | x | | | | | 1 | 4 | |
| | DB | | x | | | | | 0 | 1 | |
| | RB | x | | | | | | 0 | 1 | |
| | OE | | x | | | | | 2 | 0 | |
| | RB | | x | | | | | 3 | 9 | |
| **5** | | $\overline{1}$ | $\overline{4}$ | $\overline{0}$ | $\overline{0}$ | $\overline{0}$ | $\overline{0/0}$ | $\overline{6}$ | $\overline{15}$ | Average: 1.2 days full / 3.0 days comp |
| 1970 | DT | | x | | | | | 1 | 1 | |
| | RB | | x | | | | | 2 | 1 | |
| | DB | | | x | | | | 3 | 0 | |
| | QB | | | | x | | 2nd | 2 | 7 | Astroturf |
| | MG | | | | x | | 2nd | 3 | 1 | Astroturf |
| | OT | | | | x | | 2nd | 2 | 1 | Astroturf |
| | QB | | | | x | | 1st | 2 | 5 | |
| **7** | | $\overline{0}$ | $\overline{2}$ | $\overline{1}$ | $\overline{4}$ | $\overline{0}$ | $\overline{1/3}$ | $\overline{15}$ | $\overline{16}$ | Average: 2.1 days full / 2.1 days comp |
| TOTAL **33** | | 4 | 11 | 2 | 11 | 1 | 3/9 | 71 | 81 | Ovrll Avg: 2.1 days full / 2.4 days comp |

12.1% of total injuries
0.066 incidence rate

Table IV

Strains, Medial Collateral Ligament, Knee
*Varsity and JV Football, Yale University, 1966–1970*

| Year | Tot | Pos | Practice | | | | Games | | | Days Lost | | Comments |
| | | | Pre-sea | | Season | | | | 1st/2nd | | | |
| | | | Con | Non | Con | Non | Reg | Sub | Half | Full | Comp | |
| 1960 | | RB | x | | | | | | | 3 | 6 | |
| | | Rkl | x | | | | | | | 6 | 6 | |
| | | End | | | | | x | | 1st | 2 | 7 | |
| | 3 | | 2 | 0 | 0 | 0 | 1 | 0 | 1/0 | 11 | 19 | Average: 3.6 days full |
| | | | | | | | | | | | | 6.3 days comp |
| 1966 | 1 | LB | 1 | 0 | 0 | 0 | 0 | 0 | 0/0 | 1 | 6 | Average: 1.0 days full |
| | | | | | | | | | | | | 6.0 days comp |
| 1967 | | OG | x | | | | | | | 4 | 7 | |
| | | QB | x | | | | | | | 2 | 8 | |
| | | LB | | | | | x | | 2nd | 2 | 0 | |
| | | RB | | | | | x | | 1st | 3 | 1 | |
| | | RB | | | | | x | | 2nd | 3 | 4 | |
| | | RB | | | | | x | | 1st | 2 | 4 | |
| | | OT | | | | x | | | | 3 | 14 | poorly motivtd sub |
| | | QB | | | | x | | | | 1 | 2 | |
| | | DT | | | x | | | | | 3 | 14 | poorly motivtd sub |
| | | DT | | | | | x | | 2nd | 3 | 10 | next to last game |
| | 10 | | 2 | 0 | 1 | 2 | 5 | 0 | 2/3 | 26 | 64 | Average: 2.6 days full |
| | | | | | | | | | | | | 6.4 days comp |

| Year | Pos | | | | | | | Deg | Days (full) | Days (comp) | Notes |
|---|---|---|---|---|---|---|---|---|---|---|---|
| 1968 | DE | x | | | | | | | 3 | 7 | |
| | DT | x | | | | | | | 2 | 5 | |
| | OE | x | | | | | | | 2 | 4 | |
| | DE | | | x | | | | | 2 | 0 | |
| | RB | | | | | x | | 1st | 2 | 0 | |
| | DB | | | | | x | x | 2nd | 2 | 6 | |
| | OT | | | | | | | 2nd | 3 | 1 | |
| | OE | | | | | | x | 1st | 2 | 4 | |
| | **—8—** | **—3—** | **—0—** | **—1—** | **—0—** | **—2—** | **2** | **2/2** | **18** | **27** | Average: 2.2 days full / 3.4 days comp |
| 1969 | QB | x | | | | | | | 2 | 10 | Admin Rehab prblm |
| | OE | x | | | | | | | 2 | 2 | |
| | OE | x | | | | | | | 2 | 2 | |
| | LB | | x | | | | | | 2 | 7 | chron recurrent prob |
| | OE | x | | | | | | | 2 | 5 | |
| | OG | | | | | x | | 1st | 3 | 6 | |
| | RB | | | | | x | | 1st | 4 | 0 | |
| | **—7—** | **—4—** | **—1—** | **—0—** | **—0—** | **—2—** | **0** | **2/0** | **17** | **32** | Average: 2.4 days full / 4.6 days comp |
| 1970 | OE | x | | | | | | | 3 | 2 | severe w/o instblty |
| | QB | x | | | | | | | 3 | 14 | |
| | LB | | | | | x | | 2nd | 3 | 3 | |
| | LB | | | | | x | | 1st | 2 | 0 | |
| | RB | | x | | | x | | 2nd | 2 | 2 | |
| | DB | | | | x | x | | 2nd | 2 | 1 | |
| | DB | | | | x | | | | 0 | 2 | |
| | OT | | | | | x | | 2nd | 2 | 1 | Astroturf |
| | **—8—** | **—2—** | **—1—** | **—0—** | **—2—** | **—5—** | **0** | **1/4** | **17** | **25** | Average: 2.1 days full / 3.1 days comp |
| **TOTAL** | **34** | **12** | **2** | **2** | **2** | **14** | **2** | **7/9** | **79** | **154** | Ovrll Avg: 2.3 days full / 4.5 days comp |

12.5% of total injuries
0.068 incidence rate

[289]

Finally, some amplification seems deserved in the one prolonged time-loss injury in 1967, suffered by a defensive end during a non-contact drill. Swelling and pain were immediate, high above the lateral malleolus, and subsequent bleeding rapidly obscured the entire lateral and anterior aspect of the joint and malleolus despite immediate ice, compression, and elevation. Clinical signs and symptoms indicated either a fracture of the distal fibula or a diastasis, tibiofibular. X-rays were negative, however, hence plaster immobilization for 20 days, followed by 8 days of active rehabilitation, was the treatment of choice, on the assumption that some tibiofibular diastasis had in fact taken place despite negative x-ray findings. In any event recovery was complete, and after 28 days full competition was without any problems whatever.

## Table IV: Strain Medial Collateral Ligament, Knee

All cases in this category conformed to diagnostic criteria that sharply differentiated them from others usually listed as affecting the knee, namely surgical derangement (either ligamentous, meniscal or both), contusions, strains of the adductor tubercle, and high hyperextension strains of the gastrocnemius heads; all are frequently massed together as "knee injuries", a uselessly non-specific term. Examination in all cases was within moments of injury, preceding the usual distortion of all signs by swelling, spasm, and pain; there was in every instance full flexion, full extension, and hyperextension, without the slightest interference with joint mobility; there was abduction laxity of up to 10 degrees only with the knee in 20 degrees flexion, absolutely no laxity in full extension, and local tenderness over the medial collateral ligament and none along the joint line. Following 30 to 60 minutes of ice and elevation, felt splints and crutches were utilized in all but the mildest of cases, with ice continued constantly up to 48 hours thereafter.

During this period of careful observation a minor effusion may or may not make its appearance, usually appearing with the more severe injury, but is never comparable to effusions that characterize internal derangement. Instead, there is always a localization of tenderness to the medial collateral ligament, to the extent that its anatomical length can be easily demonstrated as perpendicular to the joint line! Therefore, as soon as swelling and pain have begun to subside (24 to 48 hours), crutch walking, then normal walking, then jogging are rapidly instituted as tolerated, progressing to sprinting and cutting full speed before returning to full activity.

As with ankle sprains, it is not surprising that analysis by position should reveal an overwhelming preponderance of mobile responsibility, either defensive or offensive, as an integral part of this particular knee injury. Of the 34 total, only three occurred in offensive tackles, and even these interior linemen had secondary downfield-blocking responsibilities requiring some mobility, though nothing comparable with the offensive guard. Of the remainder, 12 were defensive men, and of these 4 were linebackers and 2 defensive ends: thus, 6 of the 34 occurred in positions most vulnerable to the blindside "crackback" block, a suggestive though not dramatic indictment of this dangerous, soon-to-be-outlawed maneuver.

It is not surprising that all injuries were a result of contact either in practice or in games, and the consistent balance between games and practice as a source of injury, though not directly proportional to the greater number of practices, is striking not only from year to year but overall. The equally striking balance between half distribution (7 to 9) must have similar meaning, possibly that purposeful occurrence of that particular impact, necessary to produce this injury, remains uniformly scattered from half to half, game to game, and practice to game, but less between friends in practice.

The relative consistency of time-loss figures not only confirms the uniformity of diagnosis and treatment response but also highlights a problem encountered in all knee injuries of this magnitude, that is, the effect of an average overall time loss of 6.8 days; as brought out by this figure, it has been our experience that any game-incurred medial collateral strain will almost certainly miss the next week's game, no matter how hard the athlete may try, simply because the time required for complete recovery effectively keeps him from necessary practice time during rehabilitation despite his arriving successfully at that physical milestone on game day!

### Table V: Quadriceps Contusions

The so-called "charlie-horse" constitutes the third most frequent cause of time loss, a figure that may prove surprising to some. Contusion of the quadriceps, despite the thigh pad, is indeed a common problem to team physician and trainer alike, but not because of any alarming degree of overall disability or chronicity; it is the omnipresent threat of the rare yet unpredictable massive contusion and its season-long disability, its ofttimes permanent scarring and calcification, always without a single dependable factor to differentiate it at the outset from all the others. In our series 22 proved to be of the usual

## Table V
### Quadriceps Contusions
*Varsity and JV Football, Yale University, 1966–1970*

| Year | Tot | Pos | Practice Pre-sea Con | Non | Season Con | Non | Games Reg | Sub | 1st/2nd Half | Days Lost Full | Comp | Comments |
|------|-----|-----|------|-----|-----|-----|-----|-----|-----|-----|-----|----------|
| 1960 | 0 |    | 0 | 0 | 0 | 0 | 0 | 0 | 0/0 | 0 | 0 | A lucky year |
| 1966 |    | DE | x |   |   |   |   |   |   | 0 | 2 |  |
|      |    | OE |   | x |   |   |   |   |   | 3 | 1 |  |
|      |    | RB | x |   |   |   |   |   |   | 0 | 1 |  |
|      |    | MG | x |   |   |   |   |   |   | 2 | 0 |  |
|      |    | OT | x |   |   |   |   |   |   | 0 | 1 |  |
|      | 5 |    | 4 | 1 | 0 | 0 | 0 | 0 | 0/0 | 5 | 5 | Average: 1.0 days full / 2.8 days comp |
| 1967 |    | QB | x |   |   |   |   |   |   | 0 | 1 |  |
|      |    | RB | x |   |   |   |   |   |   | 0 | 2 |  |
|      |    | RB | x |   |   |   |   |   |   | 2 | 4 |  |
|      |    | MG | x |   |   |   |   |   |   | 3 | 6 |  |
|      |    | RB |   |   | x |   |   |   |   | 3 | 1 |  |
|      | 5 |    | 4 | 0 | 1 | 0 | 0 | 0 | 0/0 | 8 | 14 | Average: 1.6 days full / 2.8 days comp |
| 1968 |    | DE | x |   |   |   |   |   |   | 0 | 2 |  |
|      |    | RB | x |   |   |   |   |   |   | 2 | 2 |  |
|      |    | QB |   |   |   |   |   | x | 2nd | 3 | 0 |  |
|      |    | DB |   |   |   |   |   | x | 1st | 3 | 3 |  |
|      |    | DT |   |   |   |   | x |   | 1st | 2 | 0 |  |
|      | 5 |    | 2 | 0 | 0 | 0 | 1 | 2 | 2/1 | 10 | 7 | Average: 2.0 days full / 1.4 days comp |

severe, ext calcifctn

| Year | Type | A | B | C | D | E | 1st/2nd | grade | days full | days comp |
|---|---|---|---|---|---|---|---|---|---|---|
| 1969 | DB | x | | | | | | | 0 | 2 |
| | DB | x | | | | | | | 13 | 20 |
| | DB | x | | | | | | | 2 | 6 |
| | **3** | 3 | 0 | 0 | | | | 0/0 | 15 | 28 |

Average: 5.0 days full
7.0 days comp
(corr) 1.0 days full
4.0 days comp

| Year | Type | A | B | C | D | E | 1st/2nd | grade | days full | days comp |
|---|---|---|---|---|---|---|---|---|---|---|
| 1970 | MG | x | | | | | | | 1 | 0 |
| | OE | | | x | | | 1st | | 2 | 0 |
| | DB | | | x | | | 1st | | 3 | 0 |
| | DB | | | | x | | 2nd | | 2 | 0 |
| | DB | | | | x | | 2nd | | 2 | 0 |
| | **5** | 1 | 0 | 2 | 2 | | | 2/2 | 10 | 0 |

Average: 2.0 days full
0.0 days comp

| TOTAL | **23** | 14 | 1 | 0 | 3 | 4 | | 4/3 | 48 | 54 |
|---|---|---|---|---|---|---|---|---|---|---|

8.4% of total injuries, (0.36% severe; 1 case/5yrs)
0.046 incidence rate

Ovrll Avg: 2.1 days full
2.3 days comp
(corr) 1.6 days full
1.5 days comp

type with disability lasting 3 to 4 days, while the one remaining of the 23 total, despite an onset and initial course indistinguishable from all the others, proceeded on to massive bleeding from groin to knee, with subsequent fibrosis, stippled calcification by x-ray in 6 weeks, and a total time loss of over a month. Consequently, all contusions of the quadriceps are treated carefully and expectantly in our program, with ice, elevation and compression for as long as bleeding can be reasonably anticipated and with active rehabilitation measures carefully graduated thereafter to tolerance, without the use of any external heat modalities whatever.

Since this is by definition an impact injury, only one occurred during non-contact drills (accidental collision), which must be considered a stretch of good fortune in view of the myriad accidental collisions with one another and with fixed equipment, that do occur and do cause injury during non-contact drills. Position-wise, it is also apparent that, as might be expected, these particular injuries require considerable inherent mobility, possibly to build up the momentum necessary to penetrate the thigh pad. But the 16 practice injuries vs. 7 game injuries is not so easily explained: more frequent exposure in 60 practices vs. 9 games is a tempting solution, but Tables III and IV show an almost equal distribution of injury between practices and games, despite differing only in that both are simple counterjoint injuries as against the pure impact involved here; equally puzzling is the even distribution of quadriceps contusions between halves of games (2 to 2). It would therefore appear that contusions of the quadriceps are more directly related to the total length of exposure to random violence, game or practice, than are ankle sprains or medial collateral strains of the knee, with intrasquad friendship no longer a possible contributing factor.

Finally, the figures for overall and average time loss re-emphasize the foregoing; an intensive and expectant treatment of all such injuries results in a corrected average time loss of 3 days, with but 1 case in 5 years proceeding to more serious complication and time loss regardless of precautions.

### Table VI: Cerebral Concussions

Any study of injuries suffered in football must pay close attention to head and neck injuries, the nation-wide lethal factor year after year.[4] Fortunately, neck injuries, as summarized in Table II, totalled no more than 6 over the 5 years under study, and of these 3 were

Table VI

Cerebral Concussions

*Varsity and JV Football, Yale University, 1966–1970*

| Year | Tot | Pos | Pre-sea Con | Pre-sea Non | Season Con | Season Non | Reg | Sub | 1st/2nd Half | Full | Comp | Comments |
|---|---|---|---|---|---|---|---|---|---|---|---|---|
| 1966 | | RB | — | 0 | x | 0 | 0 | 0 | | 1 | 9 | 10 days non-contact: Absolute |
| | 1 | | — | 0 | 1 | 0 | 0 | 0 | 0/0 | 1 | 9 | |
| 1967 | | DB | | | | | | x | 1st | 3 | 7 | |
| | | RB | | | | | x | | 2nd | 3 | 7 | Occiput to ground |
| | 2 | | 0 | 0 | 0 | 0 | 1 | 1 | 1/1 | 6 | 14 | |
| 1968 | | QB | x | | | | | | | 3 | 8 | |
| | | RB | | | x | | | | | 1 | 9 | FOOTBALL BAN: Mltpl conc & amnes |
| | | RB | | | | | x | | 2nd | 0 | 10 | |
| | | DB | | | | | | x | 2nd | | | |
| | 4 | | 1 | 0 | 1 | 0 | 1 | 1 | 0/2 | 4 | 27 | |
| 1969 | 0 | | 0 | 0 | 0 | 0 | 0 | 0 | 0/0 | 0 | 0 | |
| 1970 | | QB | x | | | | | | 1st | 3 | 7 | |
| | | DB | | | | | x | | | 2 | 8 | Occiput to ground |
| | 2 | | 1 | 0 | 0 | 0 | 1 | 0 | 1/0 | 5 | 15 | |
| TOTAL | 9 | | 2 | 0 | 2 | 0 | 3 | 2 | 2/3 | 16 | 65 | |

3.26% of total injuries
0.018 incidence rate

minor strains of the trapezius and the remainder minor longissimus capitis strains of little import. In fact, there has been but one serious neck injury—a 1961 fracture of C1 and C2 without neurological deficit, complications, or sequelae—since a single fatal fracture dislocation on the field in 1931 (a West Point end), hence in our experience serious cervical injury, catastrophic though it may be when it occurs, is of such rarity as to render any statistical evaluation thereof worthless.

In contrast, head injuries or, as usually encountered in football, cerebral concussions, do show a significant incidence in all series reported, and Table VI summarizes the experience in our series. Included therein are any and all instances of loss of consciousness beyond a momentary interruption of affect as well as all cases of retrograde amnesia with or without loss of consciousness. These criteria are admittedly arbitrary and rigid, allowing for flexibility only in those cases where impact of almost any kind may for a brief few seconds cause disorientation that clears completely in less than a minute. Yet the dire possibility of serious intracranial injury must always be kept in mind, and, accordingly, all so diagnosed concussions are arbitrarily barred from contact for no less than 10 days; even the protean subdural hematoma will have made itself known within this arbitrary period, hence contact can then be resumed without reservation.

Of the nine concussions in our present series all were either defensive or running backs, since the two quarterbacks listed were definitely on the run at the time of impact. The fact that two concussions were incurred by striking the ground with the occiput may have additional significance, but the low total incidence would certainly suggest that the Riddell suspension-helmet in the face of approximately 10 impacts per play, 1200 impacts per 120 play game, or 54,000 impacts in 5 years—to say nothing of the myriad impacts in practice—must be fulfilling its function far better than it is given credit for.

As to sequelae in our series, there were none with the exception of the one tabulated instance of arbitrary medical disqualification: this particular athlete arrived as a freshman with a history of multiple concussions and amnesic episodes in high school, to the degree that his problem was well known to the bigtime football-recruiters in his area, yet with nothing official to confirm same in his medical records. In keeping with our policies, therefore, he was medically barred from freshman football despite his protestations. However, during the sum-

## Table VII
### Hamstring Injuries
*Varsity and JV Football, Yale University, 1966–1970*

| Year | Tot | Pos | Practice Pre-sea Con | Pre-sea Non | Season Con | Season Non | Games Reg | Sub | 1st/2nd Half | Days Lost Full | Comp | Comments |
|---|---|---|---|---|---|---|---|---|---|---|---|---|
| 1966 | | DT | | x | | | | | | 1 | 4 | Obese, (265 plus lbs) |
| | | RB | | x | | | | | | 0 | 3 | Chronic scarring |
| | | OT | | | | x | | | | 3 | 0 | Inactive sub |
| | 3 | | 0 | 2 | 0 | 1 | 0 | 0 | 0/0 | 4 | 7 | Average: 1.3 days full / 2.3 days comp |
| 1967 | 0 | | 0 | 0 | 0 | 0 | 0 | 0 | 0/0 | 0 | 0 | |
| 1968 | | DE | | x | | | | | | 2 | 5 | Eager sub |
| | 1 | | 0 | 1 | 0 | 0 | 0 | 0 | 0/0 | 2 | 5 | Average: 2.0 days full / 5.0 days comp |
| 1969 | | DE | | x | | | | | | 1 | 0 | Capable regular |
| | | DT | | x | | | | | | 2 | 3 | Chronic scarring |
| | | RB | | x | | | | | | 0 | 1 | Chronic scarring |
| | 3 | | 0 | 3 | 0 | 0 | 0 | 0 | 0/0 | 3 | 4 | Average: 1.0 days full / 1.3 days comp |
| 1970 | | FB | | x | | | | | | 1 | 3 | Poorly condtnd sub |
| | | DT | | x | | | | | | 3 | 1 | Poorly condtnd sub |
| | | DE | | | | | | x | 2nd | 2 | 1 | No motivatn, quit |
| | | rb | | | | x | | | | 3 | 0 | Eager sub |
| | 4 | | 0 | 2 | 0 | 1 | 0 | 1 | 0/1 | 9 | 5 | Average: 2.5 days full / 1.25 days comp |
| TOTAL | 11 | | 0 | 8 | 0 | 2 | 0 | 1 | 0/1 | 18 | 21 | Ovrll Avg: 1.6 days full / 1.9 days comp |

4.1% of total injuries
0.022 incidence rate

mer preceding his sophomore year he single-mindedly demanded and underwent a complete diagnostic work up at a world famous clinic in his home state, as a result of which he returned for pre-season practice with a written clearance for football, unequivocal and official, from said clinic, stating that no neurological problem had or did exist. In the face thereof the medical ban was lifted, but within a few weeks a minimal impact resulted in complete disorientation for 2 hours or more; a total ban on all contact sports was immediately reimposed, not, however, without some concerned misgivings over what worse tragedy might have occurred!

### Table VII: Hamstring Injuries

The tight, painful hamstring is a perennial problem of imposing magnitude among track athletes, but to a lesser degree football is likewise a running sport and the 11 cases here tabulated were equally disabled. By definition hamstring injury is a result of overexerting, hence tearing the muscle either grossly or microscopically, and its uniform occurrence as a result of non-contact activities simply confirms this definition and mechanism; in fact, the lone game injury occurred in a substitute on the "bomb-squad," who was in and out of the game so fast that none of the staff saw the actual injury take place!

Also noteable is the fact that in the total listed all but one were either cases with chronic, palpable scarring and multiple episodes of hamstring symptomatology or were substitutes, who were poorly conditioned, overeager, or, worse, poorly motivated and looking for some way out of the rigors of athletic conditioning.

The consistency of time loss and the low overall average figure tells little of the cajoling, wheedling effort necessary to restore the chronic scarred case to full activity, an effort devoted, first, to stopping any bleeding with ice and compression, then to a progressive rehabilitation that focuses on restoration of functional length in the shortened muscle. Yet, in the end the results have been worth the effort, and the low overall average of time loss remains a source of encouragement to doctor and trainer alike.

### Table VIII: Acromioclavicular Contusion, (The Shoulder "Pointer")

Injuries comprising this total are strictly confined to pure contusions, penetrating the shoulder pad by direct impact, hence clinically separate from 1st, 2nd, and 3rd degree A-C separations both by history and by clearly defined tenderness in the contiguous trapezius

## Table VIII
### Acromio-Clavicular Contusion, (the Shoulder "Pointer")
### Varsity and JV Football, Yale University, 1966–1970

| Year | Tot | Pos | Practice Pre-sea Con | Pre-sea Non | Season Con | Season Non | Games Reg | Sub | 1st/2nd Half | Days Lost Full | Comp | Comments |
|---|---|---|---|---|---|---|---|---|---|---|---|---|
| 1966 | | DE | | | x | | | | | 3 | 7 | |
| | | RB | | | x | | | | | 2 | 8 | |
| | 2 | | 0 | 0 | 2 | 0 | 0 | 0 | 0/0 | 5 | 15 | Average: 2.5 days full / 7.5 days comp |
| 1967 | | DB | x | | | | | | | 0 | 2 | |
| | 1 | | 1 | 0 | 0 | 0 | 0 | 0 | 0/0 | 0 | 2 | Average: 0.0 days full / 2.0 days comp |
| 1968 | | QB | | | x | | | | | 3 | 4 | |
| | | DB | | | x | | | | | 3 | 2 | |
| | 2 | | 0 | 0 | 2 | 0 | 0 | 0 | 0/0 | 6 | 6 | Average: 3.0 days full / 3.0 days comp |
| 1969 | | OG | x | | | | | | | 2 | 5 | |
| | | LB | x | | | | | | | 1 | 7 | |
| | | OE | | | | | x | | 1st | 2 | 3 | |
| | 3 | | 2 | 0 | 0 | 0 | 1 | 0 | 1/0 | 5 | 15 | Average: 1.6 days full / 5.0 days comp; Simultns cerebral conc |
| 1970 | | QB | x | | | | x | | 2nd | 3 | 7 | |
| | | OG | | | x | | | | | 3 | 3 | |
| | | OG | | | | | | | | 1 | 1 | |
| | | OG | x | | | | | | | 2 | 6 | |
| | 4 | | 2 | 0 | 1 | 0 | 1 | 0 | 0/1 | 9 | 17 | Average: 2.2 days full / 4.2 days comp |
| TOTAL | 12 | | 5 | 0 | 5 | 0 | 2 | 0 | 1/1 | 25 | 55 | Ovrll Avg: 2.1 days full / 4.6 days comp |

4.4% of total injuries
0.024 incidence rate

and/or deltoid muscle insertions as well as over the subcutaneous A-C joint. To make the diagnosis, thorough examination must demonstrate complete stability in the joint and must elicit acute tenderness beyond the anatomical limits of the A-C joint itself, to eliminate the 1st degree A-C strain. Such arbitrary criteria are essential to this particular injury because of its consistent time loss of at least 2 days of full disability and the average rehabilitation of 4.6 days, both essential factors in an accurate prognosis; in short, accurate initial evaluation, followed by constant application of ice, compression with strapping, and a sling will together assure a reliable estimation of total time loss at roughly 7 days, in contrast to the longer lasting disability from true A-C separations. With proper local padding, full contact activity can be confidently resumed after this time without fear of complications or functional disability.

Further examination of the figures will confirm that this is, indeed, a contact injury, occurring with equal frequency in pre-season and season practices and proportionately less in games. Aside from the 2 quarterbacks, both of whom were running with the ball at the time, all other instances were in "hard-hitters" (4 of the 12 in offensive guards). The persistent local soreness in what is after all a "bone bruise", together with the associated muscle soreness and limitation in the trapezius and deltoid groups, can be discouraging to these athletes, whose responsibilities are so predominantly directed toward impacting the same area repeatedly, but patient encouragement and, particularly, that first "hit" restore them to full effectiveness within the time loss anticipated statistically.

### Table IX: Groin Strains

Included within this broad category are all strains of the gracilis, sartorius, adductors, ilio-psoas, and pectineus, each of which is diagnostically separable by careful palpatory and functional examination, but all of which for the purpose of this study have been consolidated into a collective group of similar injuries, all functionally disabling but all rapidly responsive to local ice, elastic-bandage spica, and a carefully graduated rehabilitation program. As might be expected, all injuries under study occurred in the running positions, line-backers, defensive backs, running backs, and ends, and the incidence was confined almost entirely to practice, mostly pre-season; in fact, the lone game injury was a traumatic adductor strain from a forcible "split", with symptoms primarily distal over the femoral adductor

Table IX

"Groin Strains"

*Varsity and JV Football, Yale University, 1966–1970*

| Year | Tot | Pos | Practice Pre-sea Con | Pre-sea Non | Season Con | Season Non | Games Reg | Sub | 1st/2nd Half | Days Lost Full | Comp | Comments |
|---|---|---|---|---|---|---|---|---|---|---|---|---|
| 1966 | 0 | | 0 | 0 | 0 | 0 | 0 | 0 | 0/0 | 0 | 0 | |
| 1967 | | DB | | x | | | | | | 1 | 2 | |
| | | DE | | x | | | | | | 0 | 1 | |
| | | LB | | | | x | | | | 0 | 1 | |
| | | LB | | | | x | | | | 3 | 3 | Ilio-psoas w back pain |
| | 4 | | 0 | 2 | 0 | 2 | 0 | 0 | 0/0 | 4 | 7 | Average: 1.0 days full 1.75 days comp |
| 1968 | 0 | | 0 | 0 | 0 | 0 | 0 | 0 | 0/0 | 0 | 0 | |
| 1969 | | RB | | x | | | | | | 0 | 1 | |
| | | DB | | x | | | | | | 0 | 2 | |
| | | OE | | x | | | | | | 2 | 0 | |
| | | DB | | | | | x | | | 2 | 0 | |
| | | DB | | x | | | | | 2nd | 1 | 0 | |
| | 5 | | 0 | 4 | 0 | 0 | 1 | 0 | 0/1 | 5 | 3 | Average: 1.25 days full 0.5 days comp |
| 1970 | | DB | | x | | | | | | 1 | 0 | |
| | | DE | | | x | | | | | 3 | 2 | |
| | 2 | | 0 | 1 | 1 | 0 | 0 | 0 | 0/0 | 4 | 2 | Average: 2.0 days full 0.5 days comp |
| TOTAL | 11 | | 0 | 7 | 1 | 2 | 1 | 0 | 0/1 | 13 | 12 | Ovrll Avg: 1.2 days full 1.0 days comp |

4.1% of total injuries

0.022 incidence rate

tubercle but included in this group for convenience of classification. It is generally believed that groin strains are more likely in wet, slippery weather, and the high pre-season incidence in 1969 confirms this adage with 4 of the year's 5 instances confined to the wettest pre-season that the author and the training staff have endured! Finally, the short average time loss may be surprising to some, accustomed to season-long nagging disability, but the important factor here may be our strict control over all activity, never allowing an injured athlete to forcibly "run out" the spasmodic muscle group, as did the one prolonged time loss, a substitute who belatedly reported a full blown iliopsoas strain, with acute back pain, palpable spasm, and limitation extending up above the ilio-pectineal line, deep to the inguinal ligament; even in this case 3 days of intensive local treatment with ice, compression, and full disability, followed by 3 days of gradual rehabilitation, completely controlled symptoms and restored the athlete to full activity within an overall total of 6 days.

### Table X: Contusion of the Iliac Crest, (The Hip "Pointer")

Analogous to the shoulder "pointer" above is the iliac crest contusion. Of identical anatomical character, it involves a subcutaneous bony area, the iliac rim, and a contiguous muscle group of essential functional importance for continued athletic endeavour, in this instance the abdominal muscles as they sweep around from the flank anteriorward toward the inguinal triangle. Characteristically, therefore, it is an injury that combines exquisite bony tenderness on the iliac crest with swelling, spasm, and totally disabling pain with every trunk motion when coughing, when sneezing, and in the severe cases, when evacuating. Immediate and prolonged application of ice promptly relieves local pain, but, nonetheless, bed observation is often necessary during the initial period of acute disability. Only repeated and detailed examinations can accurately determine the true extent of soft-tissue injury and correctly gauge the proper moment, first, to discontinue supportive local measures, then with hemostasis assured, to start a graduated program of activity that will bring the athlete, step by step, through jogging, sprinting, cutting, twisting, then hitting, and finally to full activity.

From the above, it is clear that diagnosis of the injury is basically simple, namely a history of painful impact in the area either through or, more often, over the top of the hip pad—which, all too often, has slipped down too low—and increasing local pain and muscle spasm,

Table X

Contusion of the Iliac Crest

*Varsity and JV Football, Yale University, 1966–1970*

| Year | Tot | Pos | Practice Pre-sea Con | Pre-sea Non | Season Con | Season Non | Games Reg | Sub | 1st/2nd Half | Days Lost Full | Comp | Comments |
|---|---|---|---|---|---|---|---|---|---|---|---|---|
| 1966 | 0 | | 0 | 0 | 0 | 0 | 0 | 0 | 0/0 | 0 | 0 | |
| 1967 | | DE | | | | | x | | 2nd | 2 | 4 | Last game, rehab limited |
| | | RB | | | | | x | | 1st | 10 | 0 | Average: 6.0 days full |
| | 2 | | 0 | 0 | 0 | 0 | 2 | 0 | 1/1 | 12 | 4 | 2.0 days comp |
| | | | | | | | | | | | | (corr) 2.0 days full |
| | | | | | | | | | | | | 4.0 days comp |
| 1968 | | RB | | | | | x | | 2nd | 4 | 0 | |
| | | RB | | | | | x | | 1st | 3 | 1 | |
| | | LB | | | | | x | | 2nd | 3 | 1 | |
| | 3 | | 0 | 0 | 0 | 0 | 3 | 0 | 1/2 | 10 | 2 | Average: 3.3 days full |
| | | | | | | | | | | | | 0.6 days comp |
| 1969 | | OG | x | | | | x | | 1st | 2 | 3 | |
| | | OE | | | | | | | | 4 | 0 | |
| | 2 | | 1 | 0 | 0 | 0 | 1 | 0 | 1/0 | 6 | 3 | Average: 3.0 days full |
| | | | | | | | | | | | | 1.5 days comp |
| 1970 | | OG | | | | | x | | 1st | 2 | 0 | |
| | | DB | | | x | | | | | 2 | 1 | |
| | 2 | | 0 | 0 | 1 | 0 | 1 | 0 | 1/0 | 4 | 1 | Average: 2.0 days full |
| | | | | | | | | | | | | 0.5 days comp |
| TOTAL | 9 | | 1 | 0 | 1 | 0 | 7 | 0 | 4/3 | 32 | 10 | Ovrll Avg: 3.6 days full |
| | | | | | | | | | | | | 1.1 days comp |
| | | | | | | | | | | | | (corr) 2.7 days full |
| | | | | | | | | | | | | 1.25 days comp |

3.3% of total injuries

0.018 incidence rate

that draws the athlete over toward his injured side, forcing him to grunt with every respiration. On the other hand, prognosis, as with so much in athletics, is the all important factor, not only for the injured athlete but for his coach and his teammates; in short, how long will he be out?

The figures in Table X answer this last, all important question; with treatment as outlined, time loss has been strikingly consistent, around three days of full disability, followed by 2 days of intensive rehabilitation, a total of around 5 days. Keeping in mind the absolute necessity for participation in practice by mid-week, the implications of a game-incurred hip "pointer" can then be readily appreciated, that is, the very likely possibility that an athlete so injured will be unable to play in the next game, although he has actually recovered completely, simply because there has not been sufficient time for him to participate in necessary practices during the week. Consequently, the real challenge is to somehow work out his rehabilitation schedule so he can, in fact, profit from those all important midweek practice sessions without overtaxing his as yet unresolved injury, and it is here that a close working relationship with the coaching staff is absolutely essential.

As to the incidence of this disabling injury, our study reveals a striking preponderance of game injuries, only two of the nine occurring in practice, either pre-season or season; since all padding worn is identical for game and practice, differing only in the "game pant" (the shell pant that holds the thigh and knee pads and hooks over the hip pad), the reason for this significant preponderance cannot be easily answered.

Incidence by position, on the other hand, is clearly related to impact, either as a blocker, runner, or open-field tackler, with no interior linemen in the defensive "pit" appearing in the total; it would appear that the latter are too busy inflicting hip "pointers" to incur any themselves!

## Table XI: Injuries Requiring Surgery

As stated previously, the most remarkable aspect of this particular tabulation is the strikingly low overall total of surgical cases in our series; 4 in 5 years and never more than 1 in any single season. The contrast between the 4 surgical cases in the single year, 1960—this in spite of the incredibly low overall injury total for that season—and the low surgical aggregate over the past 5 years cannot be explained by a change in orthopedic consultants; 2 of the 4 cases in 1960 were

Table XI
Injuries Requiring Surgery
*Varsity and JV Football, Yale University, 1966–1970*

| Year | Tot | Pos | Pre-sea Con | Pre-sea Non | Season Con | Season Non | Games Reg | Games Sub | Games Half | Mechanism | Diagnosis | Surgery | Return | Comments |
|---|---|---|---|---|---|---|---|---|---|---|---|---|---|---|
| 1960 | | End | | x | | | | | | Axial impact (harness intact) | Pstr disl shld | Magn-Stack Repair | Quit | Chron bilat |
| | | Grd | | | | | x | | 2nd | Headon impct | Impct med men. | Meniscect | Senior | Chronic |
| | | QB | | | | x | | | | Impct, addctn & flexn | Torn med men. | Meniscect | Senior | Rtn polo |
| | | FB | | | | | | x | 1st | Headon impct | Torn med men. | Meniscect | Senior | Rtn bsbll |
| | 4 | | 0 | 1 | 1 | 0 | 1 | 1 | 1/1 | | | | | |
| 1966 | | QB | | | | | x | | 1st | Lat impct abdct extsn | Lat men & ant cruc | Meniscect | Season | Rtn bsbll |
| | 1 | | 0 | 0 | 0 | 0 | 1 | 0 | 1/0 | | | | | |
| 1967 | | RB | | | x | | | | | Lat impct abdct extsn | Torn med coll | Lig rpr | Barred | Unstbl |
| | 1 | | 0 | 0 | 1 | 0 | 0 | 0 | 0/0 | | | | | |
| 1968 | | QB | | x | | | | | | Headon impct | Torn med men. | Meniscect | 60 days | Full recovery |
| | | RB | | | | | x | | 1st | Lat impct in extensn | Torn med coll | Lig rpr | Season | Rtn 1 yr |
| | 2 | | 1 | 1 | 0 | 0 | 1 | 0 | 1/0 | | | | | |
| 1969 | 0 | | 0 | 0 | 0 | 0 | 0 | 0 | 0/0 | | | | | |
| 1970 | 0 | | 0 | 0 | 0 | 0 | 0 | 0 | 0/0 | | | | | |
| 1966–70 (1.4%) 0.008 incidence rate | 4 | 2QB 2RB | 1 | 0 | 1 | 0 | 2 | 0 | 2/0 | | | | | |

done by the same man who performed the single case in 1966, and subsequent thereto our orthopedists have, if anything, been more radical. Hence the answer must lie in the platooning of present-day football, with the same total impacts per season now more widely distributed through offensive and defensive platoons totalling around 30 men, who see regular service in scrimmages and games, in striking

Table XII
Fractures and Dislocations
*Varsity and JV Football, Yale University, 1966–1970*

| Year | Tot | Pos | Pre-sea Con | Pre-sea Non | Season Con | Season Non | Reg | Sub | Half |
|------|-----|-----|-----|-----|-----|-----|-----|-----|-----|
| 1960 | | End | x | | | | | | |
| | | Cnt | x | | | | | | |
| | | QB | | x | x | | | | |
| | | HB | | x | x | | | | |
| | 4F | | 2 | 0 | 2 | 0 | 0 | 0 | 0/0 |
| 1966 | | OG | | x | | | | | |
| | | RB | | | | | x | | 2nd |
| | 1F/1D | | 0 | 1 | 0 | 0 | 1 | 0 | 0/1 |
| 1967 | | OG | | x | | | | | |
| | | QB | | | | x | | | |
| | 2F | | 0 | 1 | 0 | 1 | 0 | 0 | 0/0 |
| 1968 | | DE | | | | | | x | 2nd |
| | 1F | | 0 | 0 | 0 | 0 | 0 | 1 | 0/1 |
| 1969 | | RB | x | | | | | | |
| | | RB | | | | | x | | 2nd |
| | 1F/1D | | 1 | 0 | 0 | 0 | 1 | 0 | 0/1 |
| 1970 | | DT | x | | | | | | |
| | | RB | | | x | | | | |
| | | OG | | | | | x | | 2nd |
| | 3F | | 1 | 0 | 1 | 0 | 1 | 0 | 0/1 |
| 1966–70 | 8F/2D | | 2F | 2F | 1F | 1F | 1F/2D | 1F | 0/2F |

2.8%/0.7% of total injuries        2D
0.016/0.004 incidence rate

contrast to the 15 or 16 two-way players in 1960, who survived pre-season and season scrimmages and contact drills as well as all 9 games without relief except by way of injury.

With but four total cases, it is dangerous to draw any conclusions, yet, valid or not, all 4 were backs, 2 running backs, and 2 quarter-backs who were running the ball on "keepers". One occurred during

| Mechanism | Diagnosis | Surgery | Return | Comments |
|---|---|---|---|---|
| Impct elbow | Lin fx maxilla | None | 3 days | Thru face mask |
| Stppd on | Fx MCiii,iv | Plstr 8 wks | Season | Snr, no return |
| Hit helmet | Fx MCii,iii | Plstr 4 wks | 33 days | Fnl gm, flt spl |
| Fell on hnd | Fx MCii,iii | Plstr 12 wks | Season | Delayed union |
| Fell on hnd | Fx MC iv | Plstr 8 wks | Season | Quit football |
| Hyperextens | Post Dsl elb | Splnt-slng | Season | Return 1 yr |
| Fell on hnd | Fx, cp; scaph | Plstr 10 wks | Season | Return 1 yr |
| Fell on hnd | Fx MC iii | Plstr 3 wks | | |
| | | Flt spl 2 wk | 31 days | Full recovery |
| Hit helmet | Fx MC ii,iii | Plstr 5 wks | 45 days | Full recovery |
| | | Flt spl 2 wk | | |
| Impct lat leg | Fx fib, lwr third | Plstr 4 wks | 38 days | Full recovery |
| Hyperabdctn | Gleno-hum disloc | Sling & swthe | Season | Quit football |
| Impct | Fx MC iii | Plstr 4 wks | 34 days | Full recovery |
| Impct | Fx nose | Reduced | 10 days | Full recovery |
| Lat impct | Fx fib lwr third | Plstr 10 wks | Season | Return 1 yr |

pre-season practice, 1 during season practice, and all 4 were due to direct impact, either head on or from the side; none were due to torsion in the open field. In no instance was diagnosis difficult even from the start; in the two cases of medial ligament disruption that required primary repair within hours, the diagnosis was unquestionable, so totally unstable were the injured knees, not only in 20 degrees flexion, but in full extension as well!

Our experience with knee surgery, however, has not been as encouraging as other studies have indicated. Of the 4 operative procedures, 2 were simple meniscectomies, which, as should be expected, returned to action promptly, depending only on whether enough of the football season remained. On the other hand, of the 2 primary ligament repairs only 1 returned to full activity, but, even with a demonstrable stability described by one observer as "like a rock", he was never the same as before; the second proved permanently unstable for football, as have over the past fifteen years 3 others from our freshman football program and two varsity hockey players, all repaired surgically less than 4 hours after injury. Some authorities will insist that such results cannot possibly be true, but so be it!

### Table XII: Fractures and Dislocations

Included herein are all fractures and dislocations suffered between 1966 and 1970, excluding only a few minor subluxations of fingers. The total is low, far lower than most orthopedists might anticipate, diagnosis was simple, and treatment no different than for any such injury, athletic or not. The position distribution suggests some preponderance of mobile positions, but this may be illusory, since metacarpal fractures, our most frequent bony injury (4 out of the 8 total), were incurred in such disparate ways as hitting other helmets or, as amply demonstrated by a star quarterback, by simply falling on a hand in an agility drill! Similarly, the 2nd half predominance in both fractures and dislocations is probably not significant, although with the dislocations fatigue might conceivably have led to increased susceptibility; however, this last seems unlikely, if only because both dislocations were from massive impact and counterjoint leverage that went far beyond what mere muscular strength might reasonably counteract. Finally, the 6 of 8 total fractures that occurred during practice sessions make the required presence of an orthopedist "on-the-bench" for games *only* a rather futile gesture.

## DISCUSSION

Conclusions that can be safely drawn from a study such as this are admittedly limited. However, although there is nothing startlingly new revealed by these statistics in bulk or in detail and certainly nothing overwhelming about their implications, the striking confirmation of everything that experienced team-physicians and trainers have been reiterating year after year cannot be denied. Broad statements by specialist "experts", who work only in one or another small segment of the football-injury spectrum, have certainly not been confirmed by these figures. Instead, it is apparent that many more studies of a similar nature must be undertaken by other team-physicians, who with their trainers maintain and control similar athletic programs elsewhere, team-physicians who can detail personal working diagnoses, treatments, and all ancillary details as they apply to all squad members under their medical control. As pointed out, rules-changes prevent any meaningful analysis of figures back beyond 5 years, no matter how accurate these may be, hence more team-physicians must pool their individual samples for these last 5 years in order to amass a truly significant total. Such an undertaking might well counterbalance and nullify many of the conclusions and implications in this report by sheer weight of significant numbers, but until then such conclusions and implications must stand.

# REFERENCES

1. Allen, M. A.: Air Force Football Injuries: A Statistical Study. JAMA *206*: 1053–1055, 1966.
2. Alley, R. H.: Head and Neck Injuries in High School Football. JAMA *188*: 118–122, 1964.
3. Allman, F. L.: Problems in Diagnosis and Treatment of Athletic Injuries. J. Louisiana Med. Soc. *117*:121–125, 1965.
4. Blyth, C. S., Arnold, D. C.: Thirty-seventh Annual Survey of Football Fatalities: 1931–1968. Chapel Hill, N.C., American Football Coaches Assoc. and National Collegiate Athletic Assoc. 1969.
5. Hirata, Jr., I.: The Doctor and the Athlete. J. B. Lippincott, Philadelphia, Penn. 1968.
6. Kraus, J. F.: An Epidemiologic Investigation of Productor Variables Associated with Intramural Touch-Football Injuries, Thesis. University of Minnesota, St. Paul, 1967.
7. Krause, M. A.: The Nature and Frequency of Injuries Occurring in Oregon High-School Football, Thesis. University of Oregon, Portland, 1959.
8. Neilsen, N. P.: The Nature of Age-Incidence of Injuries in Inter-Scholastic Football. Res. Quart. *4*:78–90, 1933.
9. O'Donoghue, D. H.: An Analysis of End-results of Surgical Treatment of Major Injuries to the Ligaments of the Knee. J. Bone Joint Surg. *37-A*: 1–13, 1955.
10. ———: Management of Acute Knee Injuries: Criteria for Early Surgery. Proceedings of the Eighth National Conference on the Medical Aspects of Sports, Chicago: American Medical Assoc., 1967, pp. 89–95.
11. Robey, J. M., Blyth, C. S., Mueller, F. O.: Athletic Injuries; Application of Epidemiological Methods, JAMA *217*:184–189, July 1971.
12. Standard Nomenclature of Athletic Injuries. American Medical Association, Chicago, Illinois.
13. Thorndike, A.: Prevention of Injury in Athletes, JAMA *162*:1126–1132, 1956.

# Suggested Reading

No attempt has been made to compile a complete bibliography for so broad a field. This selection is provided for those who wish to delve more deeply into the subject. With the bibliographies contained in these selections, the entire literature should be accessible.

1. Bender, J. A., and Kaplan, H. M.: The effectiveness of isometric exercises in physical rehabilitation: A hospital study. J. Ass. Phys. Ment. Rehab. *16*: 174–175, 1962.
2. Bilik, S. R.: The Trainers' Bible. 8th Revised Edition, New York, T. J. Reed Co., 1947.
3. Blalock, J., and Ochsner, J.: Thoracic trauma. Surg. Clin. N. Amer. *46*: 1513–1524, 1966.
4. Cameron, B., and Davis, O.: The swivel football shoe: A controlled study. J. Sports Medicine *1*:16–27, 1973.
5. Chrisman, O. D., *et al.*: Lateral-flexion neck injuries in athletic competition. JAMA *192*:613–615, 1965.
6. Cureton, T. K.: New techniques of athletic training and conditioning. J. Ass. Phys. Ment. Rehab. *15*:103–107, 1961.
7. ———: Relationship of physical fitness to athletic performance and sports. *JAMA 162*:1139–1149, 1956.
8. Dayton, O. W.: Athletic Training and Conditioning. rev. ed. New York, Ronald Press, 1965.
9. DeLorme, T. L., and Watkins, A. L.: Progressive Resistance Exercises. New York, Appleton-Century-Crofts, 1951.
10. DePalma, A. F., and Flannery, G. F.: Acute anterior dislocation of the shoulder. J. Sports Medicine *1*:6–15, 1973.
11. DiStefano, V. J., and Nixon, J. E.: Ruptures of the achilles tendon. J. Sports Medicine *1*:34–37, 1973.
12. Dyke, L. M.: Skin infection in wrestlers due to herpes simplex virus. JAMA *170*:998–1000, 1965.
13. Eastwood, F. R.: Annual survey of football injuries and fatalities. Proc. Amer. Football Coaches Assn.
14. Feurig, J. S.: Legal liabilities of team physicians. Student Medicine *10*: 478–484, 1962.

15. Frankel, S. A., and Hirata, I: The Scalenus Anticus and Competitive Swimming. JAMA *215*:1796–1798, 1971.
16. Gurdjian, E. S., *et al.*: Protection of the head and neck in athletics. JAMA *182*:509–512, 1962.
17. Hanley, D. F.: Personal communication.
18. Hirata, I: Conditioning and Training of the competitive athletic. J. Sports Medicine *1*:14–17, 1972.
19. ———: Heat exhaustion and prostration. Penn. Med. J. *73*:58–60, 1970.
20. ———: Traumatic rupture of the testicle in tackle football: a case report. J. Am. Coll. Hlth. Assn. *21*:165–166, 1972.
21. ———: Pre-game meals: a discussion. J. School Health *40*:409–413, 1970.
22. Hoffman, S., *et al.*: Direct approach in management of severe facial fractures involving orbital floor. Arch. Surg. *94*:403–412, 1967.
23. Howes, E. L., and Harvey, S. C.: Clinical significance of experimental studies in wound healing. Ann. Surg. *102*:941, 1935.
24. Hughston, J. C.: Subluxation of the patella. J. Bone Joint Surg. *50*:1003–1026, 1968.
25. Hume, M.: Arm swelling due to venous obstruction. Conn. Medicine *31*:39–42, 1967.
26. Jude, J. R., Kouwenhoven, W. B., and Knickerbocker, G. G.: Cardiac arrest. Report of application of external cardiac massage on 118 patients. JAMA *178*:1063, 1962.
27. Karpovich, P., and Hale, C. J.: The effect of warming up upon physical performance. JAMA *162*:1117–1119, 1956.
28. Key, J. A., and Conwell, H. E.: The Management of Fractures, Dislocation and Sprains. ed. 5. St. Louis, C. V. Mosby, 1957.
29. Kiphuth, R. J.: How to be Fit. New Haven, Yale University Press, 1942.
30. Kobak, M.: Comparison of healing in deep and superficial layers of experimental abdominal incisions. Am. J. Surg. *91*:365–368, 1958.
31. McPhee, H. R.: A survey of knee injuries in football. Student Medicine *10*:422–430, 1962.
32. Montoye, H. S., *et al.*: A study of longevity and morbidity of college athletes. JAMA *162*:1132–1134, 1956.
33. O'Donoghue, D. H.: Treatment of Injuries to Athletes. Philadelphia, Saunders, 1962.
34. Ordman, L. J., and Gillman, T.: Studies in healing of cutaneous wounds, I, II, and III. Arch. Surg. *93*:857–928, 1966.
35. Quigley, T. J. (Ed.): Sports injuries. Am. J. Surg. *98*:315–516, 1959.
36. Reid, S.: Radio-Telemetry in the Study of Head Impacts in Football. Presented at N.A.T.A. Convention, Chicago, Ill., 1965.
37. Reindell, H.: Herz. Kreislaufkrankheiten und Sport. Band VI, J. A. Barth, München, 1960.
38. ———: Wissenschaftliche Schriftenreihe des Deutschen Sportbundes, Band III.
39. Rich, J. M.: Artificial Turf: An In-Depth Analysis, thesis. London, Ontario, The University of Western Ontario, 1971.

40. Rose, K. D.: Cardiac contusion resulting from "spearing" in football. Arch. Int. Med. *118*:129–131, 1966.
41. Rose, K. D.: *et al.*: A liquid pre-game meal for athletes. JAMA *178*:30–33, 1961.
42. Schneider, R. D., and Crisler, F.: Serious and fatal football injuries involving the head and spinal cord. JAMA *177*:362–367, 1961.
43. Slocum, D. B.: The mechanics of common football injuries. JAMA *170*: 1640–1646, 1959.
44. Thorndike, A.: Athletic Injuries, Prevention, Diagnosis, and Treatment. ed. 3. Philadelphia, Lea and Febiger, 1958.
45. ———: Prevention of injury in athletics. JAMA *162*:1126–1132, 1956.
46. Torg, J. S., and Quedenfeld, T: The effect of shoe type and cleat lengths on incidence and severity of knee injuries among high school football players. Res. Quart. *42*:203–211, 1971.
47. Van Winkle, W.: The fibroblast in wound healing. SGO *124*:369–386, 1967.
48. Von Itallie, Sinisterra, and Stare: Nutrition and athletic performance. JAMA *162*:1120–1126, 1956.
49. Watson-Jones, R.: Fractures and Joint Injuries. ed. 4. Edinburgh, Livingstone, 1952.

# Index

Trapezius, contusion of, 137, 138
  strain of, 128, 137-138
Trapezoid ligament, 140
Trismus, in swallowed tongue, 94
Trochanteric bursa, injuries to, 196-197
Trunk, injuries to, 175-190
  *See also* Abdominal wall; Chest; Dorsal
    area; Lumbosacral area
Turf, artificial, 62-63, 70
Turf sports, field for, 62-63

Unconsciousness. *See* Consciousness, loss
  of
Ungual injuries, 125-126
University of Southern California, 26, 29
Urinary tract injuries, 100-101
Urine, blood in, in contusion of kidney,
  100
Urine tests, 59
Urination, inability, in contusion of kid-
  ney, 100
  *See also* Micturation

Vascular insufficiency, in fractures and
  dislocations, 263, 264
Vasoconstriction to control bleeding, 75
Vein thrombosis, spontaneous axillary,
  97
Vessels. *See* Blood vessels
Visceral injuries, 95
  *See also* Abdominal injury
Vision, blurring of, 111
Vitamins, 54, 56-57

"Walking the wall," 148, 150
Warm-up, 45-46

Warts, plantar, 125
Water, to avoid dehydration, 50-51
Watson-Jones strapping, 143
Weighing, and heat stroke, 50
Weight control, 57-58
Weight lifter, 46-47
  back strain of, 187
  use of anabolic steroids by, 58, 59
Weight loss, as danger sign, 50
  *See also* Thrower
Weight training, 46-48
"Wind knocked out," 99
"Winging," scapular, 149-151
Wound, examination and healing of, 120
  puncture, 121
  *See also* Laceration
Wraps, ankle, 252
  *See also* Strapping
Wrestling, mat for, 64
  weight in, 57-58
Wrist, dislocation of, 170
  sprain of, 169-170

X-ray, ankle, 244, 251
  of carpal scaphoid, 170
  in facial injuries, 106-107
  for fracture, 159
  in radial head trauma, 161-162
  shoulder, 142
  "stippling of calcium" shown in, 205
Xiphisternal junction, sprain, 178

Yale University, football injury statistics
  from sample at, 276
  medical program at, summary of, 25-
    29